D1690919

Open Access Databases and Datasets for Drug Discovery

Methods and Principles in Medicinal Chemistry

Edited by
R. Mannhold, H. Buschmann, J. Holenz

Editorial Board
G. Folkers, H. Timmermann, H. van de Waterbeemd, J. Bondo Hansen

Previous Volumes of the Series

Bachhav, Y. (Ed.)

Targeted Drug Delivery

2022
ISBN: 978-3-527-34781-0
Vol. 82

Alza, E. (Ed.)

Flow and Microreactor Technology in Medicinal Chemistry

2022
ISBN: 978-3-527-34689-9
Vol. 81

Rübsamen-Schaeff, H., and Buschmann, H. (Eds.)

New Drug Development for Known and Emerging Viruses

2022
ISBN: 978-3-527-34337-9
Vol. 80

Gruss, M. (Ed.)

Solid State Development and Processing of Pharmaceutical Molecules

Salts, Cocrystals, and Polymorphism

2021
ISBN: 978-3-527-34635-6
Vol. 79

Plowright, A.T. (Ed.)

Target Discovery and Validation Methods and Strategies for Drug Discovery

2020
ISBN: 978-3-527-34529-8
Vol. 78

Swinney, D., Pollastri, M. (Eds.)

Neglected Tropical Diseases Drug Discovery and Development

2019
ISBN: 978-3-527-34304-1
Vol. 77

Bachhav, Y. (Ed.)

Innovative Dosage Forms Design and Development at Early Stage

2019
ISBN: 978-3-527-34396-6
Vol. 76

Gervasio, F. L., Spiwok, V. (Eds.)

Biomolecular Simulations in Structure-based Drug Discovery

2018
ISBN: 978-3-527-34265-5
Vol. 75

Sippl, W., Jung, M. (Eds.)

Epigenetic Drug Discovery

2018
ISBN: 978-3-527-34314-0
Vol. 74

Giordanetto, F. (Ed.)

Early Drug Development

2018
ISBN: 978-3-527-34149-8
Vol. 73

Open Access Databases and Datasets for Drug Discovery

Edited by Antoine Daina, Michael Przewosny, and Vincent Zoete

WILEY-VCH

Volume Editors

Antoine Daina
SIB Swiss Institute of Bioinformatics
1015 Lausanne
Switzerland

Michael Przewosny
Borngasse 43
52064 Aachen
Germany

Vincent Zoete
SIB Swiss Institute of Bioinformatics
UNIL University of Lausanne and
Ludwig Institute for Cancer Research
1015 Lausanne
Switzerland

Series Editors

Prof. Dr. Raimund Mannhold[†]
Rosenweg 7
40489 Düsseldorf
Germany

Dr. Helmut Buschmann
Sperberweg 15
52076 Aachen
Germany

Dr. Jörg Holenz
BIAL - Portela & C[a]., S.A.
Av. Siderurgia Nacional
4745–457 Coronado
Portugal

Cover Design and Images: SCHULZ
Grafik-Design

■ All books published by **WILEY-VCH** are carefully produced. Nevertheless, authors, editors, and publisher do not warrant the information contained in these books, including this book, to be free of errors. Readers are advised to keep in mind that statements, data, illustrations, procedural details or other items may inadvertently be inaccurate.

Library of Congress Card No.: applied for

British Library Cataloguing-in-Publication Data
A catalogue record for this book is available from the British Library.

Bibliographic information published by the Deutsche Nationalbibliothek
The Deutsche Nationalbibliothek lists this publication in the Deutsche Nationalbibliografie; detailed bibliographic data are available on the Internet at <http://dnb.d-nb.de>.

© 2024 WILEY-VCH GmbH, Boschstraße 12, 69469 Weinheim, Germany

All rights reserved (including those of translation into other languages). No part of this book may be reproduced in any form – by photoprinting, microfilm, or any other means – nor transmitted or translated into a machine language without written permission from the publishers. Registered names, trademarks, etc. used in this book, even when not specifically marked as such, are not to be considered unprotected by law.

Print ISBN: 978-3-527-34839-8
ePDF ISBN: 978-3-527-83047-3
ePub ISBN: 978-3-527-83048-0
oBook ISBN: 978-3-527-83049-7

Typesetting Straive, Chennai, India

Contents

Series Editors Preface *xiii*
Raimund Mannhold – A Personal Obituary from the Series Editors *xvii*
A Personal Foreword *xxi*

1 **Open Access Databases and Datasets for Computer-Aided Drug Design. A Short List Used in the Molecular Modelling Group of the SIB** *1*
Antoine Daina, María José Ojeda-Montes, Maiia E. Bragina, Alessandro Cuozzo, Ute F. Röhrig, Marta A.S. Perez, and Vincent Zoete
References *30*

Part I Small Molecules *39*

2 **PubChem: A Large-Scale Public Chemical Database for Drug Discovery** *41*
Sunghwan Kim and Evan E. Bolton
2.1 Introduction *41*
2.2 Data Content and Organization *42*
2.3 Tools and Services *45*
2.3.1 PubChem Search *45*
2.3.2 Summary Pages *48*
2.3.3 Literature Knowledge Panel *49*
2.3.4 2D and 3D Neighbors *50*
2.3.5 Classification Browser *51*
2.3.6 Identifier Exchange Service *52*
2.3.7 Programmatic Access *52*
2.3.8 PubChem FTP Site and PubChemRDF *53*
2.4 Drug- and Lead-Likeness of PubChem Compounds *54*
2.5 Bioactivity Data in PubChem *56*
2.6 Comparison with Other Databases *57*
2.7 Use of PubChem Data for Drug Discovery *58*
2.8 Summary *59*
Acknowledgments *60*
References *60*

3	**DrugBank Online: A How-to Guide** 67
	Christen M. Klinger, Jordan Cox, Denise So, Teira Stauth, Michael Wilson, Alex Wilson, and Craig Knox
3.1	Introduction 67
3.2	DrugBank 68
3.2.1	Overview of DrugBank 68
3.2.2	DrugBank Datasets 69
3.2.2.1	Drug Cards: An Overview and Navigation Guide 70
3.2.2.2	Identification 70
3.2.2.3	Pharmacology 71
3.2.2.4	Categories 73
3.2.2.5	Properties 73
3.2.2.6	Targets, Enzymes, Carriers, and Transporters 73
3.2.2.7	References 77
3.3	Protocols 77
3.3.1	General Workflows 77
3.3.1.1	Using DrugBank Online's Search Functionality 77
3.3.1.2	Using DrugBank Online's Advanced Search Functionality 80
3.3.1.3	Browsing Drugs Using DrugBank Online's Drug Categories 83
3.3.2	Identifying Chemicals and Relevant Sequences 86
3.3.2.1	Searching Using Chemical Structure Search 86
3.3.2.2	Using Sequence Search to Find Similar Targets 89
3.3.3	Extracting DrugBank Datasets for ML 93
3.4	Research Using DrugBank 94
3.5	Discussion and Conclusions 95
	References 96
4	**Bioisosteric Replacement for Drug Discovery Supported by the SwissBioisostere Database** 101
	Antoine Daina, Alessandro Cuozzo, Marta A.S. Perez, and Vincent Zoete
4.1	Introduction 101
4.1.1	Concept of Isosterism and Bioisosterism 101
4.1.2	Classical vs. Non-classical Bioisostere and Further Molecular Replacements 102
4.1.3	Bioisosteric Replacement in Drug Discovery 105
4.2	Construction and Dissemination of SwissBioisostere 106
4.2.1	Intention and Requirements 106
4.2.2	Bioactivity Data 107
4.2.3	Nonsupervised Matched Molecular Pair Analysis 108
4.2.4	Database 108
4.2.5	Web Interface 109
4.3	Content of SwissBioisostere 111
4.3.1	Global Content 111
4.3.2	Biological and Chemical Contexts 112
4.3.3	Fragment Shape Diversity 113

4.4	Usage of SwissBioisostere	*115*
4.4.1	Website Usage	*115*
4.4.2	Most Frequent Requests	*117*
4.4.3	Examples Related to Drug Discovery	*117*
4.4.3.1	Use Cases	*117*
4.4.3.2	Replacing Unwanted Chemical Groups	*118*
4.4.3.3	Optimization of Passive Absorption and Blood–Brain Barrier Diffusion	*122*
4.4.3.4	Reduction of Flexibility	*124*
4.4.3.5	Reduction of Aromaticity/Escape from Flatland	*128*
4.5	Conclusive Remarks	*133*
	Acknowledgment	*133*
	References	*133*

Part II   Macromolecular Targets and Diseases   *139*

5   The Protein Data Bank (PDB) and Macromolecular Structure Data Supporting Computer-Aided Drug Design   *141*
David Armstrong, John Berrisford, Preeti Choudhary, Lukas Pravda, James Tolchard, Mihaly Varadi, and Sameer Velankar

5.1	Introduction	*141*
5.2	Small Molecule Data in Protein Data Bank (PDB) Entries	*142*
5.2.1	What Data are in the PDB Archive?	*142*
5.2.2	Definition of Small Molecules in OneDep	*145*
5.3	Small Molecule Dictionaries	*146*
5.3.1	wwPDB Chemical Component Dictionary (CCD)	*146*
5.3.2	The Peptide Reference Dictionary	*147*
5.4	Additional Ligand Annotations in the PDB Archive	*148*
5.4.1	Linkage Information	*148*
5.4.2	Carbohydrates	*149*
5.5	Validation of Ligands in the Worldwide Protein Data Bank (wwPDB)	*150*
5.5.1	Various Criteria and Software Used for Validating Ligand in Validation Reports	*150*
5.5.2	Identification of Ligand of Interest (LOI)	*151*
5.5.3	Geometric and Conformational Validation	*152*
5.5.4	Ligand Fit to Experimental Electron Density Validation	*152*
5.5.5	Accessing wwPDB Validation Reports from PDBe Entry Pages	*154*
5.5.6	Other Planned Improvements to Enhance Ligand Validation	*154*
5.6	PDBe Tools for Ligand Analysis	*155*
5.6.1	Ligand Interactions	*155*
5.6.1.1	Classifying Ligand Interactions	*155*
5.6.1.2	Data Availability	*156*
5.6.2	Ligand Environment Component	*156*
5.6.3	Chemistry Process and FTP	*158*

5.6.4	PDBeChem Pages	*158*
5.7	Ligand-Related Annotations in the PDBe-KB	*158*
5.7.1	Introduction to PDBe-KB	*158*
5.7.2	Data Access Mechanisms for Ligand-Related Annotations	*160*
5.7.3	Ligand-Related Annotations on the Aggregated Views of Proteins	*162*
5.8	Case Study: Using PDB Data to Support Drug Discovery	*164*
5.9	Conclusions and Outlook	*165*
5.9.1	Upcoming Features and Improvements	*166*
	References	*167*

6 The SWISS-MODEL Repository of 3D Protein Structures and Models *175*

Xavier Robin, Andrew Mark Waterhouse, Stefan Bienert, Gabriel Studer, Leila T. Alexander, Gerardo Tauriello, Torsten Schwede, and Joana Pereira

6.1	Introduction	*175*
6.2	SMR Database Content and Model Providers	*176*
6.2.1	PDB	*177*
6.2.2	SWISS-MODEL	*177*
6.2.3	AlphaFold Database	*179*
6.2.4	ModelArchive	*180*
6.3	Protein Feature Annotation and Cross-References to Computational Resources	*181*
6.3.1	Structural Features, Ligands, and Oligomers	*181*
6.3.2	SWISS-MODEL associated tools	*182*
6.3.3	Web and API Access	*183*
6.4	Quality Estimates and Benchmarking	*188*
6.5	Binding Site Conformational States	*189*
6.6	SMR and Computer-Aided Structure-based Drug Design	*190*
6.7	Conclusion and Outlook	*191*
	References	*193*

7 PDB-REDO in Computational-Aided Drug Design (CADD) *201*

Ida de Vries, Anastassis Perrakis, and Robbie P. Joosten

7.1	History and Concepts	*201*
7.1.1	X-ray Structure Models	*201*
7.1.2	PDB-REDO Development	*202*
7.1.2.1	First Uniformity	*203*
7.1.2.2	Automatic Rebuilding of Protein Backbone and Side Chains	*203*
7.1.2.3	Automated Model Completion Approaches	*204*
7.1.2.4	Systematic Integration of Structural Knowledge	*205*
7.1.2.5	Overview of PDB-REDO Pipeline	*205*
7.2	Structure Improvements by PDB-REDO	*206*
7.2.1	Parametrization and Rebuilding Effects on Small Molecule Ligands	*206*
7.2.1.1	Re-refinement Improves Ligand Conformation	*206*
7.2.1.2	Side Chain Rebuilding Improves Ligand Binding Sites	*207*

7.2.1.3	Histidine Flip and Improved Ligand Parameterization	*208*
7.2.2	Building of Protein Loops and Ligands into Protein Structure Models	*210*
7.2.2.1	Loop Building Completes a Binding Site Region	*210*
7.2.2.2	Loop Building Results in Improved Binding Sites	*211*
7.2.2.3	Building new Compounds into Density	*212*
7.2.3	Nucleic Acid Improvements by PDB-REDO	*213*
7.2.4	Glycoprotein Structure Model Rebuilding	*214*
7.2.5	Metal Binding Sites	*214*
7.2.6	Limitations of the PDB-REDO Databank	*216*
7.3	Access the PDB-REDO Databank and Metadata	*218*
7.3.1	Downloading and Inspecting Individual PDB-REDO Entries	*218*
7.3.2	Data Available in PDB-REDO Entries	*220*
7.3.3	Usage of the Uniform and FAIR Validation Data	*220*
7.3.4	Creating Datasets from the PDB-REDO Databank	*222*
7.3.5	Submitting Structure Models to the PDB-REDO Pipeline	*223*
7.4	Conclusions *223*	
	Acknowledgments and Funding *224*	
	List of Abbreviations and Symbols *224*	
	References *225*	
8	**Pharos and TCRD: Informatics Tools for Illuminating Dark Targets** *231*	
	Keith J. Kelleher, Timothy K. Sheils, Stephen L. Mathias, Dac-Trung Nguyen, Vishal Siramshetty, Ajay Pillai, Jeremy J. Yang, Cristian G. Bologa, Jeremy S. Edwards, Tudor I. Oprea, and Ewy Mathé	
8.1	Introduction *231*	
8.2	Methods *233*	
8.2.1	Data Organization *233*	
8.2.1.1	Target Alignment *234*	
8.2.1.2	Disease Alignment *234*	
8.2.1.3	Ligand Alignment *234*	
8.2.1.4	Data and UI Updates *235*	
8.2.2	Programmatic Access and Data Download *235*	
8.2.3	UI Organization *235*	
8.2.3.1	List Pages *236*	
8.2.3.2	Details Pages *236*	
8.2.3.3	Search *238*	
8.2.3.4	Tutorials *240*	
8.2.4	Analysis Methods Within Pharos *240*	
8.2.4.1	Searching for Ligands *240*	
8.2.4.2	Finding Targets by Amino Acid Sequence *241*	
8.2.4.3	Finding Targets with Similar Annotations *241*	
8.2.4.4	Finding Targets with Predicted Activity *241*	
8.2.4.5	Enrichment Scores for Filter Values *241*	

8.3	Use Cases	242
8.3.1	Hypothesizing the Role of a Dark Target	242
8.3.1.1	Primary Documentation	242
8.3.1.2	List Analysis	247
8.3.1.3	Downloading Data	251
8.3.1.4	Variations on this Use Case	251
8.3.2	Characterizing a Novel Chemical Compound	251
8.3.2.1	Finding Predicted Targets	252
8.3.2.2	Analyzing Similar Ligands	254
8.3.2.3	Ligand Details Pages	256
8.3.2.4	Variations on this Use Case	257
8.3.3	Investigating Diseases	260
8.4	Discussion	262
	Funding	264
	References	264

Part III Users' Points of View 269

9 Mining for Bioactive Molecules in Open Databases 271
Guillem Macip, Júlia Mestres-Truyol, Pol Garcia-Segura, Bryan Saldivar-Espinoza, Santiago Garcia-Vallvé, and Gerard Pujadas

9.1	Introduction	271
9.2	Main Tools for Virtual Screening	272
9.2.1	ADMET and PAINS Filtering	272
9.2.2	Protein–Ligand Docking	274
9.2.3	Pharmacophore Search	275
9.2.4	Shape/Electrostatic Similarity	276
9.2.5	Protein-Structure Databases	277
9.2.6	The Protein Data Bank	278
9.2.7	The PDB-REDO Databank	278
9.2.8	The SWISS-MODEL Repository	279
9.2.9	The AlphaFold Protein Structure Database	279
9.3	Validating Binding Site and Ligand Coordinates in Three-Dimensional Protein Complexes	280
9.4	Databases for Searching New Drugs	281
9.4.1	COCONUT	281
9.4.2	GDBs	282
9.4.3	ZINC20	282
9.5	Databases of Bioactive Molecules	282
9.5.1	The BindingDB Database	283
9.5.2	PubChem	283
9.5.3	ChEMBL	284
9.6	Databases of Inactive/Decoy Molecules	285

9.6.1	Collecting Experimentally Inactive Compounds from PubChem	*285*
9.6.2	Collecting Presumed Inactive Compounds from Decoy Databases	*285*
9.6.3	Building Custom-Based Decoy Sets	*286*
9.7	Main Metrics for Evaluating the Success of a Virtual Screening	*286*
9.8	Concluding Remarks	*288*
	References	*289*
10	**Open Access Databases – An Industrial View**	*299*
	Michael Przewosny	
10.1	Academic vs. Industrial Research	*299*
10.2	Scaffold-Hopping	*310*
10.3	Virtual-Screening	*311*
	Abbreviations	*312*
	References	*313*
	Index	*317*

Series Editors Preface

The work of natural scientists in all scientific disciplines has changed a lot in the recent decade. Access to information and data in scientific databases has become essential for effective and efficient work. In addition to the commercial databases from professional providers, open access databases from associations and institutes have also become increasingly popular for medicinal chemists in academia and pharmaceutical industry.

The latest volume of our book series entitled "Open Access Databases and Datasets for Drug Discovery" provides an exemplary overview of some of the most important databases and applications that should be of great help to the medicinal chemistry community as information source and motivation to explore the growing and existing field of open access databases and useful datasets. The book surely will support all type of scientists working in the field of drug discovery and medicinal chemistry who need information from databases to support their work.

It all started in the late 2010s when Raimund Mannhold suggested this topic in our annual editor meetings as a long-cherished heart's desire. And in 2019 he was successful to convince Antoine Daina and Vincent Zoete, who are well-known scientists in this field, to edit such a book.

After industrial practice as computational chemist for agrochemical research and academic experience as lecturer and researcher in drug discovery, Antoine joined the SIB Swiss Institute of Bioinformatics in 2012. He is now senior scientist in the Molecular Modeling Group in charge of methodological developments in the SwissDrugDesign program, of supporting drug discovery projects and of teaching computer-aided drug design.

Vincent joined the SIB Swiss Institute of Bioinformatics in 2004. He was the associate group leader of the SIB Molecular Modeling Group until 2017 and then group leader from 2017 until now. Besides this, Vincent is Associate Professor in molecular modeling at the University of Lausanne since 2022 and coordinator/developer of SwissDock.ch, SwissParam.ch, SwissBioisostere.ch, SwissTargetPrediction.ch, SwissSimilarity.ch, and SwissADME.ch.

The Swiss Institute of Bioinformatics hosting the Click2Drug Webpage provides the most comprehensive collection of worldwide available databases and application tools in the field of drug discovery.

At the same time Helmut Buschmann remembered his old colleague Michael Przewosny from our time together at Grünenthal GmbH located in Aachen. Michael has over 20 years of experience in pharmaceutical research and drug discovery. He held several positions as laboratory manager in medicinal chemistry and process development. Michael has created a competitive intelligence department at Grünenthal in Aachen, where he was responsible for such database and application tools as service for the entire research organization. It took some time to convince Michael for such a book assignment, but finally he was motivated to join the group of Antoine and Vincent.

Together they brought many years of experience in the development of such databases, reinforced by many years of experience in using such databases in the field of drug discovery.

Jointly Antoine, Vincent, and Michael started in late 2019 with a collection of ideas and agreed after long discussions on a useful structure of such a broad research area with an enormous rapid development.

After a successful start, there was now a long, rocky, and chaotic road ahead of them accompanied by the Covid pandemic. There were many disappointments, but they never gave up. They worked very hard and were always successful to find a way forward. Then another major setback followed. Raimund died unexpectedly after a short illness on October 14, 2022, and was not able to see the successful completion. We, the series editors and the publisher, are all the more pleased that the editors have dedicated this volume to his memory. Raimund accompanied the book series from the first volume published early as 1993 until his death and was able to enjoy the publishing of volume 81 in June 2022 "Flow and Microreactor Technology in Medicinal Chemistry" edited by Esther Alza, shortly before he passed away.

The editors managed to edit a book with the support of the best authors in the field to provide the interested reader with a detailed overview of open-access databases and datasets for drugs from early to late phases of the lengthy drug discovery process. In such rapidly growing research field, the picture of open databases and datasets remains always incomplete.

It is all the more important that the authors managed to edit a volume that depicts a wide variety of resources from the most generalist to most specialized ones. Such a volume can never be a complete and encyclopedic collection of all existing databases, but it acts much more like guidance and motivation to deal with such databases and the resulting possibilities. In different chapters the most relevant tools and databases and apps are described by explaining case studies and examples to get an easy and direct introduction to use these tools.

Antoine, Vincent, and Michael have managed with great passion to persuade and encourage the authors to provide as much practical advice as possible with step-by-step guides and helpful use cases for the interested reader of all disciplines involved in drug hunting, bringing new, powerful, and safe medicines to the patients. The selected and compiled data collection of databases and apps provides a strong comprehensive basis as a kind of guided tour through the very dense jungle of public available scientific information.

The editors have structured the guidance book in 3 thematic sections and 10 chapters. Antoine, Vincent, and Michael have not only edited the book but also contributed with their long experience and great knowledge as authors and co-authors of some of the chapters.

As a general introduction to the volume edited by Antoine and Vincent themselves with the support of their coworkers, a comprehensive overview to the topic and a rich annotated list of data sources entitled "Open Access Databases and Datasets for Computer-Aided Drug Design. A Short List Used in the Molecular Modelling Group of the SIB" is provided. The core of the book presented in part I and II consists of seven diverse and high-quality resources presented by their developers, categorized in small molecules or macromolecular targets and diseases.

Part I is dedicated to small molecules and contains three chapters describing the most popular databases in this field:

- PubChem: A Large-Scale Public Chemical Database for Drug Discovery, edited by Sunghwan Kim and Evan E. Bolton.
- DrugBank Online: A How-to Guide, edited by Christen M. Klinger, Jordan Cox, Denise So, Teira Stauth, Michael Wilson, Alex Wilson, and Craig Knox
- Bioisosteric Replacement for Drug Discovery Supported by the SwissBioisostere Database, edited by Antoine Daina, Alessandro Cuozzo, Marta A.S. Perez, and Vincent Zoete

Part II focuses on macromolecular targets and diseases comprising the following chapters:

- The Protein Data Bank (PDB) and Macromolecular Structure Data Supporting Computer-Aided Drug Design, edited by David Armstrong, John Berrisford, Preeti Choudhary, Lukas Pravda, James Tolchard, Mihaly Varadi, and Sameer Velankar
- The SWISS-MODEL Repository of 3D Protein Structures and Models, edited by Xavier Robin, Andrew Waterhouse, Stefan Bienert, Gabriel Studer, Leila T. Alexander, Gerardo Tauriello, Torsten Schwede, and Joana Pereira
- PDB-REDO in Computational-Aided Drug Design (CADD), edited by Ida de Vries, Anastassis Perrakis, and Robbie P. Joosten
- Pharos and TCRD: Informatics Tools for Illuminating Dark Targets, edited by Keith J. Kelleher, Timothy K. Sheils, Stephen L. Mathias, Dac-Trung Nguyen, Vishal Siramshetty, Ajay Pillai, Jeremy J. Yang, Cristian G. Bologa, Jeremy S. Edwards, Tudor I. Oprea, and Ewy Mathé

Part III of the book is dedicated to user's point of view working in academia and pharmaceutical industry with two chapters:

- Mining for Bioactive Molecules in Open Databases, edited by Guillem Macip, Júlia Mestres-Truyol, Pol Garcia-Segura, Bryan Saldivar-Espinoza, Santiago Garcia-Vallvé, and Gerard Pujadas
- Open Access Databases – An Industrial View, edited by Michael Przewosny

Overall, after a long and difficult journey an outstanding collection of database and dataset information is provided that will enable the interested reader an easy start to use such tools or to expand their scope by an extension of the previous application.

With this, we – the series editors – sincerely believe that readers would be highly benefited from the contents of this book.

We would like to thank Antoine, Vincent, and Michael to put the brilliant contributions of the authors together and to guide them through an adventurous journey; all authors for their brilliant contributions and their patience; and Frank Weinreich, Stefanie Volk, and their coworkers, especially Aswini M. from the content analysis and refinement team, for their great support to make this book finally possible.

Aachen, Porto, and Bonn, July 2023

Helmut Buschmann
Jörg Holenz
Christa Müller

Raimund Mannhold – A Personal Obituary from the Series Editors

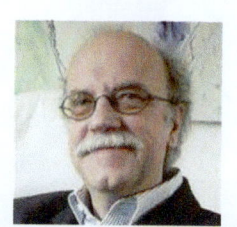

Source: http://www.raimund-mannhold.de/curriculum-vitae/

Raimund Mannhold died on October 14, 2022, after a short and serious illness at the age of 74. Nevertheless, the news of his death came as a great surprise to his immediate family and to us. Raimund accompanied the book series "Methods and Principles in Medicinal Chemistry" from the first volume published as early as 1993 until his death and was able to enjoy the publishing of volume 81 in June 2022 entitled "Flow and Microreactor Technology in Medicinal Chemistry" edited by Esther Alza, shortly before he passed away.

Established in 1993, the series "Methods and Principles in Medicinal Chemistry" has become a crucial source of information within the medicinal chemistry community and beyond. Authors and editors of the series come from pharmaceutical industry as well as from academic institutions, fostering a more active exchange between these domains.

Over time, Raimund found support from a number of internationally renowned experts and entrepreneurs in medicinal chemistry. Povl Krogsgaard-Larsen, Hendrik Timmerman, Hugo Kubinyi, and Gerd Folkers as retired series editors had a decisive influence on the book series and, like Raimund, have contributed to it becoming a figurehead for medicinal chemistry worldwide.

The following picture shows Raimund (middle) with Gerd Folkers (left) and Hugo Kubinyi during the celebration of the 25th volume of the book series in 2005.

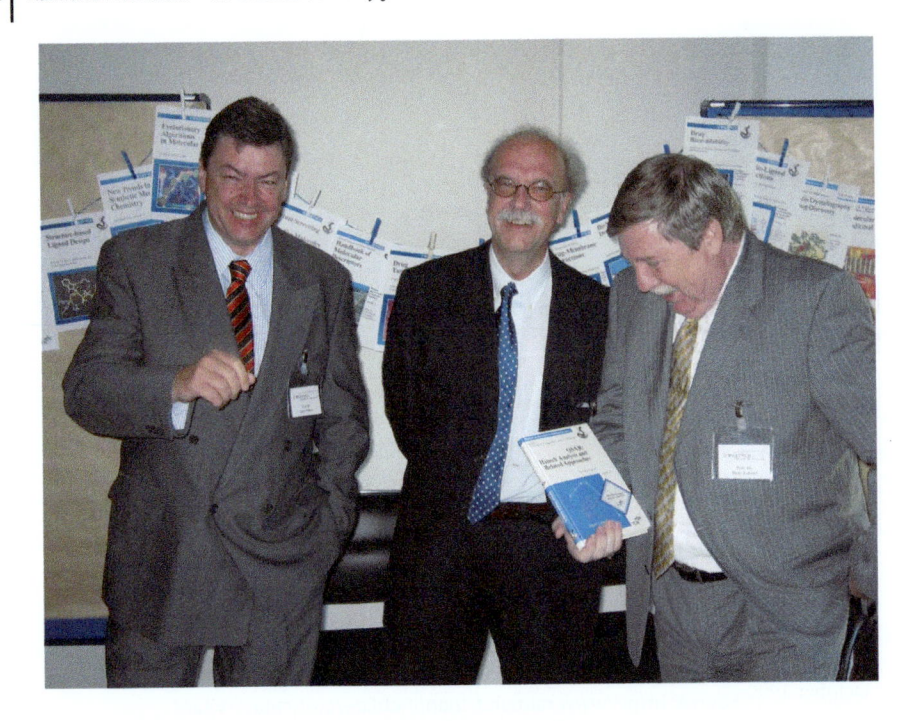

Source: Wiley-VCH

From the very beginning, the series focused on topical volumes covering hot concepts and technologies, and the reader will not miss any important topic in the field. The range of topics is as diverse as are the challenges facing modern drug developers, spanning the fields of organic chemistry, pharmacology, toxicology, life science, and analytics, the latter also including bioinformatics, chemoinformatics, and proteomics.

Raimund's heart beat for his book series, and he was now the only founding editor since the publication of the first volume 30 years ago (1993); now it must live on without Raimund, not as before, but it will continue to live on in order to preserve his legacy. That is the obligation of the current series editors Christa Müller, Jörg Holenz, and Helmut Buschmann.

Our common goal was to be able to celebrate volume 100 together; we were just able to publish volume 81 together, but without Raimund, without his commitment, and without his strong will to document the knowledge of medicinal chemistry of our time, it will be not an easy task to continue as usual. Without him there is a hard road ahead of us to fulfill his legacy and with great sadness to continue without him. But we see at the same time it as a great obligation to continue the book series in his spirit.

Raimund's life was shaped by pharmaceutical science. He was born in 1948 in Haltern (North Rhine Westphalia, Germany). From 1970 to 1973 he studied pharmacy at the Frankfurt University, received his doctorate in 1977 from the University of Düsseldorf, and in 1982 Raimund received the Venia Legendi for the subject

Physiology. In 1990 he was promoted to the professor of Molecular Drug Research at Heinrich-Heine University in Düsseldorf until his retirement on July 9, 2012.

The most important stages of his scientific career can be summarized as follows[1]:

1970–1973	Study of Pharmaceutical Sciences at the Johann-Wolfgang von Goethe Universität Frankfurt/Main
October 1973– September 1987	Scientific assistant at the Department of Clinical Physiology, Heinrich-Heine-Universität Düsseldorf
July 1977	PhD at the Department of Clinical Physiology (Heinrich-Heine-Universität Düsseldorf, Prof. Dr. R. Kaufmann). Thesis: Investigations on the Ca-antagonistic mode of action and the structure-activity relationships of verapamil
December 1982	Habilitation, conferred by the Medical Faculty of the Heinrich-Heine-Universität Düsseldorf. Title of monograph: Ca-antagonists of the aliphatic amine type and structurally related heart-active drugs – investigations on pharmacological and physicochemical properties
Since 1984	Contributing Editor of "Drugs of Today" and "Drugs of the Future"
January 1989– October 1990	Guest scientist at the Department for Pharmacochemistry, Vrije Universiteit, Amsterdam, NL (Prof. Dr. Henk Timmerman)
November 1990– July 2012	Professorship for Molecular Drug Research at the Heinrich-Heine-Universität Düsseldorf until his retirement on July 9, 2012
Since 1993	Editor of the book series "Methods and Principles in Medicinal Chemistry," Wiley-VCH, Weinheim, together with Hugo Kubinyi and Henk Timmerman (and since 2001 with Gerd Folkers)
Since 2001	Regional editor of Mini-Reviews in Medicinal Chemistry
Since 2005	Editorial board member of Medicinal Chemistry and Current Computer-Aided Drug Design
October– November 2011	Visiting professor at the School of Pharmaceutical Sciences, University of Geneva, University of Lausanne, Switzerland

His work as the serial editor of his book series will perpetuate his memory in the pharmaceutical community worldwide. His book series has now established itself as an internationally recognized standard, and millions of scientists will continue to see his name and appreciate his works in the future.

With the death of Raimund we lose a part of the spirit of the book series, which is very difficult to get over. But his footprint on the volumes published so far will be documented forever and thus remain a valuable part of scholarship.

---

1 http://www.raimund-mannhold.de/curriculum-vitae/

Dear Raimund, in addition to your content-related input, we will also miss the extremely precise planning for your beloved book series.

We promise to continue your and now our book series "Methods and Principles in Medicinal Chemistry" in your spirit, even beyond volume 100.

With deep sadness, but filled with the thought of carrying your spirit on,

Bonn, Porto, and Aachen, July 2023 *Christa, Jörg, and Helmut*

A Personal Foreword

When we think about computers to assist drug discovery, what comes to mind for most of us are the algorithms and graphics to calculate and visualize all sorts of molecular properties. What is less obvious is the knowledge that can be produced from the data itself. Today, a large amount and a vast diversity of data related to medicinal chemistry and drug discovery are available. With a few clicks, anyone can freely access downloadable raw datasets or browse more sophisticated structured databases.

This book aims to provide the reader with a detailed overview of open-access databases and datasets for drug discovery. While the picture is inevitably incomplete, it depicts a wide variety of resources from the most generalist to the most specialized. The volume begins with a rich annotated list of data sources considered of importance for (computer-aided) drug discovery and concludes with argued user perspectives. The core of the book consists of seven diverse and high-quality resources presented by their developers, categorized in *Small molecules* or *Macromolecular targets and diseases*. We have encouraged the authors to provide as much practical advice as possible with step-by-step guides and helpful use cases for medicinal chemists. Here we would like to express our deep gratitude to all the expert contributors for their remarkable commitment and admirable patience.

It all started in 2019 when the late Professor Raimund Mannhold contacted us for this project. The book is dedicated to his memory.

The process itself has been a long and chaotic journey through the COVID-19 pandemic.

Let us warmly thank the series editor, Dr. Helmut Buschmann and people at Wiley-VCH without whom this would not have been possible, in particular, Dr. Frank Weinreich, Stefany Volk, Satvinder Kaur, and Aswini Murugadass.

We wish you a pleasant and instructive reading!

Antoine Daina, Michael Przewosny, and Vincent Zoete

1

Open Access Databases and Datasets for Computer-Aided Drug Design. A Short List Used in the Molecular Modelling Group of the SIB

Antoine Daina[1], María José Ojeda-Montes[1], Maiia E. Bragina[2], Alessandro Cuozzo[2], Ute F. Röhrig[1], Marta A.S. Perez[1], and Vincent Zoete[1,2]

[1] SIB Swiss Institute of Bioinformatics, Molecular Modeling Group, Quartier UNIL-Sorge, Bâtiment Amphipôle, CH-1015 Lausanne, Switzerland
[2] University of Lausanne, Ludwig Institute for Cancer Research, Department of Oncology UNIL-CHUV, Route de la Corniche 9A, CH-1066 Epalinges, Switzerland

The role of computer-aided drug design (CADD) in modern drug discovery [1–15] is to support its various processes, including hit finding, hit-to-lead, lead optimization, and the activities preluding to preclinical trials, through numerous in silico predictors and filters. These tools have a wide variety of objectives, such as enriching the families of molecules that will be submitted to experimental screening with potentially active compounds, identifying molecules that may be problematic such as toxic moieties or those with nonspecific activities, generating ideas on the chemical modifications to be made to the compounds to increase their affinity for the therapeutic target or to improve their pharmacokinetics [16–19], or finally assisting in the various selection processes aimed at identifying and promoting the most promising molecules. These approaches are generally divided into two main families [20].

Structure-based approaches [8, 21–23] use the three-dimensional structure of the targeted protein, for example, to estimate via the use of a docking software how and how strongly a small molecule will bind to it. Avoiding the necessity to resort solely to an experimental method (*e.g.* X-ray crystallography, NMR, or cryo-electron microscopy) to obtain this information makes it possible to process a large number of molecules very quickly and at a moderate cost. In turn, this information can be used to determine how to modify the chemical structure of a small molecule to optimize rationally the intermolecular interactions with the protein target. It is then possible to select the most promising compounds for experimental validations, creating a cyclic optimization process, thanks to this feedback loop between *in silico* and *in vitro* approaches.

Ligand-based approaches take advantage of already known molecules with certain bioactivities or physicochemical properties, in order to derive the information necessary to predict the bioactivity or properties of other compounds, real or virtual. Indeed, CADD has been a pioneering research area in the development and application of machine learning methods [24–32], with the emergence, as early as the

Open Access Databases and Datasets for Drug Discovery, First Edition.
Edited by Antoine Daina, Michael Przewosny, and Vincent Zoete.
© 2024 WILEY-VCH GmbH. Published 2024 by WILEY-VCH GmbH.

1960s [33], of quantitative structure–activity relationships (QSAR [34]) or quantitative structure–property relationships (QSPR).

To perform these tasks, CADD benefits from numerous databases and datasets of small molecules, bioactivities and biological processes, 3D structures of small compounds and biomacromolecules, or molecular properties – some of which being related to pharmacokinetics or toxicity [13, 35–38]. Created in 1971, the Protein Data Bank (PDB) [39], which stores the three-dimensional structural data of large biological molecules such as proteins and nucleic acids, is a precursor in the field of freely and publicly available databases with possible applications in CADD. Currently managed by the wwPDB [40] organization and its five members, RCSB PDB [41], PDBe [42], PDBj [43], EMDB [44] and BMRB [45], the PDB continues to provide the CADD community with numerous valuable 3D structures of therapeutically relevant proteins in the apo form or in complex with small drug-like molecules, which can be used to nurture structure-based approaches. Several subsets involving such structures have been created over time, for instance, to provide reference sets to benchmark docking software, such as the Astex [46] or the Iridium [47] datasets. For a very long time, ligand-based approaches were generally limited to the use of small datasets, collected on a case-by-case basis during specific drug design projects, thus precluding their application beyond the building of focused models with limited scope. This situation dramatically changed during the 2000s with the rise of large-scale databases created specifically for the benefit of drug discovery in general and CADD in particular. ChEMBL [48, 49] released in 2008 or PubChem [50] in 2004, which collect molecules and their activities in biological assays systematically extracted from medicinal chemistry literature, patent publications, or experimental high-throughput screening programs, are certainly among the forerunners of this trend. Such databases paved the way for CADD approaches addressing, for instance, the prediction of bioactivities on a very large scale, including ligand-based methods. ZINC [51], freely accessible from 2004, is another large-scale database of small molecules, this time prepared especially for virtual screening. This important resource focuses on the compilation and storage of commercially available chemical compounds. DrugBank [52], whose first version dates back to 2006, is an example of a database gathering numerous curated and high-quality information about a group of molecules of biological interest, in this case mainly but not exclusively, approved or developmental drugs. Although smaller than ChEMBL or PubChem for instance, this type of resources, because of the quality, the structure and the practicality of the information provided, also plays an critical role in the development of new CADD techniques and filters, or for more direct applications in virtual screening.

Researchers working in CADD can be considered to have two main activities: one consists in designing, validating, and benchmarking new *in silico* approaches, the other is applying existing tools to support drug descovery projects. The nature of the databases reflects this duality. Some are clearly oriented toward an applicative usage. With virtual screening in mind, this is the case for resources gathering a large amount of commercial or virtual molecules, such as ZINC [51] or GDB-17 [53], whose main purpose is to be used as a source of molecules to feed virtual screening campaigns. At the opposite end of the spectrum, we find molecular sets constructed specifically for benchmarking screening methods, such as DUD-E [54] or DEKOIS [55]. These contain a limited number of compounds, known to be active or inactive on certain protein targets, and carefully chosen to avoid any bias in many molecular properties that would allow a screening software to identify the active ones too easily. Between these two extremes, we can find databases, such as ChEMBL, PubChem, or TCRD/Pharos [56], containing a large number of known bioactive molecules. These generalist databases can not only be used to develop a large range of CADD methods, including screening or reverse screening approaches, such as Similarity Ensemble Approach (SEA) [57, 58] or SwissTargetPrediction [59, 60], but also constitute a source of *real* molecules to be virtually screened.

By definition, the interest for many CADD-related databases lies in their capacity to store a possibly large quantity of molecules, along with useful annotations, and in their efficient diffusion to the public. This was made possible by the development and dissemination of widely accepted specific file formats. The most common file for representing molecules as strings are in SMILES [61, 62] and InChI [63, 64] formats. These one-line formats have the great advantage of using little disk or memory resources, facilitating the storage, and rapid transfer of large numbers of molecules. It should be noted, however, that several SMILES strings can represent the same molecule. This can be problematic and potentially generate redundancy when compounds from different sources are gathered. To avoid this kind of situation, it is possible to produce canonical SMILES by a well-chosen software, which are by definition unique for each molecule, or to use the UniChem [65] database that provides pointers between the molecules of most common databases. Structure-based approaches, such as molecular docking, 3D fingerprinting [66], or pharmacophores [67, 68], require a spatial representation of small molecules. The most frequently employed file definitions, including tridimensional atomic coordinates, are the Structural Data File (SDF), the MDL Mol, and Tripos Mol2 formats. Compounds are often available in such formats in the major small-molecule databases, such as ZINC [51], Chemspider [69], or DrugBank [52], which allow their direct use in 3D-based approaches. Other formats are available to store 3D structures of biomacromolecules, taking advantage of the fact that large biomolecules are based on the repetition of a small number of residues. The PDB and mmCIF [70] formats are among the standards and provided by the wwPDB consortium, and by other major databases of 3D structures of macromolecules, including PDB Redo [71, 72], as well as the SWISS-MODEL [73], MODBASE [74], and AlphaFold [75, 76] repositories of structural models.

To be valuable in the context of CADD, a database should meet several criteria in addition to the nature of its content. These criteria are very close to the findability, accessibility, interoperability, and reuse (FAIR) principles [77].

First, a database must be maintained and made available for the long term, ideally via a persistent URL, so that it can be employed for sustainable projects and developments. Unfortunately, a large fraction of new databases and datasets disappear only a few years after their initial release, due to lack of resources to maintain them or lack of interest. Attwood and colleagues studied the 18-year survival status of 326 databases published before 1997 and found that 62.3% were dead, 14.4% were archived (and not updated), and only 23.3% were still alive under their original identity or after rebranding [78]. This first analysis was independently confirmed by Finkelstein et al. who found that of the 518 original databases published in the journal *Database* between 2009 and 2016, 35% were already no longer accessible in 2020 [79], and by Imker who observed that among the 1727 databases published between 1991 and 2016 in *Nucleic Acids Research*'s "Database Issue," 40% were dead in 2018 [80]. They found that databases with higher citation counts and from researchers with higher h-index within renowned institutions were more likely to survive. In addition to straightforward online accessibility over the long term, databases should ideally be regularly updated to include the latest useful information. In order to make this process efficient and compatible with the reproducibility of the research projects that need the databases, these updates should be clearly versioned and previous releases archived for the long term. In addition, unique identifiers should be assigned to individual database entries and maintained persistently across all versions.

Second, the database should be easily searchable and retrievable. Most of those mentioned in this chapter can be accessed via a Graphical User Interface (GUI) developed to browse and search data easily, for instance by typing keywords in a search box, providing a query molecule in SMILES format or as a file, or by drawing compounds or molecular fragments within a molecular sketcher. Such interfaces are particularly efficient to search for information about a few given molecules and to display them in a well-designed graphical representation. However, such interfaces become inefficient when a project requires a large amount of data, which will eventually have to be analyzed by the user through dedicated scripts and programs. In these cases, the information should be searchable and massively retrievable by command lines, for example, with an API through specific search and download commands. Ideally, the whole database content should be downloadable for local use by classic database management systems, such as MySQL or PostgreSQL, in order to be easily deployed and managed on the computers of advanced users.

Third, CADD databases and datasets should use renowned and well-accepted formats to store and deliver molecules to the users. As mentioned above, several strings and file formats are already available for this purpose, including SMILES, InChI, SDF, Mol, Mol2, PDB, and mmCIF. These formats are readily processed by most CADD software, making the use of the databases or datasets content straightforward.

Fourth, to make the interoperability between databases easier, they should include as much as possible well-accepted unique identifiers from long-standing key players in the field. For instance, the UniProt [81] ID provides a valuable solution to identify proteins. In addition, small molecules can be identified in many cases by one of the identifiers present in UniChem. This does not prevent the authors of new databases to create their own unique identifiers, for more flexibility. For example, ChEMBL uses its own unique identifier for proteins and ensures interoperability with other resources by providing a file mapping these ChEMBL IDs with UniProt [81] IDs.

Fifth, accurate information regarding the origin of the data stored in the database or dataset should be provided, as well as a detailed description of the manual or automatic curation processes applied to it.

Sixth, databases and datasets should have a clear usage license. Free- and open-access resources are often favored in academic environment, where funding may be limited, because they increase the visibility, maximize the use and impact of data, and facilitate the reuse of research results (Table 1.1).

Table 1.1 List of databases and datasets, along with their main usage and URL. When appropriate, the key purpose is reminded: training and validation of new approaches, or applicative usage. VS: virtual screening.

Name	Main usages	Description	Availability/URL	References
Databases of experimentally determined 3D structures of biomacromolecules and related resources				
PDBe	Docking Structure-based VS Target prediction Binding free energy estimation (Application, training, and validation)	As a member of the wwPDB, PDBe collects, organizes, and disseminates data on biological macromolecular structures. Contains more than 190,000 entries.	Can be freely searched here: https://www.ebi.ac.uk/pdbe REST API: https://www.ebi.ac.uk/pdbe/pdbe-rest-api Can be downloaded here: https://www.ebi.ac.uk/pdbe/services/ftp-access	[42]
PDB-Redo	Docking Structure-based VS Target prediction Binding free energy estimation (Application, training, and validation)	The PDB–REDO databank contains optimized versions of existing PDB entries with electron density maps, a description of model changes, and a wealth of model validation data.	Can be freely searched here: https://pdb-redo.eu API and download here: https://pdb-redo.eu/download-info.html	[71, 72]
Chemical Component Dictionary	Docking Ligand-based VS Structure-based VS (Application, training, and validation)	External reference file describing all residue and small molecule components found in PDB entries, maintained by the wwPDB Foundation.	Freely accessible here: https://www.wwpdb.org/data/ccd	[82]
Ligand Expo	Docking Ligand-based VS Structure-based VS (Application, training, and validation)	Provides chemical and structural information about small molecules within the structure entries of the Protein Data Bank (about 37,000 as of 2022). Maintained by the RCSB.	Freely accessible here: http://ligand-expo.rcsb.org Downloadable here in mmCIF, SDF, MOL, PDB, SMILES, and InChi: http://ligand-expo.rcsb.org/ld-download.html	[83]

(continued)

Table 1.1 (Continued)

Name	Main usages	Description	Availability/URL	References
PDBeChem	Docking Ligand-based VS Structure-based VS (Application, training, and validation)	Provides chemical and structural information about small molecules within the structure entries of the Protein Data Bank (more than 38,000 as of 2022). Maintained by PDB Europe.	Freely accessible here: https://www.ebi.ac.uk/pdbe-srv/pdbechem/	[84]
Databases of modeled 3D structures of biomacromolecules				
AlphaFold Protein Structure Database	Docking Structure-based VS (Application)	AlphaFold DB provides 200 million protein 3D structures predicted by AlphaFold, covering the proteomes of 48 organisms including humans.	Can be freely searched here: https://alphafold.ebi.ac.uk Sets of models can be downloaded here: https://alphafold.ebi.ac.uk/download	[75, 76]
ModBase	Docking Structure-based VS (Application)	Database of annotated comparative protein structure models obtained using the MODELLER program.	Can be freely searched here: https://modbase.compbio.ucsf.edu	[74]
SWISS-MODEL Repository	Docking Structure-based VS (Application)	Database of annotated 3D protein structure models generated by the SWISS-MODEL homology-modeling pipeline. Contains 2,250,005 models from SWISS-MODEL for UniProtKB targets as well as 180,763 structures from PDB with mapping to UniProtKB.	Can be freely searched here: https://swissmodel.expasy.org/repository	[73]

Databases of experimentally determined 3D structures of small molecules

Cambridge Structure Database (CSD)	Ligand-based VS Structure-based VS	The CSD repository contains over one million accurate 3D small molecules of organic and metal–organic structures from x-ray and neutron diffraction analysis. Simple search is free, more advanced options require a license.	Freely accessible here: https://www.ccdc.cam.ac.uk/solutions/csd-core/components/csd/	[85]
COD	Ligand-based VS Structure-based VS	COD (Crystallography Open Database) provides a collection of 491,107 crystal structures of organic, inorganic, metal–organic compounds, and minerals, excluding biopolymers.	Freely accessible here: http://www.crystallography.net/cod	[86]

Data and information on proteins

UniProtKB/Swiss-Prot	Target prediction Target validation	UniProtKB/Swiss-Prot is a manually annotated, nonredundant protein sequence database to provide all known relevant information about a particular protein. By combining numerous resources, the database became one of the major tools for biomedical research and drug target identification.	Can be freely searched here: https://www.uniprot.org Can be downloaded freely here: https://www.uniprot.org/uniprotkb?query=*	[81]

(continued)

Table 1.1 (Continued)

Name	Main usages	Description	Availability/URL	References
neXtProt	Target prediction Target validation	neXtProt is a comprehensive human-centric discovery platform, offering its users a seamless integration and navigation through protein-related data, for instance, function relationships with other diseases and molecular partners like drugs or chemicals. A section, in particular, is dedicated to protein–protein and protein–drug interaction data.	Can be freely searched here: https://www.nextprot.org	[87]
TCRD/Pharos	Ligand-based VS Structure-based VS Target prediction Binding free energy estimation (Application, training, and validation)	The Target Central Resource Database (TCRD) contains information about human targets, with special emphasis on poorly characterized proteins that can potentially be modulated using small molecules or biologics. Pharos is the web interface.	Freely accessible here: https://pharos.nih.gov/ TCRD can be downloaded here: http://juniper.health.unm.edu/tcrd/download/	[56]
Data and information on drugs				
CancerDrugs_DB	Licensed cancer drugs	Open access database of licensed cancer drugs with links to DrugBank and ChEMBL IDs as well as information on targets and associated disease.	Freely accessible here: http://www.redo-project.org/cancerdrugs-db/ A machine-readable version of this database can be downloaded here: https://acfdata.coworks.be/cancerdrugsdb.txt The ReDO database of repurposing candidates in oncology can be accessed here: https://www.anticancerfund.org/en/redo-db	[88]

DrugCentral	Target prediction Drug repurposing	DrugCentral provides information on active ingredients' chemical entities, pharmaceutical products, drug mode of action, indications, and pharmacologic action. Among others, sex-specific adverse effects are incorporated from FAERS database.	Can be freely searched here: https://drugcentral.org The database is available via Docker container: https:// dockr.ly/35G46a6 and public instance drugcentral:unmtid-dbs.net:5433 A Python API is also available at: https://bit.ly/2RAHRtV.	[89]
Drug Repurposing Hub	Ligand-based VS Structure-based VS Target prediction Drug repurposing	Curated and annotated dataset of FDA-approved drugs, clinical candidates, and preclinical compounds with the accompanying information about their mechanism of action, protein targets as well as vendor's ID. It currently stores information for 6807 compounds.	Freely accessible here: https://firedb.bioinfo.cnio.es/ The dataset can be downloaded at https://clue.io/repurposing#download-data	[90]
DrugBank	Ligand-based VS Structure-based VS Target prediction	DrugBank is a comprehensive database containing 2726 approved small molecule drugs, 1520 approved biologics (proteins, peptides, vaccines, and allergenic), 132 nutraceuticals, and over 6693 experimental (discovery-phase) drugs for a total of 14,665 drug entries. Additionally, 5278 nonredundant protein are linked to these drug entries.	Freely accessible here: https://go.drugbank.com	[52]

(continued)

Table 1.1 (Continued)

Name	Main usages	Description	Availability/URL	References
KEGG DRUG	Ligand-based VS Structure-based VS Target prediction	Comprehensive drug information resource for approved drugs in Japan, USA, and Europe unified based on the chemical structure and/or the chemical components of active ingredients. It contains 11,892 entries, including 5169 with human gene targets.	Freely accessible here: https://www.genome.jp/kegg/drug	[91]
TTD Therapeutics Target Database	Docking Structure-based VS Target prediction (Application, training, and validation)	A comprehensive collection of drugs with their corresponding targets. The database provides crosslinks to the target structure in PDB and Alphafold. Target sequences and structures are also available.	Accessible through login at: http://db.idrblab.net/ttd/	[92]
Databases of natural compounds				
COCONUT	Natural product database Virtual screening	COCONUT (COlleCtion of Open Natural ProDUcTs) online is an open-source project for Natural Products (NPs) storage, search, and analysis. It gathers data from over 50 open NP resources and is available free of charge and without any restriction. Each entry corresponds to a "flat" NP structure and is associated, when available, to their known stereochemical forms, literature, organisms that produce them, natural geographical presence, and diverse precomputed molecular properties.	https://coconut.naturalproducts.net	[93]

PSC-db	Natural product database Ligand-based	PSC-db, a unique plant metabolite database that categorizes the diverse phytochemical spaces by providing 3D-structural information along with physicochemical and pharmaceutical properties of the most relevant natural products.	http://pscdb.appsbio.utalca.cl	[94]
Super Natural II	Natural product database Ligand-based Toxicity	The database contains 325,508 natural compounds (NCs), including information about the corresponding 2D structures, physicochemical properties, predicted toxicity class, and potential vendors.	https://bioinf-applied.charite.de/supernatural_new/index.php	[95]
Databases of small molecules				
ChEBI	Ligand-based VS Structure-based VS	ChEBI (Chemical Entities of Biological Interest) is a freely available dictionary of about 122,000 molecular entities focused on "small" chemical compounds.	Freely browsable at https://www.ebi.ac.uk/chebi SDF files here: https://ftp.ebi.ac.uk/pub/databases/chebi/SDF and database files here: https://ftp.ebi.ac.uk/pub/databases/chebi	[96]
ChEMBL	Ligand-based VS Structure-based VS Target prediction Binding free energy estimation (Application, training, and validation)	Database containing 2.3 million small molecules and their experimentally measured activities on 14,000 protein targets and 2000 cells, extracted from 1.5 million assays.	https://www.ebi.ac.uk/chembl Freely accessible here: Downloadable in multiple formats: https://chembl.gitbook.io/chembl-interface-documentation/downloads	[48, 49]

(continued)

Table 1.1 (Continued)

Name	Main usages	Description	Availability/URL	References
ChemSpider	Ligand-based VS Structure-based VS	Collection of 115 million chemical structures compiled by the Royal Society of Chemistry from 277 data sources (e.g. DrugBank, BindingDB, ChEBI, vendors, etc.). It includes the conversion of chemical names to chemical structures, the generation of SMILES and InChI strings, as well as the prediction of many physicochemical parameters.	Freely searchable here: http://www.chemspider.com/Default.aspx	[69]
DrugSpaceX	Ligand-based VS Structure-based VS (Application)	101 million chemical products for virtual screening based on transformation rules with approved drug molecules as the starting points.	Freely accessible here: https://drugspacex.simm.ac.cn	[97]
FireDB	Docking Binding site prediction (Application, training, and validation)	Database of small molecule ligands and related binding residues part of a functional site. The database can be accessed by PDB codes or UniProt accession numbers.	Can be freely downloaded here: http://firedb.bioinfo.cnio.es/repository/current_FireDB_release_mysqldump/current_release.tgz	[98]
GDB-17	Ligand-based VS	GDB-17 enumerates 166.4 billion organic molecules up to 17 atoms of C, N, O, S, and halogens. Smaller sets of 50 million molecules or 11 million lead-like compounds are also available in SMILES format.	Freely accessible here: https://zenodo.org/record/7041051#.Y00Xcy0RqFo Smaller sets are available here: https://gdb.unibe.ch/downloads/	[53]
PubChem	Ligand-based VS Structure-based VS Target prediction (Application, training, and validation)	Open chemistry database at the NIH containing 112 million compounds and 301 million bioactivities, with information on chemical structures, identifiers, chemical and physical properties, biological activities, patents, health, safety, and toxicity data.	Freely accessible here: https://pubchem.ncbi.nlm.nih.gov Bulk downloads are possible from outputs or by FTP: https://ftp.ncbi.nlm.nih.gov/pubchem	[50]

SCUBIDOO	Ligand-based VS Structure-based VS (Application)	SCUBIDOO (Screenable Chemical Universe Based on Intuitive Data OrganizatiOn) 21 million virtual products originating from a small library of building blocks and a collection of organic reactions. The dataset is distributed in three representative and computationally tractable samples denoted as S, M, and L, containing 9994, 99,977, and 999,794 products, respectively.	Freely accessible here: https://scubidoo.pharmazie.uni-marburg.de/index.php Set download: https://scubidoo.pharmazie.uni-marburg.de/view/download.php [99]
Zinc	Ligand-based VS Structure-based VS (Application)	Database of commercially available compounds for virtual screening. It contains 1.3 billion molecules, sourced from 310 catalogs from 150 vendors, with 2D and (for most) 3D structures. Of the 736 million lead-like molecules following the rule-or-four, 509 million are available for download in 3D ready for docking.	Freely accessible and downloadable here: https://zinc.docking.org https://zinc21.docking.org [51]
Target-class centric database			
BiasDB	Target-class centric database	Manually curated database containing all published biased GPCR ligands.	Freely accessible here: https://biasdb.drug-design.de/ [100]
GLASS	Target-class centric database	GLASS (GPCR-Ligand Association) database is a manually curated repository for experimentally validated GPCR-ligand interactions. Contains 3056 GPCR (including 825 human ones) and 342,539 ligand entries.	Freely accessible here: https://zhanggroup.org/GLASS [101]

(continued)

Table 1.1 (Continued)

Name	Main usages	Description	Availability/URL	References
GPCRdb	Target-class centric database	GPCRdb contains all human nonolfactory GPCRs (and >27,000 orthologs) in inactive, intermediate and active states, G-proteins, and arrestins. It includes over 2000 drug and in-trial agents and nearly 200,000 ligands with activity and availability data.	Freely accessible here: https://gpcrdb.org/	[102]
KinCoRe	Target-class centric database	Provides data for protein kinase sequences, structures, and phylogeny. It contains a list of FDA-approved PK inhibitors with known structures.	Can be freely searched here: http://dunbrack.fccc.edu/kincore Can be downloaded here: http://dunbrack.fccc.edu/kincore/download	[103]
KLIFS	Target-class centric database	KLIFS (Kinase–Ligand Interaction Fingerprints and Structures) contains over 5200 annotated kinase structures comprising 307 unique kinases and more than 3300 unique inhibitors, to support structure-based kinase research.	Freely accessible here: https://klifs.net	[104]
PDEStrIAn	Target-class centric database	PDEStrIAn (PhosphoDiEsterase Structure and ligand Interaction Annotated database) is a curated and annotated database of structures of catalytic PDE domains and inhibitors, collecting 377 PDB entries and 288 unique ligands.	Freely accessible here: http://pdestrian.vu-compmedchem.nl	[105]

Datasets for binding free energy estimation

BioLiP	Docking Structure-based VS Binding site prediction	Semimanually curated database for high-quality, biologically relevant ligand–protein binding interactions. It contains 573,225 entries, involving 116,643 proteins from PDB and 327,620 ligands.	Can be freely searched here: https://zhanggroup.org/BioLiP/qsearch.html And downloaded here: https://zhanggroup.org/BioLiP/download.html	[106]
Binding MOAD	Binding free energy estimation (Training and validation)	High-quality ligand–protein structure database extracted from the PDB. Clearly identified biologically relevant ligands annotated with experimentally determined binding data extracted from literature. It contains 41,409 protein–ligand structures, 15,223 binding data, 20,387 different ligands, and 11,058 different families.	Freely accessible here: https://bindingmoad.org. Different sets to download: https://bindingmoad.org/Home/download	[107, 108]
BindingDB	Binding free energy estimation (Training and validation)	Database of measured binding affinities, focusing chiefly on the interactions of proteins considered to be drug targets with drug-like small molecules. It contains 41,296 entries, involving 2,519,702 binding data for 8810 protein targets and 1,080,101 small molecules. BindingDB lists 5988 protein–ligand crystal structures with affinity measurements for proteins with 100% sequence identity, and 11,442 crystal structures allowing proteins to have 85% sequence identity.	Freely accessible here: https://www.bindingdb.org/rwd/bind/aboutus.jsp Can be freely downloaded, mainly in SDF format, at https://www.bindingdb.org/rwd/bind/chemsearch/marvin/SDFdownload.jsp?all_download=yes	[109]

(*continued*)

Table 1.1 (Continued)

Name	Main usages	Description	Availability/URL	References
PDBbind	Binding free energy estimation (Training and validation)	Comprehensive collection of experimentally measured binding affinity data for all biomolecular complexes deposited in the Protein Data Bank. It provides binding affinity data for a total of 23,496 biomolecular complexes, including protein–ligand (19,443), protein–protein (2852), protein–nucleic acid (1052), and nucleic acid–ligand complexes (149).	Can be freely searched here: http://www.pdbbind.org.cn/browse.php Can be freely downloaded here, after registration: http://www.pdbbind.org.cn/download.php	[110, 111]
Benchmark datasets				
CCD/Astex Validation Set	Docking (Validation/benchmarking)	Test set of 85 diverse, high-quality ligand–protein complexes from the PDB, for the validation of protein–ligand docking performance.	Freely accessible here: https://www.ccdc.cam.ac.uk/support-and-resources/Downloads/?d=27	[46]
CrossDocked2020	Structure-based VS (Training and validation)	22.6 million poses of 13,839 ligands (41.9% with affinity data) cross-docked into 2922 binding pockets across the Protein Data Bank.	Freely accessible here: https://github.com/gnina/models	[112]
D3R Grand Challenges	Binding free energy estimation Docking (Validation/benchmarking)	Collection of ligand–protein datasets used to benchmark docking software and binding free energy estimators, originally in a blind test. Collections are still available for a posteriori benchmarking.	Freely accessible here: https://drugdesigndata.org/about/grand-challenge	[113]

DEKOIS	Ligand-based VS Structure-based VS (Training and validation)	DEKOIS (Demanding Evaluation Kits for Objective In silico Screening) 2.0 library includes 81 high-quality benchmark sets for 80 protein targets. Positives were taken from BindingDB. Each positive is matched by 30 structurally diverse negatives with similar physicochemical properties.	Datasets free available per target available in SDF format at http://www.pharmchem.uni-tuebingen.de/dekois Full dataset here: http://www.pharmchem.uni-tuebingen.de/dekois/data/DEKOIS2.0_library/DEKOIS2.0_library.rar	[55]
DiSCO	Structure-based VS (Training and validation)	Benchmark set for cross-docking using the targets listed in DUD-E. The completed benchmark contains 4399 ligand and receptor structures homologous to one of 95 targets, an average of 46 ligands per target.	Freely accessible here: http://disco.csb.pitt.edu/	[114]
DUD-E	Ligand-based VS Structure-based VS (Training and validation)	22,886 active compounds and their affinities against 102 targets + 50 decoys for each active having similar physicochemical properties but dissimilar 2D topology. Possibility to create decoys for user-defined ligands.	Freely accessible here: http://dude.docking.org All set archive download: http://dude.docking.org/db/subsets/all/all.tar.gz	[54]
Iridium	Docking (Validation/benchmarking)	Dataset of highly trustworthy protein–ligand 3D structures including a set of 121 structures named **Iridium-HT** for highly trustworthy and a second set of 104 structures named **Iridium-MT** for moderately trustworthy that violated some of the quality criteria. The datasets are freely available to download after registration.	Freely accessible here: https://www.eyesopen.com/iridium-database	[47]

(continued)

Table 1.1 (Continued)

Name	Main usages	Description	Availability/URL	References
LIT-PCBA	Ligand-based VS Structure-based VS (Training and validation)	PubChem Bioassay data-based set designed to incorporate actives and decoys with similar molecular properties. The dataset comprises 15 target collections with 9780 high-confidence actives and 407,839 unique inactives in total.	Freely accessible here: https://drugdesign.unistra.fr/LIT-PCBA/	[115]
Database of compounds IDs in some of the main small-molecule databases				
UniChem	Diverse	UniChem is large-scale nonredundant database of pointers between chemical structures and different databases and resources, including PubChem, ChEMBL, ZINC, BindingDB, or SwissLipids.	https://www.ebi.ac.uk/unichem/	[65]
Databases for ligand design				
sc-PDB-Frag	Ligand design	Database of protein-bound fragments for selecting bioisosteric scaffolds. It contains 12,000 fragments within 8077 ligand–protein complexes from the PDB, involving 2377 proteins and 5233 ligands.	Freely searchable at: http://bioinfo-pharma.u-strasbg.fr/scPDBFrag	[116]
SwissBioisostere	Ligand design	Open access database of >25 million unique molecular replacements with data on bioactivity, physicochemistry, chemical, and biological contexts extracted from the literature and related resources.	Freely searchable at: http://www.swissbioisostere.ch	[117]

Databases of binding sites

M-CSA	Binding site prediction	CSA (Catalytic Site Atlas) lists enzyme active sites and catalytic residues in enzymes of 3D structure. It contains 1003 hand-curated entries, with detailed mechanistic descriptions. The entries in M-CSA represent 895 EC numbers, 73,211 SwissProt sequences, and 15,541 PDB files.	Can be freely searched here https://www.ebi.ac.uk/thornton-srv/m-csa/search And downloaded here https://www.ebi.ac.uk/thornton-srv/m-csa/download	[118]
PoSSuM	Docking Ligand design Binding site prediction	Database of 515,920 known and 9,160,203 putative ligand binding sites found in the Protein Data Bank (PDB).	Search mode for finding similar binding sites to a known ligand-binding site: https://possum.cbrc.jp/PoSSuM/search_k.html Search mode for predicting ligands that potentially bind to a structure of interest: https://possum.cbrc.jp/PoSSuM/search_p.html	[119, 120]
ProBiS-Dock Database	Docking Binding site prediction	Repository of 1,406,999 small-ligand binding sites.	Freely accessible here: http://probis-dock-database.insilab.org Freely accessible here: http://probis-dock-database.insilab.org/datasets	[121]

(continued)

Table 1.1 (Continued)

Name	Main usages	Description	Availability/URL	References
Datasets and databases related to ADME				
B3DB	ADME	Benchmark dataset for Blood-Brain Barrier permeability prediction, compiled from 50 published resources and containing numerical logBB values for 1058 compounds, and categorical BBB permeability labels (BBB+ or BBB−) for 7807 compounds.	Freely downloadable here: https://github.com/theochem/B3DB	[122]
HMDB	ADME	The Human Metabolome Database (HMDB) is a freely available electronic database containing detailed information about small molecule metabolites found in the human body. It is intended to be used for applications in metabolomics, clinical chemistry, biomarker discovery, and general education. The database is designed to contain or link three kinds of data: (i) chemical data, (ii) clinical data, and (iii) molecular biology/biochemistry data. The database contains 220,945 metabolite entries including both water-soluble and lipid-soluble metabolites. Additionally, 8610 protein sequences (enzymes and transporters) are linked to these metabolite entries.	Freely downloadable here: https://hmdb.ca Downloads in FASTA, SDF, XML format here: https://hmdb.ca/downloads	[123]

iCYP-MFE	ADME	Dataset of human Cytochrome P450 inhibitors for CYP1A2 (4471 inhibitors and 4886 non-inhibitors), CYP2C9 (3036, 6208), CYP2C19 (4392, 5479), CYP2D6 (1858, 8426), and CYP3A4 (4635, 7076).	Freely downloadable here: https://github.com/ mldlproject/2021-iCYP-MFE	[124]
MetaCyc	ADME	MetaCyc is a curated database of experimentally elucidated metabolic pathways involved in both primary and secondary metabolism, as well as associated metabolites, reactions, enzymes, and genes. The goal of MetaCyc is to catalog the universe of metabolism by storing a representative sample of each pathway. MetaCyc currently contains 2937 pathways, 17,780 reactions, and 18,124 metabolites.	Freely downloadable here: https://metacyc.org	[125]
Metrabase	ADME	The **Metabolism and Transport Database** (**Metrabase**) provides structured data on interactions between proteins and compounds related to their metabolic fate and transport across biological membranes. The current version includes knowledge about 20 transporters and 13 CYPs, 3437 compounds, which represent 11,662 interaction records from 1209 literature references.	Freely searchable here: https://www-metrabase.ch .cam.ac.uk The whole MySQL and different flat files here: https://www-metrabase.ch .cam.ac.uk/metrabaseui/ pageview/download/	[126]

(continued)

Table 1.1 (Continued)

Name	Main usages	Description	Availability/URL	References
NCATS-CYP	ADME	Dataset of 5094 compounds with experimentally determined antagonistic activity on different Cytochrome P450 (1742, 1984, and 2105 actives on CYP2D6, CYP2C9, and CYP3A4, respectively).	Freely downloadable here: https://pubchem.ncbi.nlm.nih.gov/bioassay/1645840 https://pubchem.ncbi.nlm.nih.gov/bioassay/1645842 https://pubchem.ncbi.nlm.nih.gov/bioassay/1645841	[127]
NCATS PAMPA1	ADME	Dataset of 2528 compounds including 295 molecules with 'low or moderate parallel artificial membrane permeability assay (PAMPA) permeability at pH 7.4 (i.e. log P_{eff} < 2.0) and 1739 compound with 'high PAMPA permeability' (i.e. log P_{eff} > 2.5).	Freely downloadable here: https://pubchem.ncbi.nlm.nih.gov/bioassay/1508612	[128, 129]
NCATS-RLM	ADME	Dataset of 752 compounds unstable ($t_{1/2}$ ≤ 30 min) in a rat liver microsome stability profiling assay and 1774 stable ones ($t_{1/2}$ > 30 min).	Freely downloadable here: https://pubchem.ncbi.nlm.nih.gov/bioassay/1508591	[130]
SMARTCyp dataset	ADME	Dataset for the construction of CYP450 site of metabolism (SOM) predict models It contains experimental SOM for different isoforms easily browsed through substructure search or downloadable as SDF files.	Freely searchable here: https://smartcyp.sund.ku.dk/mol_to_som?prediction=Search	[131]

Tox21-CYP	ADME	Dataset of 7683 compounds with experimentally determined antagonistic activity on different Cytochrome P450 (2372, 2914, 2447, 1523, and 1999 actives on CYP2C9, CYP2C19, CYP1A2, CYP3A4, and CYP2D6, respectively).	Freely downloadable here: https://pubchem.ncbi.nlm.nih.gov/bioassay/1671198 https://pubchem.ncbi.nlm.nih.gov/bioassay/1671197 https://pubchem.ncbi.nlm.nih.gov/bioassay/1671199 https://pubchem.ncbi.nlm.nih.gov/bioassay/1671201 https://pubchem.ncbi.nlm.nih.gov/bioassay/1671196	
Wang et al.	ADME	Dataset of 2358 molecules with categorical BBB permeability labels (BBB+ or BBB−).	Freely available as Supplementary Information here: https://chemistry-europe.onlinelibrary.wiley.com/doi/10.1002/cmdc.201800533	[132]
Datasets and databases related to toxicity				
Alves et al.	Toxicity	Dataset of 387 unique compounds, including 260 skin sensitizers and 127 non-sensitizers.	Freely available as Supplementary Information at https://ars.els-cdn.com/content/image/1-s2.0-S0041008X14004529-mmc2.xlsx	[133]
AMED Cardiotoxicity Database	Toxicity	Database of 9259 hERG inhibitors (IC50≤10 µM) and 279,718 inactive compounds (IC50>10 µM). Ligands of some other ion channels are also reported, including Nav1.5, Kv1.5, and Cav1.2.	Currently freely searchable at https://drugdesign.riken.jp/hERGdb/ Could be fully downloadable in the future.	[134]

(continued)

Table 1.1 (Continued)

Name	Main usages	Description	Availability/URL	References
CarPred	Toxicity	Experimental dataset of hERG assay results from 2130 chemicals, which were carried out under the same conditions.	Chemical structures of all compounds and their experimental hERG activities are available upon request to the authors	[135]
Cheng et al. 2011	Toxicity	Dataset of 1571 diverse chemicals including 1217 positives and 354 negatives on the *Tetrahymena pyriformis* toxicity test. The dataset contains the chemical names, CAS numbers, SMILES, and $pIGC_{50}$ values.	Freely available as Supplementary Information at https://ars.els-cdn.com/content/image/1-s2.0-S0045653510013500-mmc1.xls	[136]
Cheng et al. 2012	Toxicity	Dataset of 1604 unique compounds classified as "ready biodegradability" (RB) or "not ready biodegradability" (NRB) according to the biological oxygen demand test.	Freely available as Supplementary Information at https://ndownloader.figstatic.com/files/4180324	[137]
CTD (Comparative Toxicogenomics Database)	Toxicity	CTD 2021 contains 45 million toxicogenomic relationships for 16,394 chemicals, 51,344 genes, 5507 phenotypes, 7247 diseases, and 163,541 exposure events, from 601 comparative species.	Freely downloadable here: http://ctdbase.org/downloads	[138]
DGIdb (Drug-Gene Interaction Database)	Toxicity	DGIdb 4.0 (May 2021) contains 100,273 interactions between 39,095 molecules and 4847 genes, including 54,591 drug–gene interactions.	Freely accessible here: https://www.dgidb.org Downloads at: https://www.dgidb.org/downloads	[139]

DILIrank	Toxicity	The DILIrank dataset consists of 1036 FDA-approved drugs that are divided into four classes according to their potential for causing drug-induced liver injury (DILI): three groups (vMost-, vLess-, and vNo-DILI concern) with confirmed causal evidence, including 192, 278 and 312 drugs, respectively, and one additional group (ambiguous-DILI-concern) with causality undetermined, including 254 drugs.	Freely available as a xlsx file here: https://www.fda.gov/science-research/liver-toxicity-knowledge-base-ltkb/drug-induced-liver-injury-rank-dilirank-dataset	[140]
ECOTOX	Toxicity	The ECOTOXicology Knowledgebase (ECOTOX) is a source for locating single chemical toxicity data for aquatic life, terrestrial plants, and wildlife. It provides single-chemical ecotoxicity data for over 12,540 chemicals on 13,741 with over 1.1 million test results from over 53,000 references.	https://cfpub.epa.gov/ecotox	[141]
Fan et al.	Toxicity	Dataset of 641 diverse chemicals labeled as negative or positive according to the *in vivo* micronucleus assay results, i.e. compounds able or not to induce chromosomal damage or disrupt the cell division.	Freely available as Supplementary Information at https://www.rsc.org/suppdata/c7/tx/c7tx00259a/c7tx00259a2.xlsx	[142]
FDAMDD	Toxicity	Maximum recommended daily dose (MRDD) for 1216 pharmaceuticals.	Freely available in PubChem as provided by EPA DSSTox https://pubchem.ncbi.nlm.nih.gov/bioassay/1195	

(continued)

Table 1.1 (Continued)

Name	Main usages	Description	Availability/URL	References
hERGCentral	Toxicity	hERG inhibition data obtained from a primary screen against more than 300,000 structurally diverse compounds at 1 and 10 μM.	Freely downloadable at https://www.cambridgemedchemconsulting.com/news/index_files/81f15972727e1fe70ae7f37514bdab58-362.html or at https://dataverse.harvard.edu/dataset.xhtml?persistentId=doi:10.7910/DVN/7BVDG8	[143]
Mazzatorta et al.	Toxicity	Dataset of 445 compounds with Lowest Observed Adverse Effect (LOAEL) values for oral rat chronic toxicity.	Freely available as Supplementary Information at https://pubs.acs.org/doi/suppl/10.1021/ci8001974/suppl_file/ci8001974_si_001.xls	[144]
T3DB	Toxicity	The Toxin and Toxin Target Database (T3DB), a.k.a. the Toxic Exposome Database, currently houses 3678 toxins, including pollutants, pesticides, drugs, and food toxins, which are linked to 2073 corresponding toxin target records. Altogether there are 42,374 toxin-target associations. Available as CSV files including SMILES, InChi, and SDF formats.	Freely downloadable here: http://www.t3db.ca/downloads	[145]

| Tox21 challenge dataset | Toxicity | A library of several thousands of compounds, including environmental chemicals and drugs, screened against a panel of nuclear receptor (NR) and stress response (SR) pathway assays.

NR data cover Aryl hydrocarbon receptor (950 positive and 7219 negative datapoints), aromatase (360, 6866), androgen receptor full length (380, 8982), androgen receptor LBD (303, 8296), estrogen receptor alpha full length (937, 6760), estrogen receptor alpha LBD and PPARγ (446, 8307).

SR data cover nuclear factor (erythroid-derived 2)-like 2/antioxidant responsive element (1098, 6069), ATAD5 (338, 8753), heat shock factor response element (428, 7722), and mitochondrial membrane potential (1142, 7722), p53 (537, 8097).

Data available in SMILES and SDF formats. | Freely downloadable here: https://tripod.nih.gov/tox21/challenge/data.jsp | [146] |
| Xu. et al. | Toxicity | Dataset containing 7617 diverse compounds, including 4252 mutagens and 3365 nonmutagens based on the Ames test. | Freely available as Supplementary Information at https://pubs.acs.org/doi/suppl/10.1021/ci300400a/suppl_file/ci300400a_si_001.xls | [147] |

(continued)

Table 1.1 (Continued)

Name	Main usages	Description	Availability/URL	References
Zhu et al.	Toxicity	Dataset of 7385 compounds with their lethal dose (LD_{50}) in rat acute toxicity by oral exposure.	Chemical structures of all compounds and their experimental LD_{50} values are available upon request to the authors	[148]
Datasets of aggregators				
Aggregator Advisor	Aggregation prediction	Dataset of about 12,600 experimentally known aggregators from published sources.	Data are freely available in SMILES format at: http://advisor.docking.org/rawdata/aggpage.txt	[149]
ChemAgg	Aggregation prediction	Positive set of 12,119 known aggregators from Aggregator Advisor; negative set of 24,172 approved, experimental and investigational drugs taken from DrugBank and considered as non-aggregators.	Data freely available as a xlsx file, in Supplementary Information of the publication: https://pubs.acs.org/doi/suppl/10.1021/acs.jcim.9b00541/suppl_file/ci9b00541_si_002.xlsx	[150]
Other databases and datasets				
Google Patents	Patent	Gather and give access to more than 87 million patents and patent applications from 17 patent offices. It includes advanced search capability and translation.	https://patents.google.com	

LINCS	Mechanism of action/ side effects	The Library of Integrated Network-Based Cellular Signatures collects information about responses of cell lines to compound treatment. It currently stores information for 21,231 small molecule perturbagens.	LINCS Data Portal (small molecules): http://lincsportal.ccs.miami.edu/SmallMolecules/ LINCS Signature API: http://lincsportal.ccs.miami.edu/sigc-api/swagger-ui.html#/	[151]
PharmGKB	Target prediction Target validation	PharmGKB is a comprehensive resource that curates knowledge about the impact of genetic variation on drug response for clinicians and researchers. The current version includes knowledge about 746 drugs in 201 pathways involving 25,561 variants.	Freely accessible here: https://www.pharmgkb.org Different sets are downloadable: https://www.pharmgkb.org/downloads	[152]
SMPDB	Target prediction Target validation	SMPDB (The Small Molecule Pathway Database) is an interactive, visual database containing more than 30,000 small molecule pathways found in humans only. The majority of these pathways are not found in any other pathway database. SMPDB is designed specifically to support pathway elucidation and pathway discovery. For drugs in particular, both pharmacodynamic and pharmacokinetic pathways are described.	Freely accessible here: https://www.smpdb.ca	[153]
STITCH (Search Tool for Interacting Chemicals)	Understanding drug's cellular impact	Stitch 5.0 contains 367,000 protein–chemical interactions, covering 430,000 chemicals and 9.6 million proteins from 2031 organisms.	Freely accessible here: http://stitch.embl.de Networks and flat files are downloadable at: http://stitch.embl.de/cgi/download.pl	[154]

References

1 Yu, W. and MacKerell, A.D. (2017). Computer-aided drug design methods. *Methods in Molecular Biology* 1520: 85–106.
2 Talevi, A. (2018). Computer-aided drug design: an overview. *Methods in Molecular Biology* 1762: 1–19.
3 Frye, L., Bhat, S., Akinsanya, K., and Abel, R. (2021). From computer-aided drug discovery to computer-driven drug discovery. *Drug Discovery Today: Technologies* 39: 111–117.
4 Tautermann, C.S. (2020). Current and future challenges in modern drug discovery. *Methods in Molecular Biology* 2114: 1–17.
5 Shaker, B., Ahmad, S., Lee, J. et al. (2021). In silico methods and tools for drug discovery. *Computers in Biology and Medicine* 137: 104851.
6 Liu, X., Ijzerman, A.P., and van Westen, G.J.P. (2021). Computational approaches for de novo drug design: past, present, and future. *Methods in Molecular Biology* 2190: 139–165.
7 Agoni, C., Olotu, F.A., Ramharack, P., and Soliman, M.E. (2020). Druggability and drug-likeness concepts in drug design: are biomodelling and predictive tools having their say? *Journal of Molecular Modeling* 26: 120–111.
8 Gemma, S. (2020). Structure-based design of biologically active compounds. *Molecules* 25: 3115.
9 Scotti, L. and Scotti, M.T. (2020). Recent advancement in computer-aided drug design. *Current Pharmaceutical Design* 26: 1635–1636.
10 Chen, Y. and Kirchmair, J. (2020). Cheminformatics in natural product-based drug discovery. *Molecular Informatics* 39: e2000171.
11 Wang, A. and Durrant, J.D. (2022). Open-source browser-based tools for structure-based computer-aided drug discovery. *Molecules* 27: 4623.
12 Mouchlis, V.D. et al. (2021). Advances in de novo drug design: from conventional to machine learning methods. *International Journal of Molecular Sciences* 22: 1676.
13 Velmurugan, D., Pachaiappan, R., and Ramakrishnan, C. (2020). Recent trends in drug design and discovery. *Current Topics in Medicinal Chemistry* 20: 1761–1770.
14 Zagotto, G. and Bortoli, M. (2021). Drug design: where we are and future prospects. *Molecules* 26: 7061.
15 Doytchinova, I. (2022). Drug design-past, present, future. *Molecules* 27: 1496.
16 Kar, S. and Leszczynski, J. (2020). Open access in silico tools to predict the ADMET profiling of drug candidates. *Expert Opinion on Drug Discovery* 15: 1473–1487.
17 Kar, S., Roy, K., and Leszczynski, J. (2022). In silico tools and software to predict ADMET of new drug candidates. *Methods in Molecular Biology* 2425: 85–115.
18 Kirchmair, J. et al. (2015). Predicting drug metabolism: experiment and/or computation? *Nature Reviews. Drug Discovery* 14: 387–404.

19 van de Waterbeemd, H. and Gifford, E. (2003). ADMET in silico modelling: towards prediction paradise? *Nature Reviews. Drug Discovery* 2: 192–204.

20 Wilson, G.L. and Lill, M.A. (2011). Integrating structure-based and ligand-based approaches for computational drug design. *Future Medicinal Chemistry* 3: 735–750. https://doi.org/10.4155/fmc.11.18.

21 Śledź, P. and Caflisch, A. (2018). Protein structure-based drug design: from docking to molecular dynamics. *Current Opinion in Structural Biology* 48: 93–102.

22 Wang, X., Song, K., Li, L., and Chen, L. (2018). Structure-based drug design strategies and challenges. *Current Topics in Medicinal Chemistry* 18: 998–1006.

23 Maia, E.H.B., Assis, L.C., de Oliveira, T.A. et al. (2020). Structure-based virtual screening: from classical to artificial intelligence. *Frontiers in Chemistry* 8: 343.

24 Lima, A.N. et al. (2016). Use of machine learning approaches for novel drug discovery. *Expert Opinion on Drug Discovery* 11: 225–239.

25 Anighoro, A. (2022). Deep learning in structure-based drug design. *Methods in Molecular Biology* 2390: 261–271.

26 Kimber, T.B., Chen, Y., and Volkamer, A. (2021). Deep learning in virtual screening: recent applications and developments. *International Journal of Molecular Sciences* 22: 4435.

27 Jia, L. and Gao, H. (2022). Machine learning for in sSilico ADMET prediction. *Methods in Molecular Biology* 2390: 447–460.

28 Nag, S. et al. (2022). Deep learning tools for advancing drug discovery and development. *3 Biotech* 12: 110–121.

29 Rodríguez-Pérez, R., Miljković, F., and Bajorath, J. (2022). Machine learning in chemoinformatics and medicinal chemistry. *Annual Review of Biomedical Data Science* 5: 43–65.

30 Palazzesi, F. and Pozzan, A. (2022). Deep learning applied to ligand-based de novo drug design. *Methods in Molecular Biology* 2390: 273–299.

31 Xu, Y. (2022). Deep neural networks for QSAR. *Methods in Molecular Biology* 2390: 233–260.

32 Vamathevan, J. et al. (2019). Applications of machine learning in drug discovery and development. *Nature Reviews. Drug Discovery* 18: 463–477.

33 Hansch, C., Steward, A.R., and Iwasa, J. (1965). The correlation of localization rates of benzeneboronic acids in brain and tumor tissue with substituent constants. *Molecular Pharmacology* 1: 87–92.

34 Muratov, E.N. et al. (2020). QSAR without borders. *Chemical Society Reviews* 49: 3525–3564.

35 Zhao, L., Ciallella, H.L., Aleksunes, L.M., and Zhu, H. (2020). Advancing computer-aided drug discovery (CADD) by big data and data-driven machine learning modeling. *Drug Discovery Today* 25: 1624–1638.

36 Zhu, H. (2020). Big data and artificial intelligence modeling for drug discovery. *Annual Review of Pharmacology and Toxicology* 60: 573–589.

37 Brown, N. et al. (2020). Artificial intelligence in chemistry and drug design. *Journal of Computer-Aided Molecular Design* 34: 709–715.

38 Vogt, M. (2018). Progress with modeling activity landscapes in drug discovery. *Expert Opinion on Drug Discovery* 13: 605–615.

39 PDB consortium (1971). Crystallography: Protein Data Bank. *Nature: New Biology* 233: 223–223.

40 wwPDB consortium (2019). Protein Data Bank: the single global archive for 3D macromolecular structure data. *Nucleic Acids Research* 47: D520–D528.

41 Burley, S.K. et al. (2021). RCSB Protein Data Bank: powerful new tools for exploring 3D structures of biological macromolecules for basic and applied research and education in fundamental biology, biomedicine, biotechnology, bioengineering and energy sciences. *Nucleic Acids Research* 49: D437–D451.

42 Armstrong, D.R. et al. (2020). PDBe: improved findability of macromolecular structure data in the PDB. *Nucleic Acids Research* 48: D335–D343.

43 Bekker, G.-J. et al. (2022). Protein Data Bank Japan: celebrating our 20th anniversary during a global pandemic as the Asian hub of three dimensional macromolecular structural data. *Protein Science* 31: 173–186.

44 Lawson, C.L. et al. (2016). "EMDataBank unified data resource for 3DEM." *Nucleic Acids Res.* 44: D396–D403. doi:10.1093/nar/gkv1126

45 Romero, P.R. et al. (2020). BioMagResBank (BMRB) as a resource for structural biology. *Methods in Molecular Biology* 2112: 187–218.

46 Hartshorn, M.J. et al. (2007). Diverse, high-quality test set for the validation of protein-ligand docking performance. *Journal of Medicinal Chemistry* 50: 726–741.

47 Warren, G.L., Do, T.D., Kelley, B.P. et al. (2012). Essential considerations for using protein–ligand structures in drug discovery. *Drug Discovery Today* 17: 1270–1281.

48 Mendez, D. et al. (2019). ChEMBL: towards direct deposition of bioassay data. *Nucleic Acids Research* 47: D930–D940.

49 Gaulton, A. et al. (2017). The ChEMBL database in 2017. *Nucleic Acids Research* 45: D945–D954.

50 Kim, S. et al. (2021). PubChem in 2021: new data content and improved web interfaces. *Nucleic Acids Research* 49: D1388–D1395.

51 Irwin, J.J. et al. (2020). ZINC20-A free ultralarge-scale chemical database for ligand discovery. *Journal of Chemical Information and Modeling* 60: 6065–6073.

52 Wishart, D.S. et al. (2018). DrugBank 5.0: a major update to the DrugBank database for 2018. *Nucleic Acids Research* 46: D1074–D1082.

53 Ruddigkeit, L., van Deursen, R., Blum, L.C., and Reymond, J.-L. (2012). Enumeration of 166 billion organic small molecules in the chemical universe database GDB-17. *Journal of Chemical Information and Modeling* 52: 2864–2875.

54 Mysinger, M.M., Carchia, M., Irwin, J.J., and Shoichet, B.K. (2012). Directory of useful decoys, enhanced (DUD-E): better ligands and decoys for better benchmarking. *Journal of Medicinal Chemistry* 55: 6582–6594.

55 Bauer, M.R., Ibrahim, T.M., Vogel, S.M., and Boeckler, F.M. (2013). Evaluation and optimization of virtual screening workflows with DEKOIS 2.0—a public library of challenging docking benchmark sets. *Journal of Chemical Information and Modeling* 53: 1447–1462.

56 Sheils, T.K. et al. (2021). TCRD and Pharos 2021: mining the human proteome for disease biology. *Nucleic Acids Research* 49: D1334–D1346.

57 Keiser, M.J. et al. (2009). Predicting new molecular targets for known drugs. *Nature* 462: 175–181.

58 Lounkine, E. et al. (2012). Large-scale prediction and testing of drug activity on side-effect targets. *Nature* 486: 361–367.

59 Gfeller, D. et al. (2014). SwissTargetPrediction: a web server for target prediction of bioactive small molecules. *Nucleic Acids Research* 42: W32–W38.

60 Daina, A., Michielin, O., and Zoete, V. (2019). SwissTargetPrediction: updated data and new features for efficient prediction of protein targets of small molecules. *Nucleic Acids Research* 47: W357–W364.

61 Weininger, D. (1988). SMILES, a chemical language and information system. 1. Introduction to methodology and encoding rules. *Journal of Chemical Information and Computer Sciences* 28 (1): 31–36. https://doi.org/10.1021/ci00057a005.

62 Weininger, D., Weininger, A. & Weininger, J. L. SMILES. 2. Algorithm for generation of unique SMILES notation. (2002). https://doi.org/10.1021/ci00062a008

63 Heller, S.R., McNaught, A., Pletnev, I. et al. (2015). InChI, the IUPAC international chemical identifier. *Journal of Cheminformatics* 7: 23–34.

64 Heller, S., McNaught, A., Stein, S. et al. (2013). InChI - the worldwide chemical structure identifier standard. *Journal of Cheminformatics* 5: 7–9.

65 Chambers, J. et al. (2014). UniChem: extension of InChI-based compound mapping to salt, connectivity and stereochemistry layers. *Journal of Cheminformatics* 6: 43–10.

66 Cereto-Massagué, A. et al. (2015). Molecular fingerprint similarity search in virtual screening. *Methods* 71: 58–63.

67 Seidel, T., Schuetz, D.A., Garon, A., and Langer, T. (2019). The Pharmacophore concept and its applications in computer-aided drug design. *Progress in the Chemistry of Organic Natural Products* 110: 99–141.

68 Giordano, D., Biancaniello, C., Argenio, M.A., and Facchiano, A. (2022). Drug design by pharmacophore and virtual screening approach. *Pharmaceuticals (Basel)* 15: 646.

69 Pence, H. E. & Williams, A. (2010). ChemSpider: an online chemical information resource. *J. Chem. Educ.* 87 (11): 1123–1124. https://doi.org/10.1021/ed100697w

70 Bourne, P.E. et al. (1997). Macromolecular crystallographic information file. *Methods in Enzymology* 277: 571–590.

71 Joosten, R.P., Joosten, K., Cohen, S.X. et al. (2011). Automatic rebuilding and optimization of crystallographic structures in the Protein Data Bank. *Bioinformatics* 27: 3392–3398.

72 Joosten, R.P., Long, F., Murshudov, G.N., and Perrakis, A. (2014). The PDB_REDO server for macromolecular structure model optimization. *IUCrJ* 1: 213–220.

73 Bienert, S. et al. (2017). The SWISS-MODEL Repository-new features and functionality. *Nucleic Acids Research* 45: D313–D319.

74 Pieper, U. et al. (2014). ModBase, a database of annotated comparative protein structure models and associated resources. *Nucleic Acids Research* 42: D336–D346.

75 Jumper, J. et al. (2021). Highly accurate protein structure prediction with AlphaFold. *Nature* 596: 583–589.

76 Varadi, M. et al. (2022). AlphaFold protein structure database: massively expanding the structural coverage of protein-sequence space with high-accuracy models. *Nucleic Acids Research* 50: D439–D444.

77 Wilkinson, M.D. et al. (2016). The FAIR guiding principles for scientific data management and stewardship. *Scientific data* 3: 160018–160019.

78 Attwood, T.K., Agit, B., and Ellis, L.B.M. (2015). Longevity of biological databases. *EMBnet.journal* 21: 803.

79 Finkelstein, J., Guarino, J., Huo, X. et al. (2022). Exploring determinants of longevity of biomedical databases. *Studies in Health Technology and Informatics* 290: 135–139.

80 Imker, H.J. (2018). 25 Years of molecular biology databases: a study of proliferation, impact, and maintenance. *Frontiers in Research Metrics and Analytics* 3: 18.

81 UniProt Consortium (2021). UniProt: the universal protein knowledgebase in 2021. *Nucleic Acids Research* 49: D480–D489.

82 Westbrook, J.D. et al. (2015). The chemical component dictionary: complete descriptions of constituent molecules in experimentally determined 3D macromolecules in the Protein Data Bank. *Bioinformatics* 31: 1274–1278.

83 Feng, Z. et al. (2004). Ligand depot: a data warehouse for ligands bound to macromolecules. *Bioinformatics* 20: 2153–2155.

84 Dimitropoulos, D., Ionides, J., and Henrick, K. (2006). Using PDBeChem to search the PDB ligand dictionary. In: *Current Protocols in Bioinformatics* (ed. A.D. Baxevanis, R. Page, G.A. Petsko, et al.) 14.3.1–14.3.3.

85 Groom, C.R., Bruno, I.J., Lightfoot, M.P., and Ward, S.C. (2016). The Cambridge structural database. *Acta Crystallographica. Section B: Structural Science, Crystal Engineering and Materials* 72: 171–179.

86 Vaitkus, A., Merkys, A., and Gražulis, S. (2021). Validation of the crystallography open database using the crystallographic information framework. *Journal of Applied Crystallography* 54: 661–672.

87 Zahn-Zabal, M. et al. (2020). The neXtProt knowledgebase in 2020: data, tools and usability improvements. *Nucleic Acids Research* 48: D328–D334.

88 Pantziarka, P., Capistrano, I.R., De Potter, A. et al. (2021). An open access database of licensed cancer drugs. *Frontiers in Pharmacology* 12: 627574.

89 Avram, S. et al. (2021). DrugCentral 2021 supports drug discovery and repositioning. *Nucleic Acids Research* 49: D1160–D1169.

90 Corsello, S.M. et al. (2017). The drug repurposing hub: a next-generation drug library and information resource. *Nature Medicine* 23: 405–408.

91 Kanehisa, M., Furumichi, M., Tanabe, M. et al. (2017). KEGG: new perspectives on genomes, pathways, diseases and drugs. *Nucleic Acids Research* 45: D353–D361.

92 Zhou, Y. et al. (2022). Therapeutic target database update 2022: facilitating drug discovery with enriched comparative data of targeted agents. *Nucleic Acids Research* 50: D1398–D1407.

93 Sorokina, M., Merseburger, P., Rajan, K. et al. (2021). COCONUT online: collection of open natural products database. *Journal of Cheminformatics* 13: 2–13.

94 Valdés-Jiménez, A. et al. (2021). PSC-db: a structured and searchable 3D-database for plant secondary compounds. *Molecules* 26: 1124.

95 Banerjee, P. et al. (2015). Super natural II--a database of natural products. *Nucleic Acids Research* 43: D935–D939.

96 Hastings, J. et al. (2016). ChEBI in 2016: improved services and an expanding collection of metabolites. *Nucleic Acids Research* 44: D1214–D1219.

97 Yang, T. et al. (2021). DrugSpaceX: a large screenable and synthetically tractable database extending drug space. *Nucleic Acids Research* 49: D1170–D1178.

98 Maietta, P. et al. (2014). FireDB: a compendium of biological and pharmacologically relevant ligands. *Nucleic Acids Research* 42: D267–D272.

99 Chevillard, F. and Kolb, P. (2015). SCUBIDOO: a large yet screenable and easily searchable database of computationally created chemical compounds optimized toward high likelihood of synthetic tractability. *Journal of Chemical Information and Modeling* 55: 1824–1835.

100 Bermudez, M., Nguyen, T.N., Omieczynski, C., and Wolber, G. (2019). Strategies for the discovery of biased GPCR ligands. *Drug Discovery Today* 24: 1031–1037.

101 Chan, W.K.B. et al. (2015). GLASS: a comprehensive database for experimentally validated GPCR-ligand associations. *Bioinformatics* 31: 3035–3042.

102 Kooistra, A.J. et al. (2021). GPCRdb in 2021: integrating GPCR sequence, structure and function. *Nucleic Acids Research* 49: D335–D343.

103 Modi, V. and Dunbrack, R.L. (2022). Kincore: a web resource for structural classification of protein kinases and their inhibitors. *Nucleic Acids Research* 50: D654–D664.

104 Kanev, G.K., de Graaf, C., Westerman, B.A. et al. (2021). KLIFS: an overhaul after the first 5 years of supporting kinase research. *Nucleic Acids Research* 49: D562–D569.

105 Jansen, C. et al. (2016). PDEStrIAn: a phosphodiesterase structure and ligand interaction annotated database as a tool for structure-based drug design. *Journal of Medicinal Chemistry* 59: 7029–7065.

106 Yang, J., Roy, A., and Zhang, Y. (2013). BioLiP: a semi-manually curated database for biologically relevant ligand-protein interactions. *Nucleic Acids Research* 41: D1096–D1103.

107 Smith, R.D. et al. (2019). Updates to binding MOAD (mother of all databases): polypharmacology tools and their utility in drug repurposing. *Journal of Molecular Biology* 431: 2423–2433.

108 Ahmed, A., Smith, R.D., Clark, J.J. et al. (2015). Recent improvements to Binding MOAD: a resource for protein-ligand binding affinities and structures. *Nucleic Acids Research* 43: D465–D469.

109 Liu, T., Lin, Y., Wen, X. et al. (2007). BindingDB: a web-accessible database of experimentally determined protein-ligand binding affinities. *Nucleic Acids Research* 35: D198–D201.

110 Liu, Z. et al. (2017). Forging the basis for developing protein-ligand interaction scoring functions. *Accounts of Chemical Research* 50: 302–309.

111 Liu, Z. et al. (2015). PDB-wide collection of binding data: current status of the PDBbind database. *Bioinformatics* 31: 405–412.

112 Francoeur, P.G. et al. (2020). Three-dimensional convolutional neural networks and a cross-docked data set for structure-based drug design. *Journal of Chemical Information and Modeling* 60: 4200–4215.

113 Parks, C.D. et al. (2020). D3R grand challenge 4: blind prediction of protein-ligand poses, affinity rankings, and relative binding free energies. *Journal of Computer-Aided Molecular Design* 34: 99–119.

114 Wierbowski, S.D., Wingert, B.M., Zheng, J., and Camacho, C.J. (2020). Cross-docking benchmark for automated pose and ranking prediction of ligand binding. *Protein Science* 29: 298–305.

115 Tran-Nguyen, V.-K., Jacquemard, C., and Rognan, D. (2020). LIT-PCBA: an unbiased data set for machine learning and virtual screening. *Journal of Chemical Information and Modeling* 60: 4263–4273.

116 Desaphy, J. and Rognan, D. (2014). sc-PDB-Frag: a database of protein-ligand interaction patterns for bioisosteric replacements. *Journal of Chemical Information and Modeling* 54: 1908–1918.

117 Cuozzo, A., Daina, A., Perez, M.A. et al. (2022). SwissBioisostere 2021: updated structural, bioactivity and physicochemical data delivered by a reshaped web interface. *Nucleic Acids Research* 50: D1382–D1390.

118 Ribeiro, A.J.M. et al. (2018). Mechanism and catalytic site Atlas (M-CSA): a database of enzyme reaction mechanisms and active sites. *Nucleic Acids Research* 46: D618–D623.

119 Ito, J.-I., Ikeda, K., Yamada, K. et al. (2015). PoSSuM v.2.0: data update and a new function for investigating ligand analogs and target proteins of small-molecule drugs. *Nucleic Acids Research* 43: D392–D398.

120 Tsuchiya, Y. and Tomii, K. (2020). Structural modeling and ligand-binding prediction for analysis of structure-unknown and function-unknown proteins using FORTE alignment and PoSSuM pocket search. *Methods in Molecular Biology* 2165: 1–11.

121 Konc, J., Lešnik, S., Škrlj, B., and Janezic, D. (2021). ProBiS-Dock database: a web server and interactive web repository of small ligand-protein binding sites for drug design. *Journal of Chemical Information and Modeling* 61: 4097–4107.

122 Meng, F., Xi, Y., Huang, J., and Ayers, P.W. (2021). A curated diverse molecular database of blood-brain barrier permeability with chemical descriptors. *Sci Data* 8: 289–211.

123 Wishart, D.S. et al. (2022). HMDB 5.0: the human metabolome database for 2022. *Nucleic Acids Research* 50: D622–D631.

124 Nguyen-Vo, T.-H. et al. (2021). https://doi.org/10.1021/acs.jcim.1c00628). iCYP-MFE: identifying human cytochrome P450 inhibitors using multitask learning and molecular fingerprint-embedded encoding. *Journal of Chemical Information and Modeling* 62 (21): 5059–5068.

125 Caspi, R. et al. (2020). The MetaCyc database of metabolic pathways and enzymes – a 2019 update. *Nucleic Acids Research* 48: D445–D453.

126 Mak, L. et al. (2015). Metrabase: a cheminformatics and bioinformatics database for small molecule transporter data analysis and (Q)SAR modeling. *Journal of Cheminformatics* 7: 1–12.

127 Gonzalez, E. et al. (2021). Development of robust quantitative structure-activity relationship models for CYP2C9, CYP2D6, and CYP3A4 catalysis and inhibition. *Drug Metabolism and Disposition* 49: 822–832.

128 Sun, H. et al. (2017). Highly predictive and interpretable models for PAMPA permeability. *Bioorganic & Medicinal Chemistry* 25: 1266–1276.

129 Siramshetty, V. et al. (2021). Validating ADME QSAR models using marketed drugs. *SLAS Discovery* 26: 1326–1336.

130 Siramshetty, V.B. et al. (2020). Retrospective assessment of rat liver microsomal stability at NCATS: data and QSAR models. *Scientific Reports* 10: 20713–20714.

131 Olsen, L., Montefiori, M., Tran, K.P., and Jørgensen, F.S. (2019). SMARTCyp 3.0: enhanced cytochrome P450 site-of-metabolism prediction server. *Bioinformatics* 35: 3174–3175.

132 Wang, Z. et al. (2018). In silico prediction of blood-brain barrier permeability of compounds by machine learning and resampling methods. *ChemMedChem* 13: 2189–2201.

133 Alves, V.M. et al. (2015). Predicting chemically-induced skin reactions. Part I: QSAR models of skin sensitization and their application to identify potentially hazardous compounds. *Toxicology and Applied Pharmacology* 284: 262–272.

134 Sato, T., Yuki, H., Ogura, K., and Honma, T. (2018). Construction of an integrated database for hERG blocking small molecules. *PLoS One* 13: e0199348.

135 Lee, H.-M. et al. (2019). Computational determination of hERG-related cardiotoxicity of drug candidates. *BMC Bioinformatics* 20: 250–273.

136 Cheng, F. et al. (2011). In silico prediction of Tetrahymena pyriformis toxicity for diverse industrial chemicals with substructure pattern recognition and machine learning methods. *Chemosphere* 82: 1636–1643.

137 Cheng, F. et al. (2012). In silico assessment of chemical biodegradability. *Journal of Chemical Information and Modeling* 52: 655–669.

138 Davis, A.P. et al. (2021). Comparative Toxicogenomics Database (CTD): update 2021. *Nucleic Acids Research* 49: D1138–D1143.

139 Freshour, S.L. et al. (2021). Integration of the Drug-Gene interaction database (DGIdb 4.0) with open crowdsource efforts. *Nucleic Acids Research* 49: D1144–D1151.

140 Chen, M. et al. (2016). DILIrank: the largest reference drug list ranked by the risk for developing drug-induced liver injury in humans. *Drug Discovery Today* 21: 648–653.

141 Olker, J.H. et al. (2022). The ECOTOXicology knowledgebase: a curated database of ecologically relevant toxicity tests to support environmental research and risk assessment. *Environmental Toxicology and Chemistry* 41: 1520–1539.

142 Fan, D. et al. (2018). In silico prediction of chemical genotoxicity using machine learning methods and structural alerts. *Toxicology Research* 7: 211–220.

143 Du, F. et al. (2011). hERGCentral: a large database to store, retrieve, and analyze compound-human Ether-à-go-go related gene channel interactions to facilitate cardiotoxicity assessment in drug development. *Assay and Drug Development Technologies* 9: 580–588.

144 Mazzatorta, P., Estevez, M.D., Coulet, M., and Schilter, B. (2008). Modeling oral rat chronic toxicity. *Journal of Chemical Information and Modeling* 48: 1949–1954.

145 Wishart, D. et al. (2015). T3DB: the toxic exposome database. *Nucleic Acids Research* 43: D928–D934.

146 Huang, R. et al. (2016). Tox21Challenge to build predictive models of nuclear receptor and stress response pathways as mediated by exposure to environmental chemicals and drugs. *Frontiers in Environmental Science* 3: 85.

147 Xu, C. et al. (2012). In silico prediction of chemical Ames mutagenicity. *Journal of Chemical Information and Modeling* 52: 2840–2847.

148 Zhu, H. et al. (2009). Quantitative structure-activity relationship modeling of rat acute toxicity by oral exposure. *Chemical Research in Toxicology* 22: 1913–1921.

149 Irwin, J.J. et al. (2015). An aggregation advisor for ligand discovery. *Journal of Medicinal Chemistry* 58: 7076–7087.

150 Yang, Z.-Y. et al. (2019). Structural analysis and identification of colloidal aggregators in drug discovery. *Journal of Chemical Information and Modeling* 59: 3714–3726.

151 Stathias, V. et al. (2020). LINCS data portal 2.0: next generation access point for perturbation-response signatures. *Nucleic Acids Research* 48: D431–D439.

152 Whirl-Carrillo, M. et al. (2021). An evidence-based framework for evaluating pharmacogenomics knowledge for personalized medicine. *Clinical Pharmacology and Therapeutics* 110: 563–572.

153 Jewison, T. et al. (2014). SMPDB 2.0: big improvements to the small molecule pathway database. *Nucleic Acids Research* 42: D478–D484.

154 Szklarczyk, D. et al. (2015). STITCH 5: augmenting protein–chemical interaction networks with tissue and affinity data. *Nucleic Acids Research* 44: D380–D384.

Part I

Small Molecules

2

PubChem: A Large-Scale Public Chemical Database for Drug Discovery

Sunghwan Kim and Evan E. Bolton

National Center for Biotechnology Information, National Library of Medicine, National Institutes of Health, 8600 Rockville Pike, Bethesda, MD 20894, USA

2.1 Introduction

Advances in combinatorial chemistry (CC) and high-throughput screening (HTS) technologies have made it possible to rapidly test the biological activity of millions of chemicals at a very low cost. In addition, computational approaches for named-entity recognition [1–5] and optical structure recognition [6–11] are now commonly used to extract chemical information from various documents, such as scientific articles, patents, and government reports. These technological advances have significantly increased the amount of chemical data available in the public domain, creating a demand for public information resources that can collect, organize, and disseminate this data. It led to the development of many public databases, such as PubChem [12–17], ChEMBL [18], DrugBank [19], BindingDB [20], ZINC [21], and IUPHAR/BPS Guide to Pharmacology [22].

PubChem (https://pubchem.ncbi.nlm.nih.gov) (Figure 2.1) is a public chemical database at the U.S. National Institutes of Health (NIH) [12–17]. It collects chemical information from hundreds of data sources and disseminates it to the public free of charge. With more than 110 million unique chemical structures (as of 30 January 2022), PubChem is considered as one of the largest chemical databases in the public domain. Visited by millions of unique users every month [12], PubChem serves a wide range of users, including scientists, chemical safety officers, patent agents, educators, students, and many others. Especially, PubChem is an important resource for biomedical research communities in the areas of cheminformatics, chemical biology, medicinal chemistry, and drug discovery. Importantly, PubChem data are commonly used to build machine-learning models to predict various chemical properties and biological activities [23–48].

This chapter provides an overview of PubChem, including its data contents relevant to drug discovery as well as the tools and services that use these data. The chemical space of PubChem is compared with those of other popular chemical databases. Important characteristics of bioactivity data archived in PubChem are discussed.

Open Access Databases and Datasets for Drug Discovery, First Edition.
Edited by Antoine Daina, Michael Przewosny, and Vincent Zoete.
© 2024 WILEY-VCH GmbH. Published 2024 by WILEY-VCH GmbH.

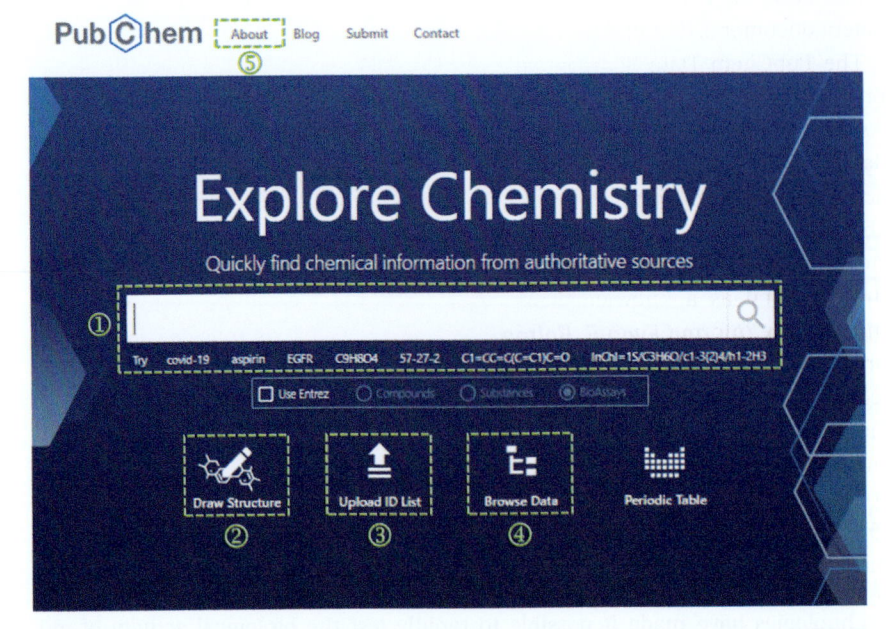

Figure 2.1 PubChem home page (https://pubchem.ncbi.nlm.nih.gov). The user can search PubChem by providing a keyword query in the search box (①). A chemical structure query can be provided using the PubChem Sketcher (②). It is also possible to provide a list of PubChem record identifiers using the "Upload ID List" button (③). The PubChem classification browser (④) allows users to get records that belong to a particular class or have a particular annotation. Clicking the "About" link (⑤) directs to PubChem's help documentation site (called PubChem Docs), where the user can also access additional tools and services.

2.2 Data Content and Organization

PubChem provides a wide range of chemical information. It contains computationally generated 3D structures of chemicals [49, 50] as well as links to experimentally determined 3D structures of chemicals available at the Protein Data Bank (PDB) [51] and the Cambridge Structural Database (CSD) [52]. Various kinds of molecular properties are available in PubChem and many of them are pertinent to drug discovery (e.g. molecular weight, solubility, octanol–water partition coefficient (log P), Caco2 permeability, acid dissociation constant (pKa), carcinogenicity, and mutagenicity). In addition, a large amount of bioactivity data submitted by data depositors are archived in PubChem. Substantial quantities of annotations on approved and investigational drugs are integrated into PubChem, such as drug labeling, indications, target genes and proteins, mechanisms of action, absorption, distribution, metabolism, excretion, and toxicity (ADMET) properties, and clinical trials carried out in the United States, Europe, and Japan. Moreover, PubChem has spectral information, including mass spectrometry (MS), infrared (IR), ultraviolet (UV), and nuclear magnetic resonance (NMR) spectroscopy data. It also provides information on synthesis and chemical vendors, as well as scientific articles and patent documents that mention chemicals.

The PubChem Data Sources page (https://pubchem.ncbi.nlm.nih.gov/sources) provides an interactive overview of organizations contributing data to PubChem. As of 30 January 2022, the data contained in PubChem are from more than 800 data sources, including U.S. government agencies, international organizations, academic institutions, pharmaceutical companies, chemical vendors, and other chemical biology databases. PubChem plays a dual role as an archive, which stores original chemical data provided by individual sources without any modification, and as a knowledgebase, which provides users with well-organized, high-quality information about chemicals. This dual role is reflected in the data organization in PubChem. PubChem data is organized into multiple data collections, including Substance, Compound, BioAssay, Gene, Protein, Pathway, Taxonomy, and Patent (Figure 2.2). Substance archives chemical descriptions submitted by individual data providers. Compound contains unique chemical structures extracted from Substance through chemical structure standardization [53]. BioAssay stores biological assay descriptions and test results, provided by assay data providers. The Gene, Protein, Pathway, and Taxonomy collections provide information on chemicals related to a given gene, protein, pathway, and taxon, respectively [17]. The Patent collection contains chemicals mentioned in a given patent document. Among these data collections, Substance and BioAssay are

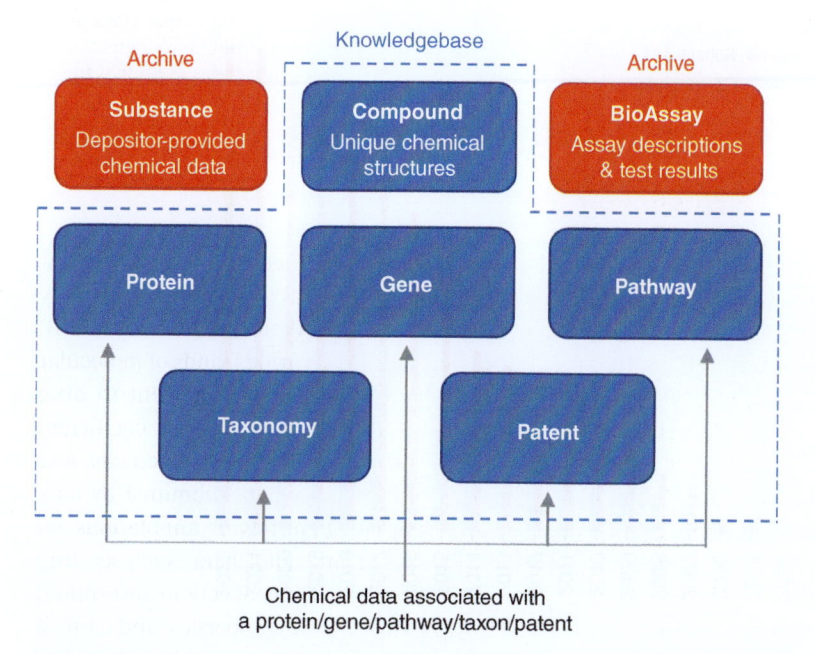

Figure 2.2 PubChem data collections. While Substance and BioAssay collections (indicated in red boxes) serve as archives, the other data collections (indicated in blue boxes) are knowledgebases.

archives that store depositor-provided data, while the other collections serve as knowledgebases.

It is noteworthy that, because of their archival nature, the data in Substance and BioAssay are kept as they were at the time of data submission by the sources. In essence, these data are owned and controlled by the data contributors. When necessary, the data source, not PubChem, may correct or update a record in Substance or BioAssay: the record will be versioned, and both the new and original ones will be retained and accessible. PubChem does, however, facilitate corrections to the data by working with the data submitter, when errors are made known to PubChem.

Each record in the Substance, Compound, and BioAssay collections is assigned a numeric identifier called Substance ID (SID), Compound ID (CID), and Assay ID (AID), respectively. Records in the Substance and Compound collections are called substances and compounds. It is worth mentioning that users are often confused with these two PubChem-specific terms. Simply put, while substances are depositor-provide descriptions of chemicals, compounds are unique chemical structures extracted from substances, meaning that a compound may be associated with multiple substances. Currently, PubChem contains 110 million compounds, extracted from 277 million substances (Figure 2.3). Detailed discussion about the substances and compounds is given in our previous paper [14] and blog post (http://go.usa.gov/x72qw).

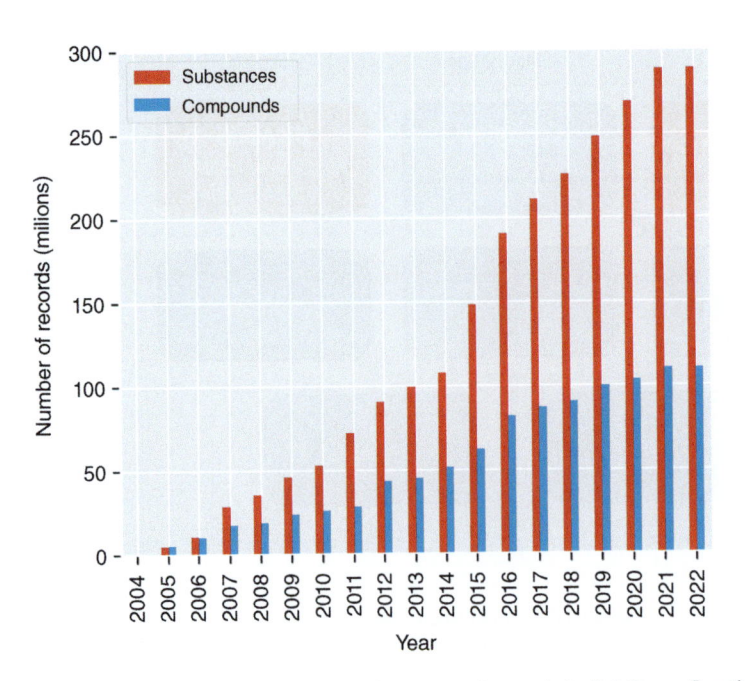

Figure 2.3 Growth of substance and compound records in PubChem. See the text for the definition of substances and compounds in PubChem. The data underlying this chart were generated on 30 January 2022.

2.3 Tools and Services

PubChem provides various tools and services to assist users in exploiting PubChem data, and they can be accessed through the PubChem homepage or the PubChem Help site (https://pubchemdocs.ncbi.nlm.nih.gov) (⑤ in Figure 2.1). This section provides a brief overview of some of these tools and services, while more details can be found at the PubChem Help site. In addition, step-by-step instructions on how to explore PubChem data through web browsers are given in our recent protocol paper [15].

2.3.1 PubChem Search

PubChem data can be searched from the PubChem home page (https://pubchem.ncbi.nlm.nih.gov) (Figure 2.1), which also serves as the entry point to various tools and services. A simple keyword search can be initiated by providing the query keyword in the search box (① in Figure 2.1). PubChem accepts various types of keywords, including chemical names, chemical abstract service (CAS) registry numbers, PubChem record identifiers (SID, CID, and AID), gene/protein names and symbols, and disease names. When a keyword query is provided, PubChem searches all data collections simultaneously and returns hit records for individual collections (Figure 2.4). It also tries to identify the most relevant record and presents it at the top of the search result page (① in Figure 2.4). The hits from a given collection can be viewed by clicking the corresponding tab (② in Figure 2.4). Users can refine this hit list based on some select attributes using filters (③ in Figure 2.4). The buttons available on the right column of the search result page (④ in Figure 2.4) allow users to perform additional tasks with the hit records, such as downloading them on a local machine, saving them for later use, or getting other records related to the hits. Clicking one of the returned hits leads to its Summary page, which displays all information available in PubChem for a given record (to be discussed in 2.3.2 Summary pages section).

The Compound collection can also be searched using a chemical structure query. The input structure can be provided using a simplified molecular-input line-entry system (SMILES) [54–56] or International Chemical Identifier (InChI) string [57]. Alternatively, it can be drawn using the PubChem Sketcher [58], which is accessible from the PubChem homepage (② in Figure 2.1). When a chemical structure input is provided, multiple types of structure searches are simultaneously performed, including identity searches, 2-dimensional (2D) and 3-dimensional (3D) similarity searches, and sub- and superstructure searches. The result for each search type can be accessed through the corresponding tab (① in Figure 2.5). Users can customize the structure search by changing the parameters and options used for the search through the Settings button (② in Figure 2.5).

It is noteworthy that PubChem supports two types of similarity search, based on fingerprint-based 2D similarity and Gaussian-shape overlay-based 3D similarity methods [59–61]. The 2D similarity between molecules is calculated by using

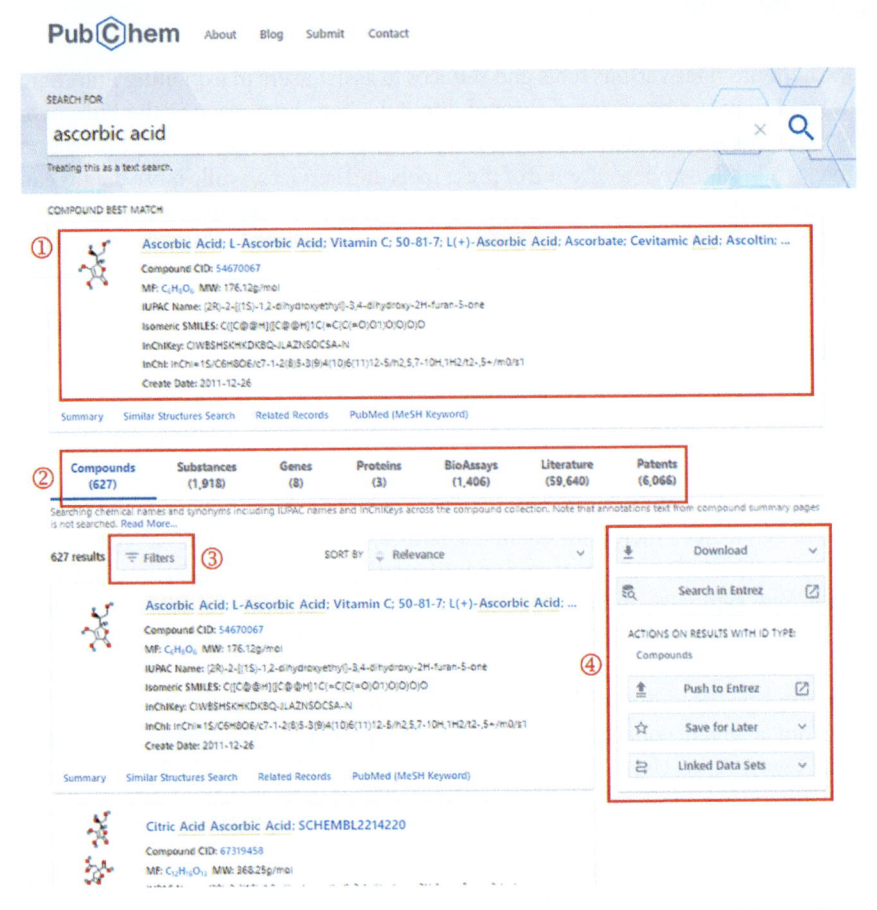

Figure 2.4 Search result page for a text query (ascorbic acid as an example) (https://pubchem.ncbi.nlm.nih.gov/#query=ascorbic%20acid). The best hit (①) will be presented at the top, and the hits from each data collection can be accessed by clicking the corresponding tab (②). The search result can be refined using the filters (③), and additional tasks can be done through the buttons on the right column of the page (④).

the PubChem subgraph fingerprints in conjunction with the Tanimoto equation [62–64]:

$$\text{Tanimoto} = \frac{N_{AB}}{N_A + N_B - N_{AB}} \qquad (2.1)$$

where N_A and N_B are the respective counts of fingerprint bits set in molecules A and B, and N_{AB} is the count of bits set in common. On the other hand, 3D molecular similarity is quantified with the shape-Tanimoto (ST) [15, 59, 60], which evaluates steric shape similarity, and color-Tanimoto (CT) [15], which quantifies functional group similarity. They are defined as:

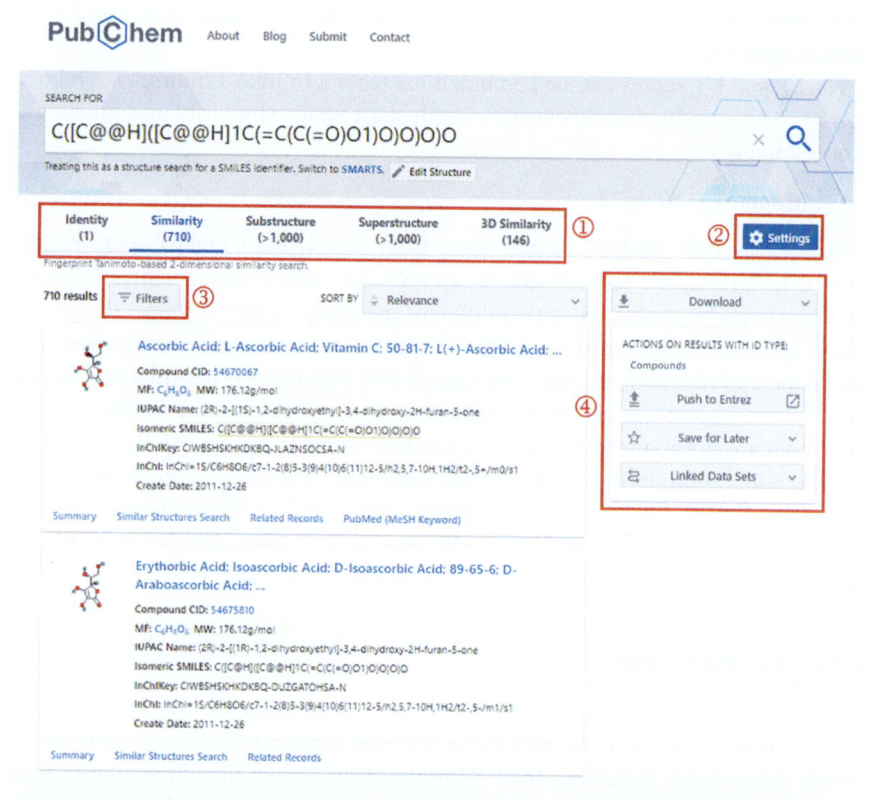

Figure 2.5 Search result page for a chemical structure query (the SMILES string for ascorbic acid as an example) (https://pubchem.ncbi.nlm.nih.gov/#query=C([C@@H] ([C@@H]1C(=C(C(=O)O1)O)O)O)O). PubChem performs multiple types of structure searches against the Compound collection, and the results for each search type can be accessed through the corresponding tab (①). The parameters and options used for structure searches can be adjusted using the Settings button (②). The search result can be refined using the filters (③), and additional tasks can be done through the buttons on the right column of the page (④).

$$ST = \frac{V_{AB}}{V_{AA} + V_{BB} - V_{AB}} \qquad (2.2)$$

$$CT = \frac{\sum_f V^f_{AB}}{\sum_f V^f_{AA} + \sum_f V^f_{BB} - \sum_f V^f_{AB}} \qquad (2.3)$$

where V_{AA} and V_{BB} are the self-overlap volumes of molecules A and B, respectively, and the V_{AB} is the overlap volume between them. In Eq (2.3), the index f indicates any of six functional group types (i.e. hydrogen-bond donors and acceptors, cations, anions, hydrophobes, and rings), represented by fictitious "feature" or "color" atoms. V^f_{AA} and V^f_{BB} are the self-overlap volumes of A and B for feature atom type f, respectively, and V_{AB}^f is the overlap volume of molecules A and B for feature atom type f.

The ST and CT scores can be combined to create a Combo-Tanimoto (ComboT) score, which simultaneously considers both steric shape similarity and functional group similarity:

$$\text{ComboT} = \text{ST} + \text{CT} \tag{2.4}$$

Because both ST and CT scores range from 0 to 1, the ComboT score ranges from 0 to 2 (without normalization). The ST, CT, and ComboT scores between molecules can be evaluated in two different molecular superpositions: the ST- or shape-optimized superposition and the CT- or feature-optimized superposition. In the shape-optimization, the superposition of two molecules is optimized to have a maximum ST score. In the feature-optimization, both shapes and features of the molecules are simultaneously considered to find the best superposition.

By default, 2D similarity search returns compounds whose Tanimoto score relative to the query molecule is equal to or greater than 0.90. For 3D similarity searches, compounds with $ST \geq 0.80$ and $CT \geq 0.50$ are returned. More detailed information on 2D and 3D similarity searches is given in our previous paper [15].

2.3.2 Summary Pages

The Summary page for a given PubChem record displays all information available for that record. For the records in the Substance and BioAssay collections, which are archival in nature, their Summary page shows the current version of depositor-provided data by default. An older version of data can be displayed by selecting the desired version from the dropdown menu (① in Figure 2.6). For the records in the other data collections, which serve as knowledgebases, the Summary page contains not only relevant depositor-provided data but also annotation data collected by the PubChem crew from external authoritative sources. These annotations are regularly updated to provide up-to-date information.

The Summary page for a given record has links to other related records (in the same or different collections), providing users with quick access to information about them. In addition, the annotation data are presented with the data sources, allowing users to go to the original data source to check the context of the data and obtain additional information. Users can quickly access the desired information by using the Table of Contents available in the right column (② in Figure 2.6). The data presented on the Summary page are downloadable using the Download button available at the top of the right column (③ in Figure 2.6). It is also possible to download the data presented under an individual (sub)section of the Summary page. Because each (sub)section of the Summary page is widgetized, it can be embedded within the user's web page. More information on PubChem Widgets is available in its help document, available at: https://pubchem.ncbi.nlm.nih.gov/docs/widgets.

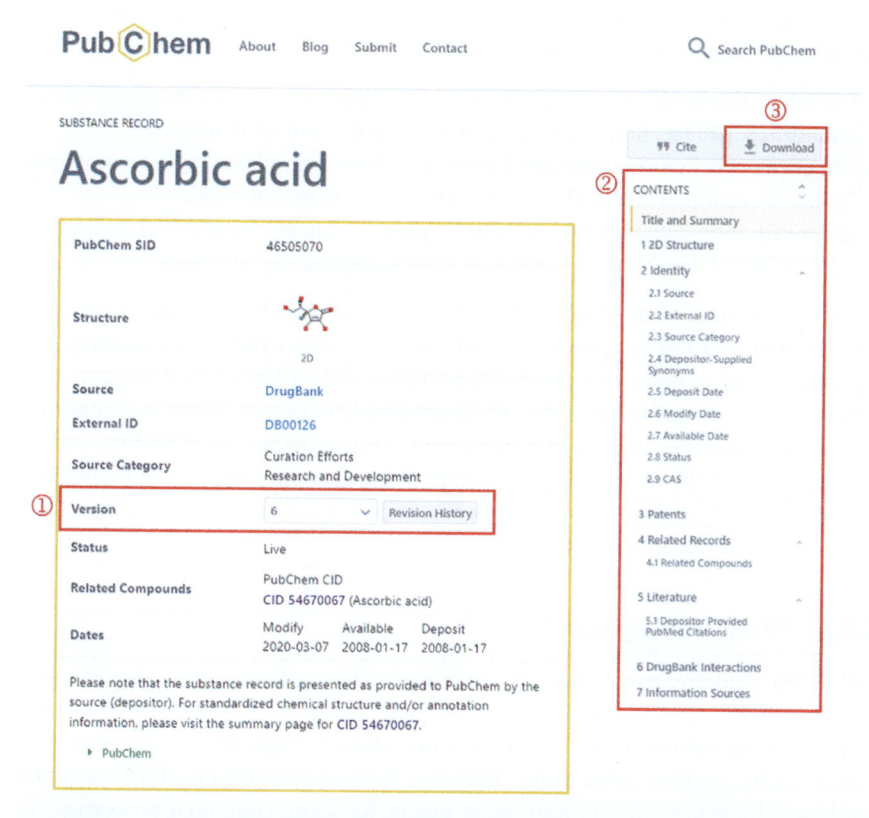

Figure 2.6 Summary page for SID 46505070 (https://pubchem.ncbi.nlm.nih.gov/substance/46505070). The dropdown menu (①) allows users to view the older version of this substance record. The Table of Contents on the right column (②) helps navigate the Summary page. The data presented on this page can be downloaded by using the Download button (③) above the Table of Contents.

2.3.3 Literature Knowledge Panel

PubChem contains a great deal of information on scientific articles and patent documents that mention chemicals and their bioactivity data [65]. Users often desire to explore these articles to learn about the relationships among chemicals, genes, proteins, and diseases, which is not trivial given the size and scope of PubChem data. To assist users in this task, the Literature Knowledge Panels [66] are presented on the Summary page of a compound, gene, or protein. The Literature Knowledge Panels for a given entity (i.e. a chemical, gene, or protein) display a few of its most relevant, nonredundant "neighbors," which are defined as other entities co-mentioned in scientific articles (e.g. chemicals, genes, proteins, and diseases). The panels also provide a sample of PubMed records co-mentioning the entity and its neighbors.

For example, the following uniform resource locators (URLs) are for the Literature Knowledge Panels for morphine (CID 5288826):

- Chemical–chemical co-occurrences: https://pubchem.ncbi.nlm.nih.gov/compound/5288826#section=Chemical-Co-Occurrences-in-Literature
- Chemical–gene co-occurrences: https://pubchem.ncbi.nlm.nih.gov/compound/5288826#section=Chemical-Gene-Co-Occurrences-in-Literature
- Chemical-disease co-occurrences: https://pubchem.ncbi.nlm.nih.gov/compound/5288826#section=Chemical-Disease-Co-Occurrences-in-Literature

The development and implementation of the Literature Knowledge Panels are described in detail in our previous paper [66]. The Knowledge Panels facilitate the quick discovery of important relationships between chemicals, genes, proteins, and diseases, as evidenced by peer-reviewed journal articles that co-mention the entities. A sample of PubMed records presented in the Panels helps understand the nature and reliability of the relationships. The underlying data presented in the Knowledge Panels can be downloaded, allowing users to gain a deeper understanding of the relationships between entities.

2.3.4 2D and 3D Neighbors

PubChem contains more than one hundred million compounds. A great deal of information is available for some of these compounds (e.g. U.S. Food and Drug Administration (FDA)-approved drugs, dietary supplements, and common solvents). In contrast, other compounds (e.g. those synthesized for HTS screening purposes) have little-to-no information except for some computed properties. To deal with this uneven degree of available information, PubChem precomputes the "neighboring" relationship between compounds based on their structural similarity. For each compound, the PubChem neighboring process identifies structurally similar compounds, which may have similar molecular properties and biological functions. Note that these "structural" neighbors should not be confused with the neighbors presented in the Literature Knowledge Panel (which refers to entities commonly mentioned together in literature).

During the neighboring process, structural similarity between compounds is evaluated using the 2D and 3D similarity methods previously described in 2.3.1 PubChem Search section, resulting in two sets of neighbors, called 2D and 3D neighbors, respectively. If two compounds have a Tanimoto score of 0.9 or greater, they are considered to be 2D neighbors of each other. On the other hand, if two compounds have an ST score of ≥ 0.8 and a CT score of ≥ 0.5, they are considered to be 3D neighbors of each other. More detailed information on 2D and 3D neighboring is explained in our previous papers [67, 68].

The precomputed neighbors of a compound can be accessed in the "Related Records" section of its Compound Summary page (Figure 2.7). The neighbors with annotations are displayed in the "Related Compounds with Annotation" section, which allows users to quickly go to the Summary pages of the neighbors and check what information is available for the neighbors (① in Figure 2.7). The lists of 2D

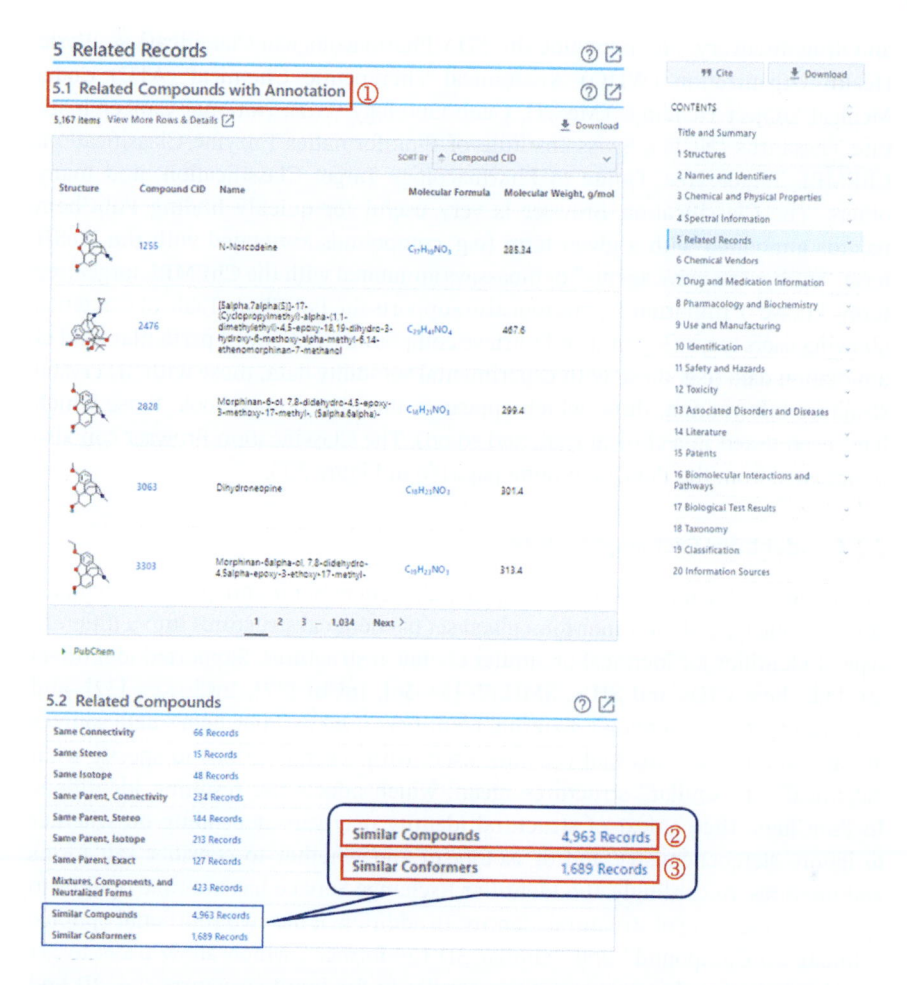

Figure 2.7 Structural neighbors are presented in the "Related Records" section of the Summary page of morphine (CID 5288826) (https://pubchem.ncbi.nlm.nih.gov/compound/5288826#section=Related-Records). Neighbors with annotations are displayed in the "Related Compounds with Annotation" subsection (①). The lists of 2D and 3D neighbors are accessible through the "Similar Compounds" (②) and "Similar Conformers" links (③), respectively, available in the "Related Compounds" subsection.

and 3D neighbors are accessible through the "Similar Compounds" and "Similar Conformers" links, respectively, available under the "Related Compounds" section of the Compound Summary page (② and ③ in Figure 2.7).

2.3.5 Classification Browser

The PubChem Classification Browser (https://pubchem.ncbi.nlm.nih.gov/classification) displays classification or ontological terms in a list or a tree structure, along with the counts of PubChem records annotated with them. It supports various classifications and ontologies, many of which are relevant to medicinal chemistry and drug discovery. These include the FDA Pharmacological Classification, World Health Organization (WHO) Anatomical Therapeutic Chemical (ATC) Code, Medical Subject Headings (MeSH), Gene Ontology (GO), National Cancer Institute Thesaurus (NCIT), Swiss Institute of Bioinformatics Enzyme Classification, ChEMBL Target Tree, Guide to Pharmacology Target Classification, and many others. The Classification Browser is very useful for quickly finding PubChem records annotated with a given term (e.g. compounds annotated with the MeSH term "antihypertensive agents" or bioassays annotated with the ChEMBL target tree term "kinase"). Importantly, this tool also supports the PubChem Table of Contents, allowing users to quickly find and retrieve compounds that have a particular kind of annotation data (e.g. those with experimental solubility data, those with 3D crystal structure information, those which appear in the FDA orange book, those which have been tested in a clinical trial, and so on). The Classification Browser can also be accessed from the PubChem homepage (④ in Figure 2.1).

2.3.6 Identifier Exchange Service

The Identifier Exchange Service (https://pubchem.ncbi.nlm.nih.gov/idexchange/) converts one type of identifier for a given set of chemical structures into a different type of identifier for identical or similar chemical structures. Supported identifiers are PubChem CIDs and SIDs, SMILES [54–56], InChI [57], InChIKey [57], and chemical names (synonyms). External identifiers used by PubChem's data sources are also supported. This tool provides users with several options to specify what "identical" or "similar" structures mean, which affects the resulting identifiers. In PubChem, the context of structural identity may vary depending on whether to ignore stereochemistry and/or isotopism and whether to consider salt forms and mixtures. Accordingly, the Identifier Exchange Service has multiple options to specify the meaning of structural identity. In addition, it has two additional options, "Similar 2D Compound" and "Similar 3D Conformer", which allow users to get the identifiers for chemical structures similar to the input structures (i.e. 2D and 3D structural neighbors, described in 2.3.4 "2D and 3D neighbors" section). When one of the two options is selected, it returns the identifiers for the precomputed structural neighbors of the input structures.

In the initial stage, the Identifier Exchange Service tries to map them with existing compound records in PubChem, and then the mapped compounds are subject to the requested operation (i.e. getting identical, related, or similar compounds), which uses precomputed relationships between compounds. Therefore, if an input identifier fails to map with any compound in PubChem, the subsequent operation cannot be performed and the input identifier will be ignored. For this reason, the Identifier Exchange Service can only work with the input identifiers that can be mapped with existing compounds.

2.3.7 Programmatic Access

PubChem provides multiple programmatic access routes [69], including Entrez Utilities (E-Utilities), Power User Gateway (PUG), PUG-SOAP [69], PUG-REST [69–71], and PUG-View [72]. Among them, PUG-REST [69–71] and PUG-View [72] are the simplest to learn and use. Both are Representational State Transfer (REST)-like interfaces, meaning that (almost) all information necessary to make a data access request through PUG-REST or PUG-View can be encoded into a single URL, which can be readily incorporated into a third-party computer program or script.

It is noteworthy that the two programmatic interfaces are designed to serve different kinds of data in general. While PUG-REST is used to access data that can be readily structured (e.g. computed properties of compounds and activity data for assays), PUG-View provides access to unstructured, textual annotation data (e.g. excerpts about the ecotoxicity of a compound). Another important difference between the two interfaces is that PUG-View cannot access multiple records in a single request, as opposed to PUG-REST. For more details about the comparison between these two interfaces, see our previous paper [72].

PubChem has a standard time limit of 30 seconds per web service request. Both PUG-REST and PUG-View are intended to handle short requests that can be completed within this time limit. In addition, PubChem also employs request volume limits, which are dynamically adjusted based on the web traffic status for the PubChem servers and the extent to which the user is approaching limits. Under normal circumstances, these limits are:

- Not more than five requests per second.
- Not more than 400 requests per minute.
- Not more than 300 seconds of running time per minute (across all running requests on PubChem)

However, at times of excessive demand, these limits may be tightened through dynamic web request throttling [70]. The user should moderate the speed at which requests are sent to PubChem based on the throttling information provided in the Hypertext Transfer Protocol (HTTP) header response. Violation of usage policies may result in users being temporarily blocked from accessing PubChem resources. See our previous paper [70] for more details about dynamic web traffic control.

2.3.8 PubChem FTP Site and PubChemRDF

PubChem data can be freely downloaded in various formats (e.g. CSV, SDF, XML, JSON, and PNG) from a search result page (Figures 2.4 and 2.5) or the Summary page of each PubChem record (Figure 2.6). It is also downloadable through programmatic access interfaces, including PUG-REST [69–71] and PUG-View [72]. In addition, the PubChem FTP site supports bulk downloads for a wide range of PubChem data. Importantly, the FTP site hosts PubChemRDF (https://pubchem.ncbi.nlm.nih.gov/rdf/) [73], PubChem data encoded using the RDF. RDF is a World Wide Web Consortium (W3C) standard model for data interchange on the web (https://www.w3.org/RDF/). PubChemRDF is very useful for integrating PubChem data with in-house data or data from other resources across scientific domains.

RDF expresses knowledge into a directed, labeled graph by breaking it down into so-called triples, each of which consists of the subject, object, and predicate. For example, the phrase "alcohol may cause liver cirrhosis" can be broken into three pieces: "alcohol" (subject), "liver cirrhosis" (object), and "may cause" (predicate). Note that the predicate defines the semantic relationship between the subject and the object.

The technical details of PubChemRDF are described in our previous paper [73] as well as the PubChemRDF Help page (https://pubchemdocs.ncbi.nlm.nih.gov/rdf). As of 30 January 2022, PubChemRDF has more than 97 billion triples, which encode semantic relationships among various entities contained in PubChem, such as compounds, substances, bioassays, proteins, genes, pathways, and endpoints. Up-to-date and more detailed RDF triple statistics are available at the PubChemRDF Statistics page (https://pubchemdocs.ncbi.nlm.nih.gov/rdf-statistics). PubChemRDF data also contains direct links to RDF-formatted data in other community resources, including MeSH RDF [74, 75], UniProtRDF [76], PDB RDF [77, 78], Reactome RDF [79], ChEMBL RDF [79], and WikiData RDF [80], making it easier to share and integrate PubChem data with data across scientific domains.

The PubChemRDF data on the FTP site are partitioned by subdomain. A subdomain refers to all RDF triples that have the same type of entity as subjects. For example, the Compound subdomain contains all triples whose subject is a compound record in PubChem. The RDF data for each subdomain is stored in its own subdirectory. This allows users to download only the desired data (rather than getting all RDF data).

The downloaded RDF data can be loaded on a local computing machine and exploited using Semantic Web Technologies. For example, the RDF data can be imported into an RDF triple store (e.g. Apache Jana TDB or OpenLink Virtuoso) and accessed using the SPARQL query interface. Alternatively, the data can be loaded into an RDF-aware graph database (e.g. Neo4j), and the graph traversal algorithm can be used to query PubChem knowledge graphs. In addition to bulk downloads via FTP, PubChemRDF can also be accessed through a REST-full interface. More detailed information on PubChemRDF can be found in our previous paper [73] as well as at the PubChemRDF help page (https://pubchemdocs.ncbi.nlm.nih.gov/rdf).

2.4 Drug- and Lead-Likeness of PubChem Compounds

Large chemical databases like PubChem often contain tens of millions of molecules, which cover various chemical classes. It would be fairly expensive to screen all these molecules during the drug discovery campaign. Therefore, in the early stage of drug discovery, it is common to filter out molecules that do not have good properties as drug candidates, based on a set of molecular properties. Examples of such filters are Lipinski's rule of five [81], the Ghose filter [82], Veber filter [83], Rapid Elimination Of Swill (REOS) filters [84], and Quantitative Estimate of Drug-likeness (QED) filters [85]. PubChem provides molecular properties that can be used to apply these filters to subset compounds. Especially, these properties are very useful for refining the search result from a query by filtering out the compounds without desired properties.

2.4 Drug- and Lead-Likeness of PubChem Compounds

One of the most popular molecular property filters is Lipinski's rule of five (Ro5) for drug-likeness [81], which is used to determine if a chemical has good solubility and permeability as a candidate for an orally administered drug in humans, based on four molecular properties: molecular weight, log P, the number of H-bond donors, and the number of H-bond acceptors. As shown in Figure 2.8, 86% of the PubChem compound records meet all four criteria or violate only one of them (68.9% and 17.2%, respectively), indicating that most compounds in PubChem are drug-like. Figure 2.8 also shows that 4.85 million compounds (4.39% of all PubChem compounds) are fragment-lead-like, satisfying all criteria of Congreve's rule of three (Ro3) [86]. There are 10.4 million compounds (9.39% of all PubChem compounds) that violate only one of the criteria of Ro3.

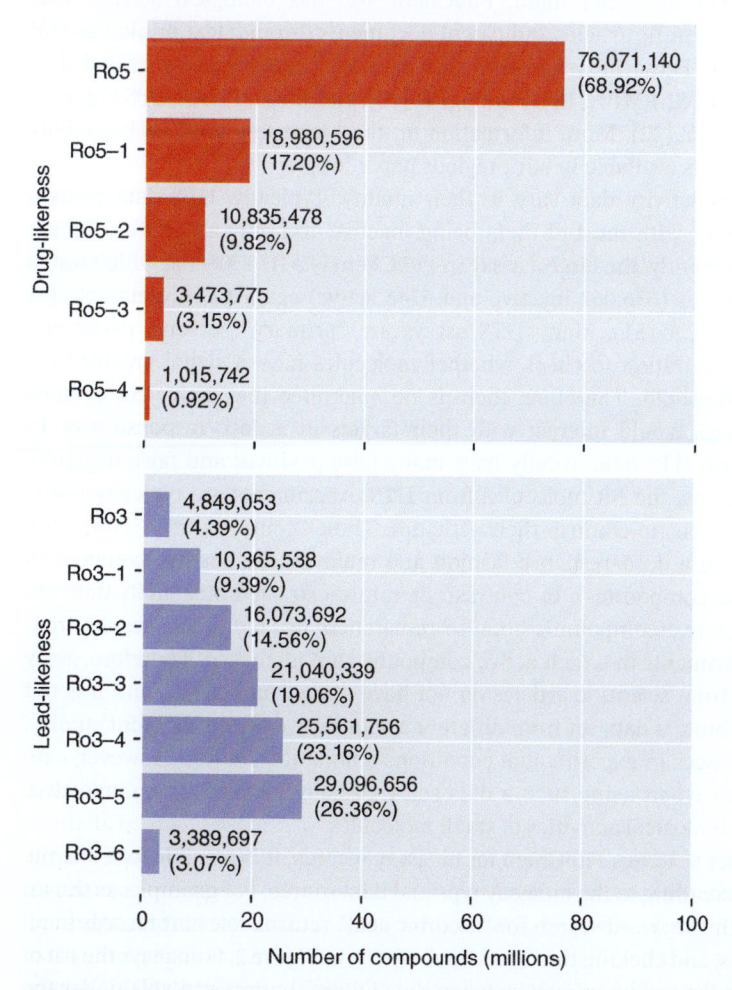

Figure 2.8 Drug-likeness and lead-likeness of compounds in PubChem, evaluated using Lipinski's rule of five (Ro5) and Congreve's rule of three (Ro3), respectively. Ro5-*n* and Ro3-*n* represent the compounds that violate *n* number of criteria of Ro5 and Ro3, respectively. The data underlying this chart was generated on 30 January 2022.

2.5 Bioactivity Data in PubChem

PubChem contains 293 million biological activity data points from 1.4 million biological assays (as of 30 January 2022). Most of these assays are small-molecule assays, with 185 RNAi screenings. Among the 110 million compounds in PubChem, 3.6 million compounds have been tested in at least one bioassay archived in PubChem, and about half of them (1.5 million compounds) have been declared active in at least one bioassay. In addition, 75,000 compounds have shown subnanomolar activity in at least one assay.

Most PubChem's bioassay data were generated through HTS from the now-concluded Molecular Libraries Initiatives at NIH and other large-scale HTS projects. On the other hand, PubChem also has biological activity data extracted from scientific articles and patent documents through text mining and/or manual curation. These literature-extracted data are contributed by several data sources, including ChEMBL [18], BindingDB [20], and the IUPHAR/BPS Guide to PHARMACOLOGY [22]. More information on the literature-extracted bioactivity data in PubChem is available in our previous paper [65].

PubChem's bioactivity data vary in their quality. Typically, HTS data contain many compounds, with most of them being inactive and only a handful of them being active. Currently, the largest assay in PubChem is AID 1508602, which tested 642,701 compounds (636,062 inactive and 6746 active) against G-protein-coupled receptor 151 (GPCR-151). Many HTS assays are "primary" screens, performed at a single concentration to check whether molecules have a signal greater than a predefined threshold. Therefore, there is no guarantee that active compounds from these assays would interact with their targets in a dose–response way. In addition, because HTS data usually have many false positives and false negatives for various reasons, the hit molecules from HTS experiments are typically tested in secondary screens to confirm their activities. These "confirmatory" screens are normally done in a dose–response fashion and remove false positive compounds (and often toxic compounds). In contrast, literature-extracted bioactivity data are dominated by active compounds because researchers usually report results from successful experiments in which active compounds are identified. Therefore, assay data extracted from scientific articles do not have many compounds, and it is not uncommon to build a data set from different assays derived from different studies, ignoring differences in experimental conditions among the studies. However, care should be taken when using such a data set, especially for developing predictive models for the biological activities of small molecules.

When the user searches PubChem for bioassay records, it is possible to refine the search result according to the bioassay type and data source. For example, as shown in Figure 2.4, the keyword search for "ascorbic acid" returns relevant records in all data collections, and clicking the "BioAssay" tab (② in Figure 2.4) displays the list of hit assays. This list can be refined by using the "Filters" button available under the tabs (③ in Figure 2.4), which allows the user to select only those assays with desired attributes (e.g. whether an assay is primary or confirmatory screening, or whether it is literature-extracted). Using the "Filters" button, it is also possible to retrieve only those assays provided by a particular data source or only those assays performed in vivo.

PubChem users often want to get all bioactivity data for a given target (e.g. a protein, gene, or organism), scattered across multiple assays from different data sources. To meet this demand, PubChem organizes bioactivity data by target and stores them in the Protein, Gene, and Taxonomy data collections (see Figure 2.2) [17]. Users can quickly access target-specific bioactivity data through the corresponding Summary page of the target, as shown in these examples:

- Chemicals and their bioactivities against the human hypoxia-inducible factor 1 subunit α (HIF1A) (NCBI Protein Accession: Q16665) https://pubchem.ncbi.nlm.nih.gov/protein/Q16665#section=Chemicals-and-Bioactivities
- Assay experiments targeting the human peroxisome proliferator-activated receptor δ (PPARD) gene (NCBI Gene ID: 5467) https://pubchem.ncbi.nlm.nih.gov/gene/5467#section=BioAssays
- Whole organism bioactivities against *Plasmodium falciparum* (NCBI Taxonomy ID: 5833) https://pubchem.ncbi.nlm.nih.gov/taxonomy/5833#section=Whole-Organism-Bioactivities

These Summary pages present the target-specific bioactivity data, along with additional information on the target, collected from authoritative sources. This target information helps users to better understand the bioactivity data. In addition, the target-specific data presented on these Summary pages can be downloaded for further analysis. More details on the PubChem Protein, Gene, and Taxonomy data collections can be found in our recent paper [17].

2.6 Comparison with Other Databases

Table 2.1 shows the overlap of the chemical structure coverage between PubChem and popular chemical databases, including ChEMBL [18], CompTox [87], BindingDB [20], ChEBI [88], PDB in Europe (PDBe) [89], DrugBank [19], Rhea [90], IUPHAR/BPS Guide to PHARMACOLOGY [22], ClinicalTrials.gov (https://clinicaltrials.gov), and DailyMed (https://dailymed.nlm.nih.gov). These overlap data were obtained from UniChem [91, 92], which is a free online chemical identifier mapping service. They were computed based on structural identity defined as FULIK (e.g. identity of the full InChIKey), meaning that two chemical structures were considered identical if their full InChIKey strings were the same as each other. Most compounds contained in the databases listed in Table 2.1 were also found in PubChem, indicating a substantial overlap between PubChem and these databases. PDBe had the smallest overlap, with only 92% of PDBe ligands also being contained in PubChem.

PubChem data sources include all information resources listed in Table 2.1, and their data are integrated within PubChem. Therefore, most chemical structures in these resources are expected to be contained in PubChem. However, a small percentage of their structures are not found in PubChem. It is primarily due to

Table 2.1 Comparison of popular chemical databases with PubChem. For a given database, N_{total} indicates the total number of chemical structures contained in that database. $N_{overlap}$ are the numbers of chemical structures that also exist in PubChem, and $N_{exclusive}$ is the number of chemical structures contained only in the given database but not in PubChem. Numbers in parentheses are the percentages of $N_{overlap}$ and $N_{exclusive}$ with respect to N_{total}. This overlap data, obtained from UniChem [91, 92] was calculated on the basis of structural identity defined as FULIK (i.e. identity of the full InChIKey).

Database	N_{total}	$N_{overlap}$		$N_{exclusive}$	
ChEMBL [18]	2,065,509	2,003,482	(97.00%)	62,027	(3.00%)
CompTox [87]	742,310	723,551	(97.47%)	18,759	(2.53%)
BindingDB [20]	673,355	649,481	(96.45%)	23,874	(3.55%)
ChEBI [88]	122,680	119,832	(97.68%)	2,848	(2.32%)
Protein Data Bank in Europe (PDBe) [89]	34,383	31,668	(92.10%)	2,715	(7.90%)
DrugBank [19]	11,161	10,727	(96.11%)	434	(3.89%)
Rhea [90]	8,964	8,596	(95.89%)	368	(4.11%)
IUPHAR/BPS Guide to PHARMACOLOGY [22]	8,411	8,200	(97.49%)	211	(2.51%)
ClinicalTrials.gov	4,678	4,510	(96.41%)	168	(3.59%)
DailyMed	2,454	2,364	(96.33%)	90	(3.67%)

a lag time between when new structures are added to a data source and when those additions are reflected in PubChem. This lag time ranges from a few days to several weeks, depending on the amount of new data and the update schedule. In addition, some molecules are too big for entry into PubChem. With the primary focus on small molecules, PubChem only considers chemical structures with fewer than 1000 explicit atoms. This limit excludes large molecules contained in other databases (such as biologics and chemically modified biopolymers).

2.7 Use of PubChem Data for Drug Discovery

PubChem is commonly used as a reference tool, enabling users to quickly find desired information on a chemical. Our recent paper [15] provides an overview of how to explore the wealth of chemical information contained in PubChem through web browsers. PubChem also serves as a resource for virtual screening in drug discovery projects, as discussed in another paper [16].

Importantly, bioactivity data contained in PubChem BioAssay are now routinely used in conjunction with machine learning algorithms to develop computational models for the identification of potential drug candidates [23–48]. It is noteworthy that these data are applied to predict not only drug-target interaction but also various properties that a good drug candidate should have. As an example, PubChem's HTS data have been used to develop computational models to predict small-molecule activities against human Cytochrome P450 (CYP) enzymes [23–27] and human Ether-a-go-go Related Gene (hERG) proteins [28–30], which are involved in drug-induced hepatotoxicity and cardiotoxicity, respectively. Svensson et al. [31] developed prediction models for cytotoxicity of chemicals using cytotoxicity data for 440,000 compounds extracted from 16 HTS assays. Russo et al. [32] extracted bioassay data for 7385 compounds from PubChem BioAssay and developed a computational approach to predict the acute oral toxicity of chemicals. Rodríguez-Pérez et al. [33] used PubChem HTS data to predict the bioactivity profiles of chemicals against 53 targets.

In addition, PubChem's bioactivity data have been used to develop algorithms to identify potential false positives in assay experiments. For instance, Matlock et al. [34] and Stork et al. [35] developed machine-learning-based models for the prediction of frequent hitters (also referred to as promiscuous molecules). Su et al. [36] developed classification models to identify autofluorescent compounds, which often result in false-positive signals in assays that use fluorescence-based detection methods.

Information contained in other PubChem data collections can also be used for drug discovery-related research. For instance, there have been several studies that developed computational algorithms to identify metabolites from MS data in metabolomics experiments [37–39]. Another example is the study by Meyer et al. [40], in which PubChem compounds annotated with MeSH therapeutic use classes were used to develop computational models that predict the therapeutic functions of a chemical only from its structure.

2.8 Summary

PubChem is one of the public chemical databases that contain a large amount of chemical information. As a data aggregator, PubChem collects a wide range of chemical information from hundreds of data sources, including molecular structures and properties, spectral information, bioactivities, drug labeling, clinical trials, chemical vendors, synthesis, journal articles, patents, and many others. These data are organized into multiple data collections (Substance, Compound, BioAssay, Gene, Protein, Pathway, Taxonomy, and Patent) and each record in these collections has a Summary page, which presents all information available in PubChem for that record.

PubChem's search interface supports various types of text queries, such as chemical names, PubChem record identifiers (SIDs, CIDs, and AIDs), CAS registry numbers, gene/protein names and symbols, disease names, and so on. The Compound collection can also be searched using a chemical structure input, which can be specified with line notations like SMILES and InChI strings or drawn using the PubChem Sketcher. Multiple types of chemical structure searches are supported, including identity search, 2D and 3D similarity searches, and sub- and super-structure searches. Using the PubChem Classification Browser, it is possible to quickly retrieve records that are annotated with a classification or ontological term. In addition, the Identifier Exchange Service allows users to convert identifiers for a given set of chemical structures into different types of identifiers for identical or similar chemical structures.

PubChem records are highly interlinked with each other. The Literature Knowledge Panels, which are embedded in the Summary page of a PubChem record, help users explore the relationship between entities contained in PubChem (e.g. chemicals, genes, proteins, and diseases). In addition, for a given compound, PubChem provides a precomputed list of 2D and 3D neighbors. These neighbors help users to predict the molecular properties and biological activities of a compound that does not have much information.

PubChem data are accessible through multiple programmatic interfaces, including PUG-REST and PUG-View. Bulk data download via FTP is also supported. Especially, the PubChem FTP site hosts PubChemRDF data, which helps users to integrate PubChem data with in-house data or data from other resources across scientific domains.

PubChem contains more than 110 million compounds, and the majority of them are drug-like, satisfying all criteria of Ro5 or violating only one criterion of Ro5. Because data from many public chemical databases (Table 2.1) are integrated within PubChem, a substantial number of compounds in these resources are also contained in PubChem. In addition, 3.6 million compounds have been tested in at least one bioassay in PubChem, and about half of them (1.5 million compounds) have been declared active in at least one bioassay. While the majority of bioactivity data in PubChem are generated from HTS, a substantial amount of data are extracted from literature through text mining and manual curation. PubChem's bioactivity data can be used to build predictive models for the bioactivities of chemicals.

Acknowledgments

This work was supported by the National Center for Biotechnology Information of the National Library of Medicine (NLM), National Institutes of Health. The authors thank Yolanda L. Jones, National Institutes of Health Library, for editing assistance.

References

1 Eltyeb, S. and Salim, N. (2014). Chemical named entities recognition: a review on approaches and applications. *Journal of Cheminformatics* 6: 17.
2 Krallinger, M., Leitner, F., Rabal, O. et al. (2015). CHEMDNER: the drugs and chemical names extraction challenge. *Journal of Cheminformatics* 7: S1.
3 Leaman, R., Wei, C.H., and Lu, Z.Y. (2015). tmChem: a high performance approach for chemical named entity recognition and normalization. *Journal of Cheminformatics* 7: S3.

4 Luo, L., Yang, Z.H., Yang, P. et al. (2018). An attention-based BiLSTM-CRF approach to document-level chemical named entity recognition. *Bioinformatics* 34 (8): 1381–1388.

5 Krallinger, M., Rabal, O., Lourenco, A. et al. (2017). Information retrieval and text mining technologies for chemistry. *Chemical Reviews* 117 (12): 7673–7761.

6 Rajan, K., Brinkhaus, H.O., Zielesny, A. et al. (2020). A review of optical chemical structure recognition tools. *Journal of Cheminformatics* 12: 60.

7 Filippov, I.V. and Nicklaus, M.C. (2009). Optical structure recognition software to recover chemical information: OSRA, an open source solution. *Journal of Chemical Information and Modeling* 49 (3): 740–743.

8 Rajan, K., Zielesny, A., and Steinbeck, C. (2021). DECIMER 1.0: deep learning for chemical image recognition using transformers. *Journal of Cheminformatics* 13: 61.

9 Staker, J., Marshall, K., Abel, R. et al. (2019). Molecular structure extraction from documents using deep learning. *Journal of Chemical Information and Modeling* 59 (3): 1017–1029.

10 Oldenhof, M., Arany, A., Moreau, Y. et al. (2020). ChemGrapher: optical graph recognition of chemical compounds by deep learning. *Journal of Chemical Information and Modeling* 60 (10): 4506–4517.

11 Frasconi, P., Gabbrielli, F., Lippi, M. et al. (2014). Markov logic networks for optical chemical structure recognition. *Journal of Chemical Information and Modeling* 54 (8): 2380–2390.

12 Kim, S., Chen, J., Cheng, T.J. et al. (2021). PubChem in 2021: new data content and improved web interfaces. *Nucleic Acids Research* 49 (D1): D1388–D1395.

13 Kim, S., Chen, J., Cheng, T.J. et al. (2019). PubChem 2019 update: improved access to chemical data. *Nucleic Acids Research* 47 (D1): D1102–D1109.

14 Kim, S., Thiessen, P.A., Bolton, E.E. et al. (2016). PubChem Substance and Compound databases. *Nucleic Acids Research* 44 (D1): D1202–D1213.

15 Kim, S. (2021). Exploring chemical information in pubChem. *Current Protocols* 1 (8): e217.

16 Kim, S. (2016). Getting the most out of PubChem for virtual screening. *Expert Opinion on Drug Discovery* 11 (9): 843–855.

17 Kim, S., Cheng, T.J., He, S.Q. et al. (2022). PubChem Protein, Gene, Pathway, and Taxonomy data collections: bridging biology and chemistry through target-centric views of pubChem data. *Journal of Molecular Biology* 434 (11): 167514.

18 Gaulton, A., Hersey, A., Nowotka, M. et al. (2017). The ChEMBL database in 2017. *Nucleic Acids Research* 45 (D1): D945–D954.

19 Southan, C., Sitzmann, M., and Muresan, S. (2013). Comparing the chemical structure and protein content of ChEMBL, drugBank, human metabolome database and the therapeutic target database. *Molecular Informatics* 32 (11-12): 881–897.

20 Gilson, M.K., Liu, T.Q., Baitaluk, M. et al. (2016). BindingDB in 2015: a public database for medicinal chemistry, computational chemistry and systems pharmacology. *Nucleic Acids Research* 44 (D1): D1045–D1053.

21 Sterling, T. and Irwin, J.J. (2015). ZINC 15-Ligand discovery for everyone. *Journal of Chemical Information and Modeling* 55 (11): 2324–2337.

22 Harding, S., Armstrong, J., Faccenda, E. et al. (2021). IUPHAR/BPS Guide to PHARMACOLOGY: expansion for anti-malarials, antibiotics and COVID-19. *British Journal of Pharmacology* 178 (2): 390–391.

23 Goldwaser, E., Laurent, C., Lagarde, N. et al. (2022). Machine learning-driven identification of drugs inhibiting cytochrome P450 2C9. *PLoS Computational Biology* 18 (1): e1009820.

24 Wu, Z.X., Lei, T.L., Shen, C. et al. (2019). ADMET evaluation in drug discovery. 19. reliable prediction of human cytochrome P450 inhibition using artificial intelligence approaches. *Journal of Chemical Information and Modeling* 59 (11): 4587–4601.

25 Li, X., Xu, Y.J., Lai, L.H. et al. (2018). Prediction of human cytochrome P450 inhibition using a multitask deep autoencoder neural network. *Molecular Pharmaceutics* 15 (10): 4336–4345.

26 Lee, J.H., Basith, S., Cui, M. et al. (2017). In silico prediction of multiple-category classification model for cytochrome P450 inhibitors and non-inhibitors using machine-learning method. *SAR and QSAR in Environmental Research* 28 (10): 863–874.

27 Su, B.H., Tu, Y.S., Lin, C. et al. (2015). Rule-based prediction models of cytochrome P450 inhibition. *Journal of Chemical Information and Modeling* 55 (7): 1426–1434.

28 Kim, H. and Nam, H. (2020). hERG-Att: self-attention-based deep neural network for predicting hERG blockers. *Computational Biology and Chemistry* 87: 107286.

29 Ogura, K., Sato, T., Tuki, H. et al. (2019). Support vector machine model for hERG inhibitory activities based on the integrated hERG database using descriptor selection by NSGA-II. *Scientific Reports* 9: 12220.

30 Shen, M.Y., Su, B.H., Esposito, E.X. et al. (2011). A comprehensive support vector machine binary hERG classification model based on extensive but biased end point hERG data sets. *Chemical Research in Toxicology* 24 (6): 934–949.

31 Svensson, F., Norinder, U., and Bender, A. (2017). Modelling compound cytotoxicity using conformal prediction and PubChem HTS data. *Toxicology Research* 6 (1): 73–80.

32 Russo, D.P., Strickland, J., Karmaus, A.L. et al. (2019). Nonanimal models for acute toxicity evaluations: applying data-driven profiling and read-across. *Environmental Health Perspectives* 127 (4): 047001.

33 Rodríguez-Pérez, R., Miyao, T., Jasial, S. et al. (2018). Prediction of compound profiling matrices using machine learning. *ACS Omega* 3 (4): 4713–4723.

34 Matlock, M.K., Hughes, T.B., Dahlin, J.L. et al. (2018). Modeling small-molecule reactivity identifies promiscuous bioactive compounds. *Journal of Chemical Information and Modeling* 58 (8): 1483–1500.

35 Stork, C., Wagner, J., Friedrich, N.O. et al. (2018). Hit dexter: a machine-learning model for the prediction of frequent hitters. *ChemMedChem* 13 (6): 564–571.

36 Su, B.H., Tu, Y.S., Lin, O.A. et al. (2015). Rule-based classification models of molecular autofluorescence. *Journal of Chemical Information and Modeling* 55 (2): 434–445.

37 Ludwig, M., Dührkop, K., and Böcker, S. (2018). Bayesian networks for mass spectrometric metabolite identification via molecular fingerprints. *Bioinformatics* 34 (13): 333–340.

38 Dührkop, K., Shen, H.B., Meusel, M. et al. (2015). Searching molecular structure databases with tandem mass spectra using CSI:FingerID. *Proceedings of the National Academy of Sciences of the United States of America* 112 (41): 12580–12585.

39 Qiu, F., Lei, Z.T., and Sumner, L.W. (2018). MetExpert: an expert system to enhance gas chromatography-mass spectrometry-based metabolite identifications. *Analytica Chimica Acta* 1037: 316–326.

40 Meyer, J.G., Liu, S.C., Miller, I.J. et al. (2019). Learning drug functions from chemical structures with convolutional neural networks and random forests. *Journal of Chemical Information and Modeling* 59 (10): 4438–4449.

41 Korkmaz, S. (2020). Deep learning-based imbalanced data classification for drug discovery. *Journal of Chemical Information and Modeling* 60 (9): 4180–4190.

42 Ancuceanu, R., Dinu, M., Neaga, I. et al. (2019). Development of QSAR machine learning-based models to forecast the effect of substances on malignant melanoma cells. *Oncology Letters* 17 (5): 4188–4196.

43 Ciallella, H.L. and Zhu, H. (2019). Advancing computational toxicology in the big data era by artificial intelligence: data-driven and mechanism-driven modeling for chemical toxicity. *Chemical Research in Toxicology* 32 (4): 536–547.

44 Danishuddin, Madhukar, G., Malik, M.Z. et al. (2019). Development and rigorous validation of antimalarial predictive models using machine learning approaches. *SAR and QSAR in Environmental Research* 30 (8): 543–560.

45 Laufkötter, O., Sturm, N., Bajorath, J. et al. (2019). Combining structural and bioactivity-based fingerprints improves prediction performance and scaffold hopping capability. *Journal of Cheminformatics* 11 (1): 54.

46 Capuzzi, S.J., Sun, W., Muratov, E.N. et al. (2018). Computer-aided discovery and characterization of Novel Ebola virus inhibitors. *Journal of Medicinal Chemistry* 61 (8): 3582–3594.

47 Chen, J.J.F. and Visco, D.P. (2017). Identifying novel factor XIIa inhibitors with PCA-GA-SVM developed vHTS models. *European Journal of Medicinal Chemistry* 140: 31–41.

48 Deshmukh, A.L., Chandra, S., Singh, D.K. et al. (2017). Identification of human flap endonuclease 1 (FEN1) inhibitors using a machine learning based consensus virtual screening. *Molecular BioSystems* 13 (8): 1630–1639.

49 Bolton, E.E., Kim, S., and Bryant, S.H. (2011). PubChem3D: conformer generation. *Journal of Cheminformatics* 3: 4.

50 Kim, S., Bolton, E.E., and Bryant, S.H. (2013). PubChem3D: conformer ensemble accuracy. *Journal of Cheminformatics* 5: 1.

51 Berman, H., Henrick, K., and Nakamura, H. (2003). Announcing the worldwide protein data bank. *Nature Structural Biology* 10 (12): 980–980.

52 Groom, C.R., Bruno, I.J., Lightfoot, M.P. et al. (2016). The cambridge structural database. *Acta Crystallographica. Section B: Structural Science, Crystal Engineering and Materials* 72: 171–179.

53 Hähnke, V.D., Kim, S., and Bolton, E.E. (2018). PubChem chemical structure standardization. *Journal of Cheminformatics* 10: 36.

54 Weininger, D. (1990). SMILES .3. DEPICT – graphical depiction of chemical structures. *Journal of Chemical Information and Computer Sciences* 30 (3): 237–243.

55 Weininger, D., Weininger, A., and Weininger, J.L. (1989). SMILES .2. Algorithm for generation of unique smiles notation. *Journal of Chemical Information and Computer Sciences* 29 (2): 97–101.

56 Weininger, D. (1988). SMILES, a chemical language and information-system .1. Introduction to methodology and encoding rules. *Journal of Chemical Information and Computer Sciences* 28 (1): 31–36.

57 Heller, S.R., McNaught, A., Pletnev, I. et al. (2015). InChI, the IUPAC international chemical identifier. *Journal of Cheminformatics* 7: 23.

58 Ihlenfeldt, W.D., Bolton, E.E., and Bryant, S.H. (2009). The PubChem chemical structure sketcher. *Journal of Cheminformatics* 1: 20.

59 Grant, J.A., Gallardo, M.A., and Pickup, B.T. (1996). A fast method of molecular shape comparison: a simple application of a Gaussian description of molecular shape. *Journal of Computational Chemistry* 17 (14): 1653–1666.

60 Grant, J.A. and Pickup, B.T. (1995). A gaussian description of molecular shape. *The Journal of Physical Chemistry* 99 (11): 3503–3510.

61 Rush, T.S., Grant, J.A., Mosyak, L. et al. (2005). A shape-based 3-D scaffold hopping method and its application to a bacterial protein-protein interaction. *Journal of Medicinal Chemistry* 48 (5): 1489–1495.

62 Holliday, J.D., Salim, N., Whittle, M. et al. (2003). Analysis and display of the size dependence of chemical similarity coefficients. *Journal of Chemical Information and Computer Sciences* 43 (3): 819–828.

63 Holliday, J.D., Hu, C.Y., and Willett, P. (2002). Grouping of coefficients for the calculation of inter-molecular similarity and dissimilarity using 2D fragment bit-strings. *Combinatorial Chemistry & High Throughput Screening* 5 (2): 155–166.

64 Chen, X. and Reynolds, C.H. (2002). Performance of similarity measures in 2D fragment-based similarity searching: comparison of structural descriptors and similarity coefficients. *Journal of Chemical Information and Computer Sciences* 42 (6): 1407–1414.

65 Kim, S., Thiessen, P.A., Cheng, T. et al. (2016). Literature information in PubChem: associations between PubChem records and scientific articles. *Journal of Cheminformatics* 8: 32.

66 Zaslavsky, L., Cheng, T., Gindulyte, A. et al. (2021). Discovering and summarizing relationships between chemicals, genes, proteins, and diseases in PubChem. *Frontiers in Research Metrics and Analytics* 6: 689059.

67 Bolton, E.E., Kim, S., and Bryant, S.H. (2011). PubChem3D: similar conformers. *Journal of Cheminformatics* 3: 13.

68 Kim, S., Bolton, E.E., and Bryant, S.H. (2016). Similar compounds versus similar conformers: complementarity between PubChem 2-D and 3-D neighboring sets. *Journal of Cheminformatics* 8: 62.

69 Kim, S., Thiessen, P.A., Bolton, E.E. et al. (2015). PUG-SOAP and PUG-REST: web services for programmatic access to chemical information in PubChem. *Nucleic Acids Research* 43 (W1): W605–W611.

70 Kim, S., Thiessen, P.A., Cheng, T.J. et al. (2018). An update on PUG-REST: RESTful interface for programmatic access to PubChem. *Nucleic Acids Research* 46 (W1): W563–W570.

71 Kim, S., Shoemaker, B.A., Bolton, E.E. et al. (2018). Finding potential multitarget ligands using PubChem. In: *Computational Chemogenomics* (ed. J.B. Brown), 63–91. Totowa: Humana Press Inc.

72 Kim, S., Thiessen, P.A., Cheng, T.J. et al. (2019). PUG-View: programmatic access to chemical annotations integrated in PubChem. *Journal of Cheminformatics* 11: 56.

73 Fu, G., Batchelor, C., Dumontier, M. et al. (2015). PubChemRDF: towards the semantic annotation of PubChem Compound and Substance databases. *Journal of Cheminformatics* 7: 34.

74 Boehr, D.L. and Bushman, B. (2018). Preparing for the future: National Library of Medicine's® project to add MeSH® RDF URIs to its bibliographic and authority records. *Cataloging and Classification Quarterly* 56 (2-3): 262–272.

75 Bushman, B., Anderson, D., and Fu, G. (2015). Transforming the medical subject headings into linked data: creating the authorized version of MeSH in RDF. *Journal of Library Metadata* 15 (3-4): 157–176.

76 Redaschi, N. and Uniprot Consortium (2009). UniProt in RDF: tackling data integration and distributed annotation with the semantic web. *Nature Precedings* https://doi.org/10.1038/npre.2009.3193.1.

77 Kinjo, A.R., Bekker, G.-J., Suzuki, H. et al. (2016). Protein Data Bank Japan (PDBj): updated user interfaces, resource description framework, analysis tools for large structures. *Nucleic Acids Research* 45 (D1): D282–D288.

78 Kinjo, A.R., Suzuki, H., Yamashita, R. et al. (2011). Protein Data Bank Japan (PDBj): maintaining a structural data archive and resource description framework format. *Nucleic Acids Research* 40 (D1): D453–D460.

79 Jupp, S., Malone, J., Bolleman, J. et al. (2014). The EBI RDF platform: linked open data for the life sciences. *Bioinformatics* 30 (9): 1338–1339.

80 Erxleben, F., Günther, M., Krötzsch, M. et al. (2014). *Introducing Wikidata to the Linked Data Web*, 50–65. Cham: Springer International Publishing.

81 Lipinski, C.A., Lombardo, F., Dominy, B.W. et al. (1997). Experimental and computational approaches to estimate solubility and permeability in drug discovery and development settings. *Advanced Drug Delivery Reviews* 23 (1-3): 3–25.

82 Ghose, A.K., Viswanadhan, V.N., and Wendoloski, J.J. (1999). A knowledge-based approach in designing combinatorial or medicinal chemistry libraries for drug discovery. 1. A qualitative and quantitative characterization of known drug databases. *Journal of Combinatorial Chemistry* 1 (1): 55–68.

83 Veber, D.F., Johnson, S.R., Cheng, H.Y. et al. (2002). Molecular properties that influence the oral bioavailability of drug candidates. *Journal of Medicinal Chemistry* 45 (12): 2615–2623.

84 Walters, W.P. and Namchuk, M. (2003). Designing screens: How to make your hits a hit. *Nature Reviews Drug Discovery* 2 (4): 259–266.

85 Bickerton, G.R., Paolini, G.V., Besnard, J. et al. (2012). Quantifying the chemical beauty of drugs. *Nature Chemistry* 4 (2): 90–98.

86 Congreve, M., Carr, R., Murray, C. et al. (2003). A rule of three for fragment-based lead discovery? *Drug Discovery Today* 8 (19): 876–877.

87 Williams, A.J., Grulke, C.M., Edwards, J. et al. (2017). The CompTox chemistry dashboard: a community data resource for environmental chemistry. *Journal of Cheminformatics* 9: 61.

88 Hastings, J., Owen, G., Dekker, A. et al. (2016). ChEBI in 2016: improved services and an expanding collection of metabolites. *Nucleic Acids Research* 44 (D1): D1214–D1219.

89 Armstrong, D.R., Berrisford, J.M., Conroy, M.J. et al. (2019). PDBe: improved findability of macromolecular structure data in the PDB. *Nucleic Acids Research* 48 (D1): D335–D343.

90 Bansal, P., Morgat, A., Axelsen, K.B. et al. (2021). Rhea, the reaction knowledgebase in 2022. *Nucleic Acids Research* 50 (D1): D693–D700.

91 Chambers, J., Davies, M., Gaulton, A. et al. (2014). UniChem: extension of InChI-based compound mapping to salt, connectivity and stereochemistry layers. *Journal of Cheminformatics* 6: 43.

92 Chambers, J., Davies, M., Gaulton, A. et al. (2013). UniChem: a unified chemical structure cross-referencing and identifier tracking system. *Journal of Cheminformatics* 5: 3.

3

DrugBank Online: A How-to Guide

Christen M. Klinger[1], Jordan Cox[1], Denise So[2], Teira Stauth[3], Michael Wilson[1], Alex Wilson[1], and Craig Knox[1]

[1] *University of Alberta, Edmonton, AB, Canada*
[2] *University of Ottawa, Ottawa, ON, Canada*
[3] *University of Calgary, Calgary, AB, Canada*

3.1 Introduction

The process of discovering new drugs has undergone substantial changes from the historical paradigm of directly using natural products to high-throughput screening (HTS) to the modern state-of-the-art that melds HTS and computational approaches [1, 2]. Despite these advancements, drug discovery remains challenging; high attrition rates and costs remain barriers to entry for smaller biotech companies and academic institutions [3]. In addition, the promise of HTS as a means for overcoming the practical limitations of smaller-scale molecular interaction studies has fallen short. Antibiotics remain an illustrative example where, despite expansive library screening, few truly novel chemical scaffolds have been discovered since the 1960s [4].

Modern drug discovery follows a "target-centric" paradigm, wherein both a drug candidate and at least one validated target will be identified prior to proceeding to clinical studies [5]. This not only ensures a conceptual mechanistic rationale for drug action but also facilitates refinement of the candidate molecule through the iterative application of structure–activity relationship studies [6, 7]. Regardless of the exact technologies used, the process of identifying both candidate molecules and targets can be conceptually divided into two schemes, depending on the order in which they are sought [2].

In so-called "target-based" discovery [2], the first step is the identification of one or more putative targets, whose properties may be manipulated through the addition of specific molecules in order to achieve a therapeutic effect. These targets may be prioritized based on previous data, by genetic signals linking the target to the condition in question (e.g. in genome-wide association studies), or may represent promising hits identified in large-scale screening efforts [5]. Each putative target might then serve as the basis for the development of one or more candidate molecules.

Open Access Databases and Datasets for Drug Discovery, First Edition.
Edited by Antoine Daina, Michael Przewosny, and Vincent Zoete.
© 2024 WILEY-VCH GmbH. Published 2024 by WILEY-VCH GmbH.

In contrast, "phenotypic-based" (sometimes referred to as "molecule-based") discovery [2] takes advantage of biological screening platforms with a well-characterized phenotypic readout to screen large compound libraries. High-scoring hits are then deconvoluted to identify the putative target(s) prior to more direct target validation [8].

As the end result, a set of candidate molecules and known targets, remains unchanged between these schemes, the choice of which approach to use is largely contextual. More recent advances in the last approximately two decades have also seen an increasing dependency across both schemes for computational tools. The ability to investigate intermolecular interactions between putative candidate molecules and proteins (e.g. by molecular docking) and to simulate these interactions in a temporal manner (e.g. by molecular dynamics) have significantly increased the size of screening libraries from $\sim 10^6$ compounds to virtual libraries of $\sim 10^{13}$ compounds [9]. More recently, artificial intelligence/machine learning (AI/ML) tools that assist in target prediction, compound identification/design, high-content screening, candidate retrosynthesis, and other areas have been developed [10, 11].

The potential for computational methods to revolutionize drug discovery is undoubtedly exciting, but it brings new challenges with it. Computational approaches require highly structured and accurate data in order to work effectively. However, data within the biomedical space are often unstructured and diffuse, being scattered across a collection of publications and databases, each with its own specific schemas and formats.

In this chapter, we present an updated view of the DrugBank database. We explore the nature and kinds of data within DrugBank, with an emphasis on the structured nature of the data. Protocols are provided for the use of the free online data and tools available through our website. Some examples of published research using DrugBank are provided for further context and as starting points for further exploration of the myriad ways in which this resource may assist those working in the drug discovery field. Lastly, we discuss our current outlook and possible avenues for future development.

3.2 DrugBank

3.2.1 Overview of DrugBank

DrugBank maintains a comprehensive database of drugs and related information, which we will explore further in Section 3.2.2. Data within DrugBank are a mixture of data imported from relevant databases, novel content authored by an in-house curation team of pharmacists, doctors, and biomedical experts, and insights generated from proprietary ML-based workflows (Figure 3.1). Regardless of the source, data within DrugBank are highly structured, such that they can be used to train ML models or form the basis for novel algorithms and pipelines.

Although commercialized in 2015, DrugBank started as an academic research project and is committed to supporting the research community through access

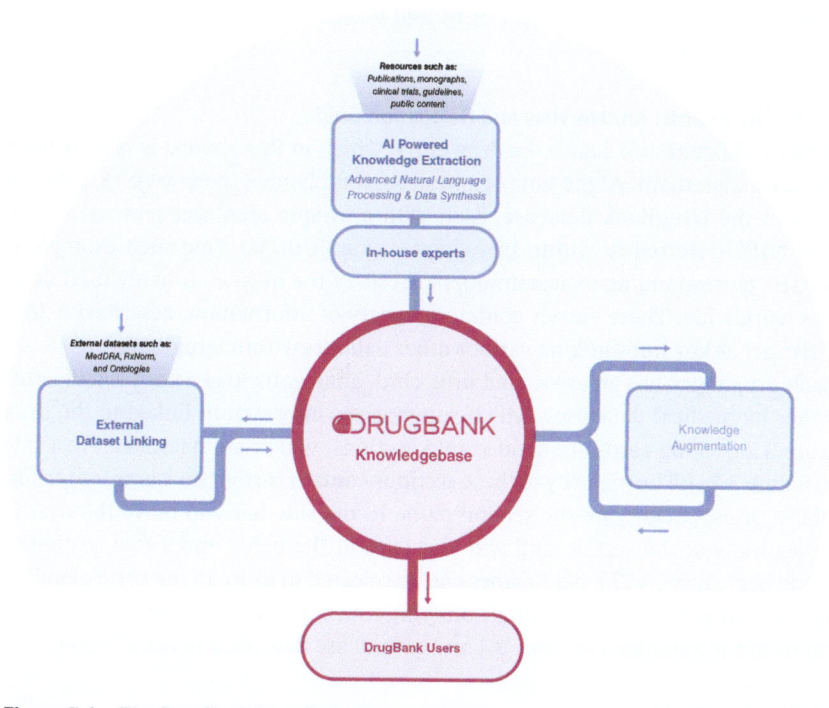

Figure 3.1 The DrugBank knowledgebase. This figure shows a graphical overview of the DrugBank knowledgebase, which powers DrugBank Online and our other product offerings. Proprietary ML tools scour literary resources such as publications, monographs, public data resources, and others to bring relevant content to an in-house curation team (top). This team then vets the content, synthesizes multiple pieces, and authors novel information for inclusion in the knowledgebase. Concurrently, recognized external datasets in the biomedical space, such as ontologies related to drug products and their possible medical effects, are imported and processed for inclusion into the knowledgebase (left). All of these data together provide the potential for cyclical knowledge augmentation, wherein the combination of information can yield new insights that are "larger than the sum of their parts" (right). The combined information from all of these sources is provided to users in a highly structured and usable format (bottom).

to free datasets and tools. Public-facing content is available as part of DrugBank Online (https://go.drugbank.com/) and will form the bulk of this chapter. Further support for academic (through our Academic + program) and commercial users, including structured data downloads in a variety of formats, will not be discussed in detail here but may be obtained through the "Solutions" tab at the top of this webpage.

3.2.2 DrugBank Datasets

DrugBank contains a wide variety of datasets for use in both clinical and scientific applications, not all of which will be discussed here. The primary purpose of this section is to provide an overview of key datasets within DrugBank, including their attributes and connections. Navigating to, and practical use of, these datasets will be covered in Section 3.3.

3.2.2.1 Drug Cards: An Overview and Navigation Guide

The heart of DrugBank data is the drug entry, which in this context is synonymous with active ingredient. At the time of authoring this chapter, there were 15,234 such entries in the DrugBank database, each with a unique identifier prefixed by the letters "DB" (referred to within this chapter as a "DBID"). One such example is DB00316, corresponding to acetaminophen, one of the most commonly used analgesics worldwide. These entries contain a variety of information, described below, but also act as key hubs linking various other datasets within DrugBank.

Each drug entry has an associated drug card, analogous to gene or protein cards in other biomedical databases, which summarizes information linked to the drug (Figure 3.2a). Drug cards are divided into sections, which are navigated via a side bar (Figure 3.2a). The majority of these sections contain further divisions into fields. In these cases, clicking on the section name in the side bar will move the user to the beginning of the section and will also expand the fields under that section in the side bar (Figure 3.2b); field names can be selected to move to the corresponding field. Each section represents a single unifying concept associated with a drug. These sections are summarized in Table 3.1 and several are described in detail below.

3.2.2.2 Identification

The Identification section is the first information a user will see when navigating to a drug card. As the name implies, this section is primarily concerned with providing an overview of the drug and the various ways in which it may be referred to. The **Summary** field provides a one- or two-sentence overview appropriate for a clinician or scientist while the **Background** field provides a more in-depth explanation of the drug, including its primary use and approval information; both fields are authored in-house.

Below the **Background** field, there are several important identifiers associated with the drug, such as the chemical structure, formula, and external identifiers in other databases. The **Type** field categorizes the drug based on its chemical properties and source, and its value will be either "Small Molecule" or "Biotech." Similarly, the **Groups** field summarizes the approval status of the drug, either "Approved," "Investigational," "Experimental," "Illicit," "Vet Approved," "Nutraceutical," or "Withdrawn." Investigational drugs are those that have not yet been approved but are currently in clinical trials, whereas experimental drugs have not yet reached clinical trials. The remaining field values are less common but correspond to drugs that are approved for veterinary use, those that are primarily based on natural products (nutraceutical), and those for which approved indications do not exist (illicit/withdrawn). As approved drugs may also be investigated for other indications, it is possible for a drug to have multiple values in this field.

The last notable field is **Synonyms**, which provide alternative names for the drug in question. One obvious application of these is to assist in regional localization by language, but drugs will often have several English synonyms as well. As an example,

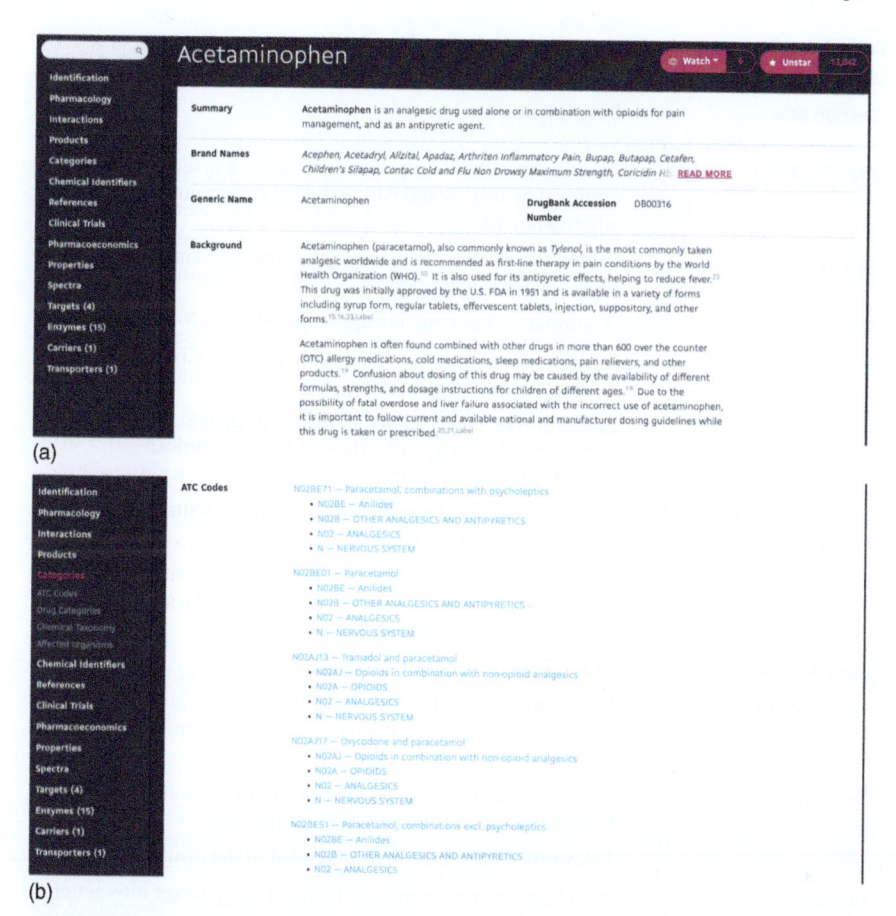

Figure 3.2 Overview of DrugBank drug cards. This figure shows an example drug card for DB00316 (acetaminophen). (a) The view a user would see after navigating to the drug card. Note the side navigation bar containing the drug card sections (also see Table 3.1). The search widget at the top of this side bar allows users to search for specific sections or fields. (b) An example of clicking on one of the section names (in this case, Categories). Note that the view is centered on the first field within the section (**ATC Codes**) and that the four fields available within Categories are shown in the side bar; these may be selected directly.

acetaminophen is usually referred to as paracetamol in the United Kingdom and Europe. Searching any of these synonyms within DrugBank will retrieve the same entry.

3.2.2.3 Pharmacology

The Pharmacology section contains a combination of unstructured text and links to related structured data surrounding a drug's pharmacodynamic and pharmacokinetic properties. The pharmacodynamic properties include the drug indication(s) along with linked structured entries of the conditions for which the drug is indicated (under **Associated Conditions**). If the drug is used in specific therapies or

Table 3.1 Summary of relevant sections within a DrugBank drug card.

Section title	Description
Identification	An overview of the drug: what it is, what it is used for, and its approval history. Brand names and synonyms are provided, where available.
Pharmacology	Information related to a drug's pharmacodynamic and pharmacokinetic properties.
Interactions	A summary of potential drug–drug and drug–food interactions.
Products	Information related to prescription, generic, mixture, and other products containing the drug.
Categories	Relevant ATC codes related to the drug, DrugBank categories containing the drug, and structure-based chemical classification of the drug.
Chemical Identifiers	Identifiers for the drug, including UNII, CAS number, InChI, InChI key, IUPAC name, and SMILES.
References	Journal, textbook, and link references used throughout the drug card. Links to relevant external resources and a specific reference for the drug's synthesis.
Clinical Trials	Clinical trials involving the drug.
Pharmacoeconomics	Information related to the sale of the drug, including manufacturers, packaging, product routes/forms, prices, and patents.
Properties	Chemical and pharmacokinetic properties of a drug, including both experimental and predicted properties.
Spectra	Relevant spectral information related to the drug.
Targets	Structured entries representing direct drug–target interactions (may be absent).
Enzymes	Structured entries representing direct interactions between the drug and enzymes (may be absent).
Carriers	Structured entries representing direct interactions between the drug and blood proteins (may be absent).
Transporters	Structured entries representing direct interactions between the drug and transmembrane transport proteins (may be absent).

procedures, these will also be linked in **Associated Therapies**. The **Pharmacodynamics** field includes information on the high-level view of the drug's mechanism of action (MoA) together with other notable effects the drug may have on the body. Lastly, the MoA field provides a detailed view of the drug–biomolecule (usually protein) interactions that result in the observed therapeutic effect. Those targets (see Section 3.2.2.6) relevant to the MoA are summarized below with links to the full entries.

The included pharmacokinetic properties are largely focused on Absorption, Distribution, Metabolism, Excretion, and Toxicity (ADMET) properties, which are further summarized elsewhere (see Section 3.2.2.5). Of special interest is the **Metabolism** field, which provides both a detailed description of the metabolic pathways as well as a graphical depiction of the possible routes from starting compounds to excreted metabolites (Figure 3.3). The final two fields in this section, **Pathways** and **Pharmacogenomic Effects/ADRs**, provide links to structured entries describing known pathways the drug is involved in and known genetic associations related to drug action or safety, respectively.

3.2.2.4 Categories

The Categories section is primarily concerned with the ways in which the drug can be classified. All relevant ATC codes [12] are provided; each listed code is a hyperlink that, when clicked, will navigate to a representation of the ATC code hierarchy focused on the code in question.

The **Drug Categories** field contains a tabular list of associated DrugBank categories, each of which has a unique identifier prefixed with "DBCAT." These categories are a union of external sources, including ATC [12], MeSH [13], and EPC [14], with our own proprietary in-house curation. Navigating to the individual category page yields more detailed information for each, including a description, a list of drugs categorized into the category, and targets (see Section 3.2.2.6) for each of these drugs. In this way, it is possible to easily discern, which targets represent possible drug targets for a given category of drugs.

The **Chemical Taxonomy** field provides a classification on the basis of chemical structure, powered by the ClassyFire tool [15]. In keeping with the output of ClassyFire itself, the first four levels of taxonomy, "Kingdom," "Super Class," "Class," and "Sub Class," are provided, together with the direct parent and alternative parents. These categories are hyperlinked to the relevant entry within the ClassyFire website [15] and a description of each is provided as hover text. Links to the classification in other taxonomies/ontologies are provided, when available. In addition, a full list of the extracted substituents, including functional groups, is provided under the **Substituents** field, which may be useful in grouping or comparing chemicals (see Section 3.3.2.2).

3.2.2.5 Properties

The Properties section compiles experimental and predicted properties. The **State** and the **Experimental Properties** fields are curated based on Material Safety Data Sheets (MSDS) and other relevant literature. A number of chemical properties are predicted using ALOGPS [16] or ChemAxon (https://chemaxon.com/; Figure 3.4a), and a selection of ADMET properties are predicted using admetSAR [17] (Figure 3.4b).

3.2.2.6 Targets, Enzymes, Carriers, and Transporters

Four (possibly absent) sections of a drug card include the associated targets, enzymes, carriers, and transporters. The Targets section contains entries for each biomolecule that the drug is known to directly bind; the type of biomolecule is denoted by the **Kind** field, which may hold a value of "protein," "protein

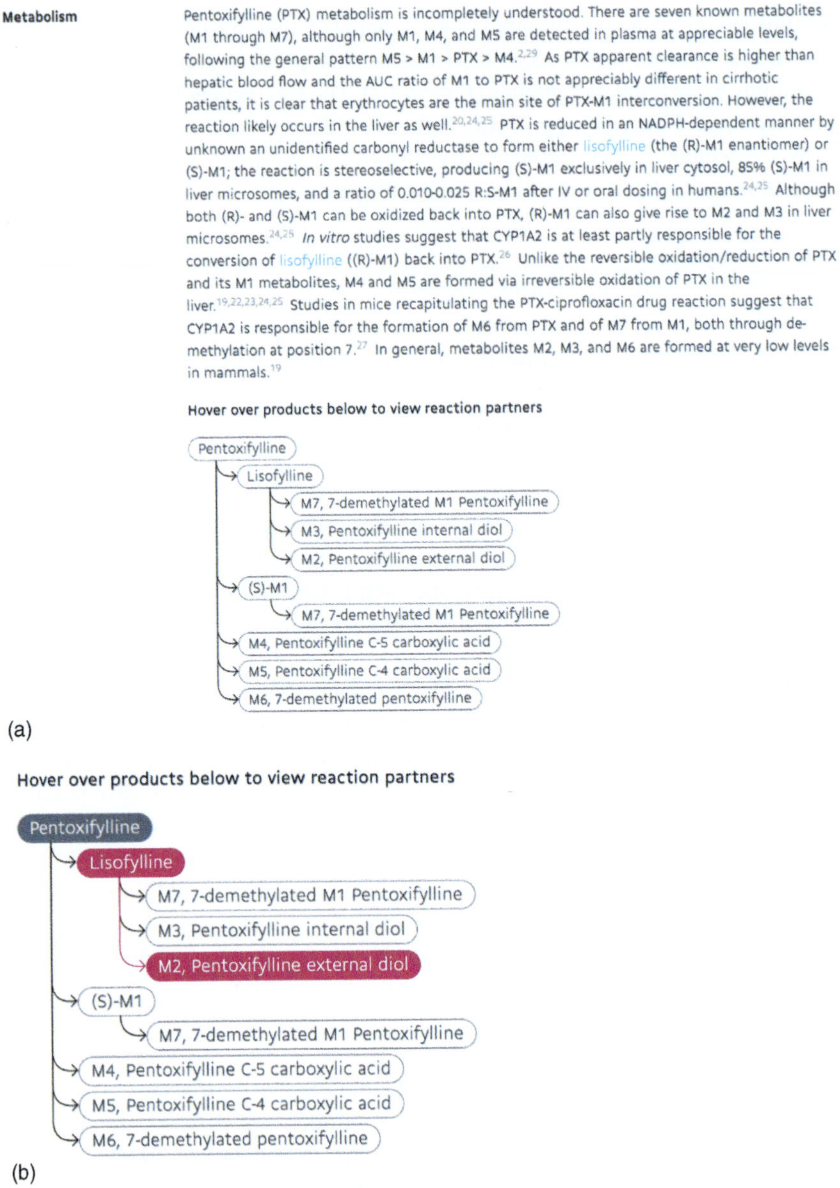

Metabolism

Pentoxifylline (PTX) metabolism is incompletely understood. There are seven known metabolites (M1 through M7), although only M1, M4, and M5 are detected in plasma at appreciable levels, following the general pattern M5 > M1 > PTX > M4.[2,29] As PTX apparent clearance is higher than hepatic blood flow and the AUC ratio of M1 to PTX is not appreciably different in cirrhotic patients, it is clear that erythrocytes are the main site of PTX-M1 interconversion. However, the reaction likely occurs in the liver as well.[20,24,25] PTX is reduced in an NADPH-dependent manner by unknown an unidentified carbonyl reductase to form either lisofylline (the (R)-M1 enantiomer) or (S)-M1; the reaction is stereoselective, producing (S)-M1 exclusively in liver cytosol, 85% (S)-M1 in liver microsomes, and a ratio of 0.010-0.025 R:S-M1 after IV or oral dosing in humans.[24,25] Although both (R)- and (S)-M1 can be oxidized back into PTX, (R)-M1 can also give rise to M2 and M3 in liver microsomes.[24,25] In vitro studies suggest that CYP1A2 is at least partly responsible for the conversion of lisofylline ((R)-M1) back into PTX.[26] Unlike the reversible oxidation/reduction of PTX and its M1 metabolites, M4 and M5 are formed via irreversible oxidation of PTX in the liver.[19,22,23,24,25] Studies in mice recapitulating the PTX-ciprofloxacin drug reaction suggest that CYP1A2 is responsible for the formation of M6 from PTX and of M7 from M1, both through demethylation at position 7.[27] In general, metabolites M2, M3, and M6 are formed at very low levels in mammals.[19]

Hover over products below to view reaction partners

- Pentoxifylline
  - Lisofylline
    - M7, 7-demethylated M1 Pentoxifylline
    - M3, Pentoxifylline internal diol
    - M2, Pentoxifylline external diol
  - (S)-M1
    - M7, 7-demethylated M1 Pentoxifylline
  - M4, Pentoxifylline C-5 carboxylic acid
  - M5, Pentoxifylline C-4 carboxylic acid
  - M6, 7-demethylated pentoxifylline

(a)

Hover over products below to view reaction partners

- **Pentoxifylline**
  - **Lisofylline**
    - M7, 7-demethylated M1 Pentoxifylline
    - M3, Pentoxifylline internal diol
    - **M2, Pentoxifylline external diol**
  - (S)-M1
    - M7, 7-demethylated M1 Pentoxifylline
  - M4, Pentoxifylline C-5 carboxylic acid
  - M5, Pentoxifylline C-4 carboxylic acid
  - M6, 7-demethylated pentoxifylline

(b)

Figure 3.3   The drug card metabolism section. This figure shows the available information within the **Metabolism** field of a DrugBank drug card. (a) An exemplar **Metabolism** entry (DB00806, pentoxifylline) is shown. Note the detailed description of the reactions and the acknowledgment of uncertainty for some steps within the scientific literature. The graphic at the bottom of the panel shows the known pathways by which the starting drug may be transformed into terminal metabolites. (b) An enhanced view of the graphic shown in (a), demonstrating its interactive nature by placing the cursor over "M2, pentoxifylline external diol." The currently selected metabolite and its direct parent are highlighted in pink, while other ancestors are highlighted in grey, including the starting drug.

(a) Predicted Properties

PROPERTY	VALUE	SOURCE
Water Solubility	4.15 mg/mL	ALOGPS
logP	0.51	ALOGPS
logP	0.91	ChemAxon
logS	-1.6	ALOGPS
pKa (Strongest Acidic)	9.46	ChemAxon
pKa (Strongest Basic)	-4.4	ChemAxon
Physiological Charge	0	ChemAxon
Hydrogen Acceptor Count	2	ChemAxon
Hydrogen Donor Count	2	ChemAxon
Polar Surface Area	49.33 Å^2	ChemAxon
Rotatable Bond Count	1	ChemAxon
Refractivity	42.9 m^3·mol^{-1}	ChemAxon
Polarizability	15.52 Å^3	ChemAxon
Number of Rings	1	ChemAxon
Bioavailability	1	ChemAxon
Rule of Five	Yes	ChemAxon
Ghose Filter	No	ChemAxon
Veber's Rule	No	ChemAxon
MDDR-like Rule	No	ChemAxon

(b) Predicted ADMET Features

PROPERTY	VALUE	PROBABILITY
Human Intestinal Absorption	+	0.9921
Blood Brain Barrier	+	0.9544
Caco-2 permeable	+	0.8285
P-glycoprotein substrate	Non-substrate	0.8202
P-glycoprotein inhibitor I	Non-inhibitor	0.982
P-glycoprotein inhibitor II	Non-inhibitor	0.9781
Renal organic cation transporter	Non-inhibitor	0.9292
CYP450 2C9 substrate	Non-substrate	0.7259
CYP450 2D6 substrate	Substrate	0.8918
CYP450 3A4 substrate	Non-substrate	0.5554
CYP450 1A2 substrate	Non-inhibitor	0.9045
CYP450 2C9 inhibitor	Non-inhibitor	0.907
CYP450 2D6 inhibitor	Non-inhibitor	0.9755
CYP450 2C19 inhibitor	Non-inhibitor	0.9161
CYP450 3A4 inhibitor	Non-inhibitor	0.8496
CYP450 inhibitory promiscuity	Low CYP Inhibitory Promiscuity	0.8842
Ames test	Non AMES toxic	0.8767
Carcinogenicity	Non-carcinogens	0.7654
Biodegradation	Ready biodegradable	0.6342
Rat acute toxicity	1.8596 LD50, mol/kg	Not applicable
hERG inhibition (predictor I)	Weak inhibitor	0.9717
hERG inhibition (predictor II)	Non-inhibitor	0.9597

Figure 3.4 Predicted properties available within drug cards. This figure shows the predicted properties, both chemical (a) and pharmacokinetic (b) available for DrugBank entries through the drug card (acetaminophen shown here). Each chemical property has a hyperlink to its specific source (either ALOGPS or ChemAxon) while all pharmacokinetic properties are predicted by admetSAR. See the main text for more information.

group," "nucleotide," "small molecule," or "group." Proteins are the most common kind of target and include information pulled from UniProt [18]. More detailed information can be obtained by clicking on the hyperlinked UniProt ID. Protein groups are a collection of proteins; target entries of this kind have an additional table, "components," that lists the constituent proteins. Protein groups are used in cases where the drug targets a protein complex, where experimental evidence cannot adequately discern between specific members of a protein family, or where the presumed target is deduced on the basis of phenotype rather than detailed molecular studies. Nucleotides, small molecules, and groups have different sets of included information, but will not be discussed in detail here.

Each target will be associated with an organism. This is usually humans but, in other cases such as anti-infectives, may correspond to a different organism. The **Pharmacological Action** field will hold one of three possible values: "yes," "no," or "unknown." A value of "yes" indicates that this drug–biomolecule interaction is known to contribute to the drug's therapeutic effect while "no" indicates the opposite; a value of "unknown" indicates that there is insufficient evidence to either demonstrate or rule out a therapeutic effect. If the value is "yes," the target will also be mentioned in the MoA field under the Pharmacology section (see Section 3.2.2.3). The **Actions** field contains one or more entries capturing the effect of the drug on the biomolecule. This can be as simple as "binder," but is often more specific. A list of common possible actions is given in Table 3.2.

The Enzymes section captures information for enzymes known to participate in the drug's metabolism. If an enzyme is the target of a drug action (e.g. suicide inhibitors), it will be listed in the Targets section instead. Similar to protein

Table 3.2 List of common actions within DrugBank.

Action	Description
Agonist	The drug promotes the activity of the target (usually a receptor).
Antagonist	The drug reduces the activity of the target (usually a receptor).
Partial Agonist	As above, but the drug does not fully promote the activity.
Activator	The drug activates the target, increasing its ability to induce a given effect or promote a specific process.
Inhibitor	The drug inhibits the target, preventing it from carrying out its normal function.
Inducer	The drug induces the target, either directly or by increasing its transcription or translation (usually relevant with enzymes).
Binder	The drug binds to the target.
Ligand	The drug forms a complex with the target.
Cofactor	The drug serves as a cofactor for the target.
Potentiator	The drug does not directly activate the target but alters its activation threshold for another molecule.
Antibody	The drug is an antibody (or derivative) that specifically binds the target.
Modulator	The drug alters the activity of the target.
Positive Allosteric Modulator	The drug increases the activity of the target by binding to a site removed from the main active site.
Product of	The drug is a product of the target (usually an enzyme).
Regulator	The drug regulates the target.

This table lists the most frequent (used at least 50 times) actions between drugs and biomolecules within DrugBank and a description of their meaning.

targets, enzyme entries contain additional information associated with the relevant UniProt entry. The **Pharmacological Action** field for an enzyme is usually either "no" or "unknown," but maybe "yes" in some cases, such as if an enzyme is known to activate a prodrug. Common actions include "substrate," "inducer," and "inhibitor." Induction and inhibition of common metabolic enzymes, or the identification of the drug as a substrate of such enzymes, including those of the CYP superfamily, are usually mirrored with corresponding DBCAT category entries (see Section 3.2.2.4).

Carriers and Transporters are additional sections that relate to blood protein binding and cross-membrane transport of the drug, respectively. Both sections will similarly relate to UniProt entries. The **Pharmacological Action** field for carriers and transporters is usually either "no" or "unknown." Rare exceptions may be found though, such as when induction/inhibition of a transporter is the intended mechanistic action of the drug, or when a drug requires a transporter to reach its intended therapeutic target.

3.2.2.7 References

An important trait for all data within DrugBank is the presence of associated references. These references may correspond to published literature indexed in PubMed, other published literature such as textbooks, or links to online resources. The **Synthesis Reference** field provides either a patent or other literature reference that describes in detail how to synthesize the drug. The **General References** field contains references that are cited throughout the drug card. Each in-text reference callout is formatted to match this section and is available as hover text on the callout itself. Also included in this section are external links to related page entries and any related protein structures in the PDB [19, 20].

3.3 Protocols

3.3.1 General Workflows

Described below are several general protocols for utilizing DrugBank Online. Readers will be shown how to conduct both a basic and advanced search of DrugBank and how to browse drugs via DrugBank's drug categories. These protocols and their accompanying descriptions are intended to provide users with a practical guide for a handful of DrugBank Online's numerous functionalities, with a focus on features useful in the realm of drug discovery.

3.3.1.1 Using DrugBank Online's Search Functionality

The landing page of DrugBank Online has search functionality allowing users to search across more than 15,000 drugs and 500,000 drug products. Entering the name of a drug, or a branded drug product, will pull up the relevant drug card and all of its associated data (described in Section 3.2.2). Searching via unique chemical identifiers (e.g. CAS or UNII) is also supported. Additionally, users can search via

3 DrugBank Online: A How-to Guide

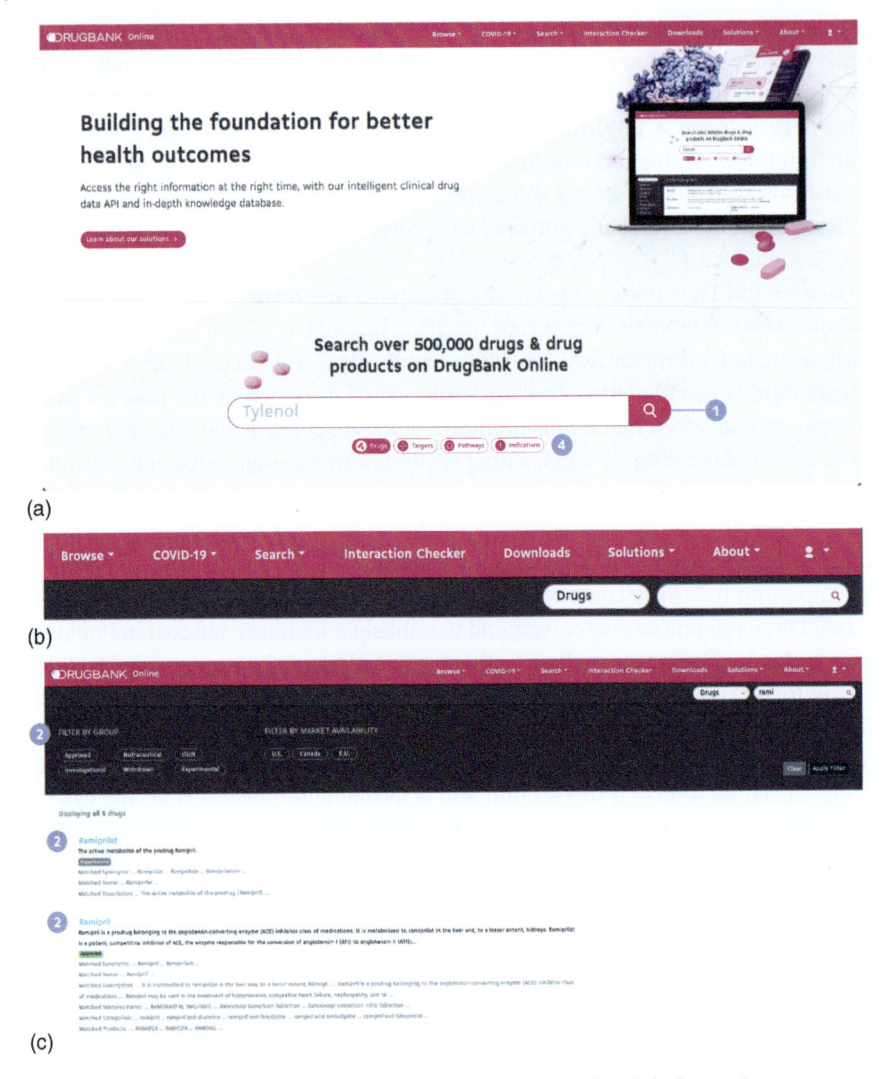

Figure 3.5 Using DrugBank Online's basic search functionality. This figure shows a screenshot of the landing page search bar (a) and the smaller search bar accessible below the upper navigation bar (b). Searches that return a single match will jump the user directly to the relevant page, while searches with multiple results (c) will display in list format.

keywords – for example, "tricyclic" or "glycopeptide" – to find any drugs relevant to those terms. The search bar also allows users to search through DrugBank's drug targets, pathways, and indications (Figure 3.5).

In this first protocol, we will perform a simple search for a drug molecule. To begin, navigate to the DrugBank Online search bar found centered in the landing page near the bottom of the window (Figure 3.5a) or in the top right of the window beneath the navigation bar (Figure 3.5b). Next:

1. Enter a drug, drug product, or keyword for which to search. Ensure the filter is set appropriately (in this case to "Drugs") and click the magnifying glass or press "Enter" to run the search.
    a. As discussed above, DrugBank Online's search function also supports searches using unique chemical identifiers, e.g. CAS numbers, DBIDs, or UNIIs.
2. Searches returning an exact match will direct the user immediately to the relevant drug card (Section 3.2.2.1). If an exact match is not found, or if the user is searching via keyword, any relevant results will be displayed in list format (Figure 3.5c).
    a. Each result will display the name of the drug, an excerpt from its **Background** data (see Section 3.2.2.2), and a list of drug card sections within which the search term was matched.
    b. This list can be further filtered by market availability and/or **Group** (discussed in Section 3.2.2.2) using the buttons at the top of the page.
3. Individual drug cards can be viewed by clicking the name of the desired drug from the list of search results.
    a. See Section 3.2.2 of this document for detailed information regarding the content of each section of the drug card.
4. The search bar additionally allows users to search through DrugBank's targets, pathways, and indications data.
    a. **Targets,** as described in Section 3.2.2.6, are proteins or other biomolecules with which a drug may interact to exert its pharmacologic effect(s). After selecting the "Target" filter under the search bar, users can enter the name of a protein (e.g. "Angiotensin-converting enzyme (ACE)") to return a list of targets matching that name. Each result will display the name of the matched target and the specific sections of the target's data to which the search term was matched. Clicking the hyperlinked name of the target will direct the user to a page containing more detailed information about the target in question, including the **Kind** of the target (e.g. "protein"), the organism in which it is present, its UniProt ID, and a list of drugs with which it is known to interact.
    b. **Pathways** are visual representations of physiologic or pharmacologic processes. DrugBank Online allows users to search through the Small Molecule Pathway Database (SMPDB) [21, 22], which contains more than 48,000 pathways comprising drug-specific pathways illustrating the metabolism and MoA of a given drug, as well as various biological processes involved in disease pathogenesis, signaling, and metabolism. After selecting the "Pathways" filter under the search bar, users can search for relevant pathways by entering the name of a drug, disease, or other physiological phenomena. For example, searching for the term "Insulin" returns a pathway illustrating endogenous insulin signaling, and also returns several results illustrating mechanistic pathways for drugs affecting insulin secretion and production. Each search result displays a truncated description of the pathway along with a list of drugs and enzymes relevant to that pathway. Clicking the hyperlinked pathway name will open a new window wherein the pathway and its description can be viewed in full.

c. **Indications**, discussed briefly in Section 3.2.2.3, are the diseases or conditions for which a given drug may be used. After selecting the "Indications" filter under the search bar, users can enter the name of a condition (e.g. "migraine") to return a list of matching conditions. Each search result displays the name of the condition, the section of the condition's data within which the search term was matched, and a list of drugs indicated for the given condition. Clicking the hyperlinked condition name will direct the user to a page containing additional information about the condition, including potential synonyms, additional information about any indicated drugs, a list of targets for the indicated drugs, and a list of clinical trials examining the condition in question.
   i. Alternatively, users can search through "Indications" data by searching for a drug of interest rather than a condition. Selecting the "Indications" filter and searching for the name of a drug will return a list of conditions for which the queried drug may be used.

DrugBank Online's basic search functionality provides a simple and intuitive means of searching through DrugBank data. It is simple enough for a member of the general public to use, while simultaneously providing enough detail and flexibility to meet the needs of healthcare practitioners, academics, and other professionals requiring detailed and comprehensive drug data. For users wanting to build more complicated queries, DrugBank Online has an advanced search functionality discussed in detail below.

3.3.1.2 Using DrugBank Online's Advanced Search Functionality

The advanced search function provides an additional means of searching DrugBank's data. Users can build powerful queries using search conditions, predicates, and operators to fine-tune their search criteria and the displayed results. The advanced search function supports searches of both drug and target data and allows for the use of wildcard matching (using * or ?) and exact matching (using quotation marks) in addition to the built-in search conditions and predicates (Figure 3.6).

In this protocol, we will perform an advanced search of DrugBank's data. From the DrugBank Online landing page, navigate to the advanced search page (https://go.drugbank.com/unearth/advanced/drugs) by clicking the **Search** button in the navigation bar at the top of the window and selecting **Advanced Search.** Next:

1. To start building our advanced search query, scroll down to the Search Conditions section and select **Add Search Condition**. Users can input as many search conditions as required to achieve the desired results.
    a. By default, the search will be set to match all of the specified search conditions (i.e. condition 1 and condition 2). Alternatively, selecting the "all" dropdown and changing it to "any" will search for drugs or targets matching any of the specified search conditions (i.e. condition 1 or condition 2).
2. For this exercise, we will use the advanced search to generate a list of approved ACE inhibitor drugs along with the CAS number, UNII, and average mass for each. ACE inhibitors are a class of antihypertensive drugs used in the treatment

3.3 Protocols | 81

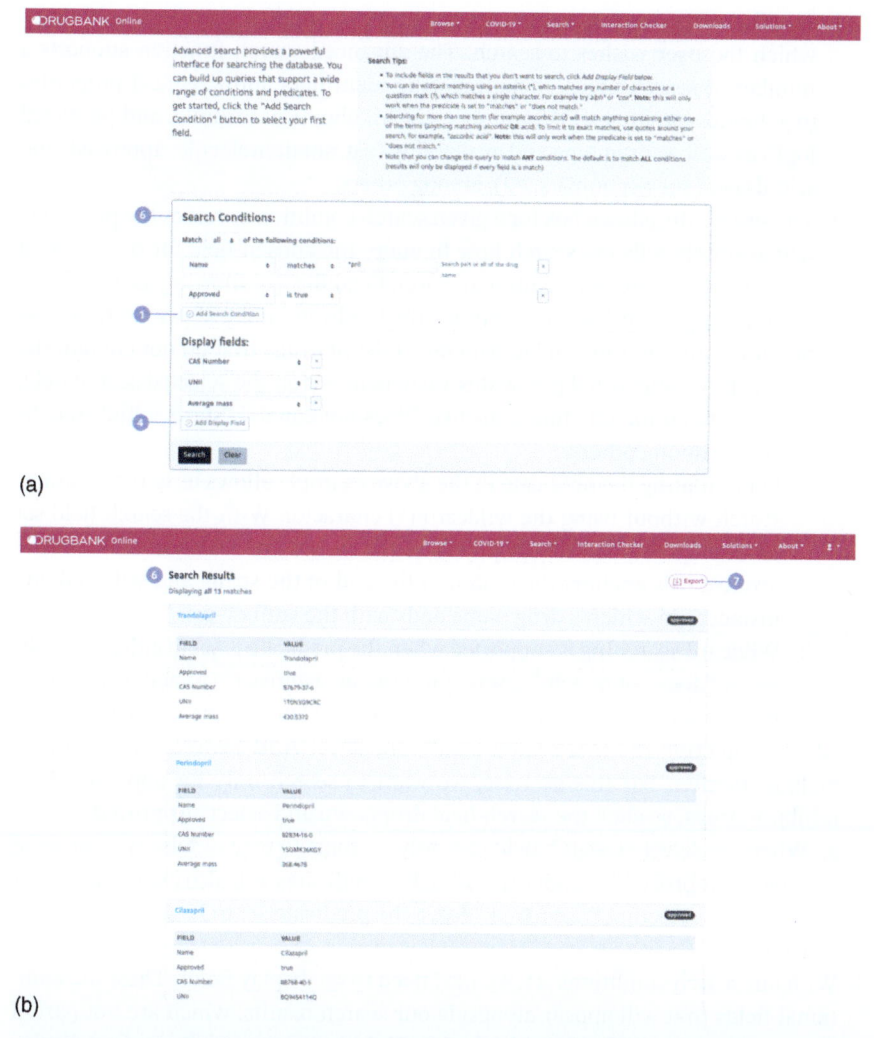

Figure 3.6 Using DrugBank Online's advanced search functionality. This figure shows the process of conducting an advanced search. (a) The completed advanced query includes multiple search conditions and display fields. (b) Search results are displayed in list format, with each result containing the fields used in the search conditions and requested in the display fields.

and management of cardiovascular diseases. As per World Health Organization (WHO) guidance around International Nonproprietary Names (INN), inhibitors of ACE are given the suffix "-pril" [23]. For the first search condition, the field and predicate can remain in their default state ("Name" and "matches") – this will search through drug names in DrugBank and return any results that match the query entered in the "search drug name" textbox. To complete the first search condition, type *pril into the textbox – because the asterisk can be used as a wildcard matching any number of characters, this search term will find any drug names that end with the string "pril."

a. The first dropdown box for a given search condition specifies the field in which the user wishes to search. The advanced search function supports a number of search fields, including drug identifiers and chemical properties (e.g. brands/products, CAS number, InChI, chemical formula, and predicted logP) as well as drug type and availability (e.g. small molecule, approved, and withdrawn; see Section 3.2.2.2), among others.
b. The second dropdown box for a given search condition specifies the predicate, which simply tells the search how to query the chosen field for the inputted text. Predicates provide additional search flexibility by allowing users to build more complex queries – for example, the predicate in the above exercise may be set to "does not match" to generate a list of drugs that do not contain the string "pril." Supported predicates are dependent on the selected search field, and in general include functions like "does not equal," "starts with," and "is present," among others.
  i. Manipulating the predicate in the above example allows us to run a similar search without using the wildcard (*) character. With the search field set to "Name," we can set the predicate to "ends with" and type "pril" in the textbox, this anchors the search to the end of the string and will find any instances in which a drug name ends with the suffix "-pril."
  ii. Wildcard searching is supported when the predicate is set to either "matches" or "does not match." Users can input an asterisk (*) to match any number of characters or a question mark (?) to match a single character.
3. After completing the first search condition, select **Add Search Condition** to include another. For this exercise, we want to search only for approved ACE inhibitor drugs, so click the search field dropdown and select "Approved."
  a. When the selected search field can only evaluate to true or false (i.e. the drug is either approved or is not), the available predicates will also change to reflect this. After selecting "Approved," leave the predicate set to its default state, "is true."
4. With our search conditions set, we next need to set display fields. These are additional fields that will appear alongside our search results, which are not part of the actual query. Click the **Add Display Field** button to create our first display field.
  a. Display fields can be selected from the same list available for search fields (e.g. Name, CAS number, and InChI). They do not require a predicate or the input of a query, as they are simply additional pieces of data that we would like to display alongside our search results.
5. We will set three display fields: one each for CAS number, UNII, and average mass. First, create two more display fields by clicking the **Add Display Field** button two more times. In the first display field, select "CAS Number." In the second, select "UNII," and in the third select "Average mass."
  a. Similar to creating search conditions, users can add as many display fields as necessary to achieve the desired results.
6. Once the appropriate search conditions and display fields are set (Figure 3.6a), clicking the **Search** button will generate the search results below the search

widget. Each result will first display the data found by the search conditions – in this case, "Name" and whether the drug is "Approved" – followed by the specified display fields. By default, each returned drug will also populate with its approval status (e.g. approved, withdrawn, and investigational) in its top-right corner (Figure 3.6b).

7. Users with a free DrugBank Online account can export the results of an advanced search as a CSV file.
    a. To create a new DrugBank Online account, click the **Sign Up** button near the top of the advanced search page and follow the instructions provided. If you have an existing DrugBank Online account, click **Login** and enter your username and password.
    b. Once signed in, users can export their search results in CSV format by clicking the **Export** button found at the top-right of the search results.
8. The advanced search function also supports searches of DrugBank's drug target data. To search through targets instead of drugs, click the **Target Advanced Search** button in the top-right of the advanced search page.
    a. The functionality of the target advanced search is essentially identical to that of the drug search. Users can add one or more search conditions, specifying a search field and, if necessary, a predicate and text query for each. Display fields can also be added to target searches, and search results can be exported using the method described in Step 7.
    b. Rather than returning a list of drugs, target searches return a list of biomolecules that may interact with drugs (e.g. receptors and enzymes). The available search fields for this dataset are different than those available for the advanced drug search, with more focus on target-specific data like UniProt ID and taxonomy.

DrugBank Online's advanced search functionality serves to illustrate the power and potential of DrugBank data. The flexibility afforded by this advanced search, as well as the ability to export its results, means that users can generate highly focused and specific datasets for use in a variety of applications, such as ML (see Section 3.3.3). A less focused exploration of drugs and compounds with similar traits can be achieved by browsing through DrugBank Online's drug categories as described in the following section.

3.3.1.3 Browsing Drugs Using DrugBank Online's Drug Categories

As described in Section 3.2.2.4, drugs in DrugBank are assigned categories that serve to group similar drugs together based on shared characteristics. Drugs may be grouped into categories based on mechanistic similarities (e.g. "Proton Pump Inhibitors"), pharmacokinetic properties (e.g. "CYP3A4 Substrates"), structural similarities (e.g. "Catecholamines"), or clinical use (e.g. "Antifungal Agents"). Grouping like drugs together within drug categories can help to elucidate commonalities between member drugs, for example, a common target that might represent an MoA or a common metabolic pathway through which member drugs may be metabolized.

1. From the DrugBank Online landing page, navigate to the drug category browser (https://go.drugbank.com/categories) by clicking the **Browse** tab in the navigation bar at the top of the page and selecting **Categories.**
    a. Individual categories can also be accessed directly from a drug card by clicking the hyperlinked title of the category of interest from the "Categories" section of the drug card (see Section 3.2.2.4).
2. Drug categories are presented as a searchable table that can be filtered by the approval status and/or market availability of the drugs within them.
    a. Each category in the table contains the name of the category, a truncated description of the category, the number of drugs within the category, and the total number of targets associated with those drugs.
        i. The category table can be additionally filtered via these columns. Users can search through category names and descriptions by inputting their search term(s) in the text boxes at the top of each column. Inputting a value into the text box at the top of the "# of drugs" or "# of targets" column will filter the table to show only the categories, which contain a number of drugs or targets greater than or equal to the value input at the top of the column.
    b. Clicking the hyperlinked category name will direct the user to a category-specific page with additional information about the selected category.
3. For this exercise, we will navigate to the "ACE inhibitors" category in order to view the same drugs returned in the advanced search query outlined in Section 3.3.1.2. In the textbox at the top of the category column, type "enzyme inhibitors" and click the magnifying glass or hit "Enter" to filter the list down to a handful of categories (Figure 3.7a). Navigate to the category page for "ACE inhibitors" by clicking the hyperlinked category name in the leftmost column.
4. Every category in DrugBank has a number of data fields that can be viewed from the page of that specific category. Information about the category as a whole includes its name, accession number (a 6-digit number prefixed with "DBCAT"), a description of the category, and its equivalent ATC classification [12] (Figure 3.7a).
    a. Some categories in DrugBank are associated with multiple accession numbers, which will be indicated by additional bracketed accession numbers following the first. This means that two (or more) categories were, at some point, deemed synonymous and merged together.
    b. Within each category, users can browse through its member drugs and their associated targets, or search through drugs and targets using the search bar in the top right of the respective sections. In the "Drugs" section of the page, each drug contained within the category will populate with its name (hyperlinked to the relevant drug card) and a brief description of the drug. In the "Drug & Drug Targets" section, the targets for each drug will display alongside the name of the drug and the type of relationship between the drug and its target (see Section 3.2.2.6 for more information on types of drug–target interactions). Both the drug name and the target names in this section are hyperlinked to their respective pages on DrugBank Online.

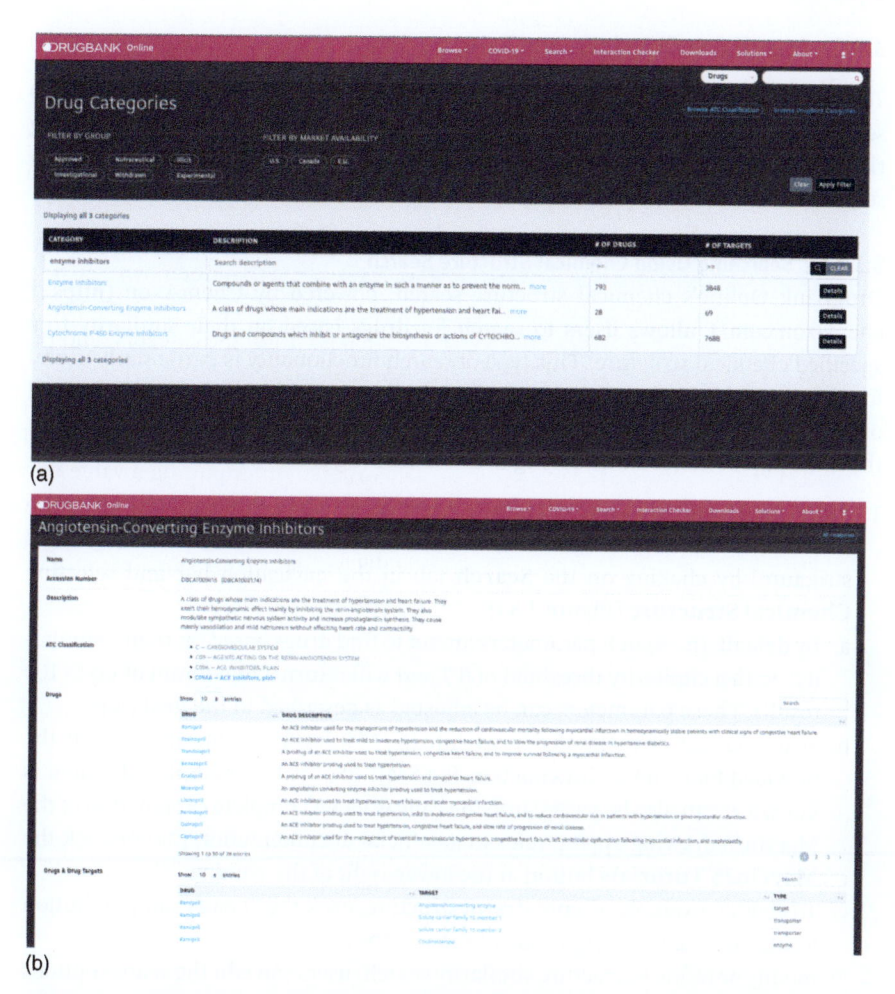

Figure 3.7 Browsing drug categories using DrugBank Online. This figure shows an example of DrugBank's browsing feature for drug categories. (a) The drug category browser with search results narrowed to show only categories with "enzyme inhibitor" in the title. Categories can be broadly filtered by group or market availability (of the drugs within them), or more specifically searched via the text boxes at the top of each column.
(b) DrugBank's drug category page for ACE inhibitors. Note that both the "Drugs" and "Drugs and Drug Targets" lists can be searched using the search box to the upper-right of each list, and can be reordered using the up-down arrow icons at the top of each column.

Organizing drugs into categories allows users to examine groups of similar drugs at a higher level of abstraction. Previously hidden relationships might become apparent when browsing drugs in this way – for example, we may notice a target or enzyme common to several members of a given drug category that can provide clues or additional context in the process of drug discovery or in the evaluation of a newly synthesized molecule.

3.3.2 Identifying Chemicals and Relevant Sequences

Text searching, including both basic (Section 3.3.1.1) and advanced (Section 3.3.1.2) searching, was covered in Section 3.3. It is also possible to query DrugBank using richer data structures including chemical structures and nucleic acid or protein sequences.

3.3.2.1 Searching Using Chemical Structure Search

DrugBank Online's chemical structure search, powered by ChemAxon (https://chemaxon.com/), allows users to search for drugs based on their similarity to a specified chemical structure. This type of search functionality is particularly useful for chemists who are interested in finding similar molecules to newly synthesized or identified compounds. It is also useful for searching for compounds that have the same parent molecule or belong to the same drug class.

1. From the DrugBank Online landing page, navigate to the chemical structure search (https://go.drugbank.com/structures/search/small_molecule_drugs/structure) by clicking on the **Search** tab in the navigation bar and selecting **Chemical Structure** (Figure 3.8a).
    a. By default, the search parameters are set to find drugs based on their "Similarity" with a similarity threshold of 0.7 and will return a maximum of up to 100 results. These parameters can be adjusted as described in the next step.
    b. Structures can be manually drawn into the MarvinJS drawing applet using the provided tools in the drawing box. If a SMILES, InChI, or similar identifier is known, it can also be pasted into the canvas. For a complete explanation of the MarvinJS drawing applet, refer to its official documentation [24] or click the **MarvinJS Tutorials** button at the lower-right of the window.
    c. To view an example of a pre-drawn structure, click the "Load example" button located on the lower right side of the window.
2. To modify or refine a structure similarity search, users can edit the search options located to the right of the drawing canvas.
    a. Users can use radio buttons to specify that a query structure be searched based on its "Similarity" to other molecules, whether it is a "Substructure" contained within other drugs, or to specify that it must be an "Exact" match to other drugs in DrugBank.
    b. Additionally, users can adjust query parameters to specify a similarity threshold, a minimum and maximum molecular weight, the maximum number of displayed results, and the types of drugs returned.
    c. The similarity threshold allows users to set a minimum similarity score for the results of a chemical structure similarity search. A similarity score is a value between 0 and 1 that represents the degree of similarity between the queried structure and each returned structure, with a greater value indicating greater similarity. These scores are generated by first creating a chemical hashed fingerprint – a bit string encoding structural features – of the structure being queried, which by default is a 1024-bit fingerprint with a maximum pattern length of seven. Using this fingerprint, the Tanimoto similarity

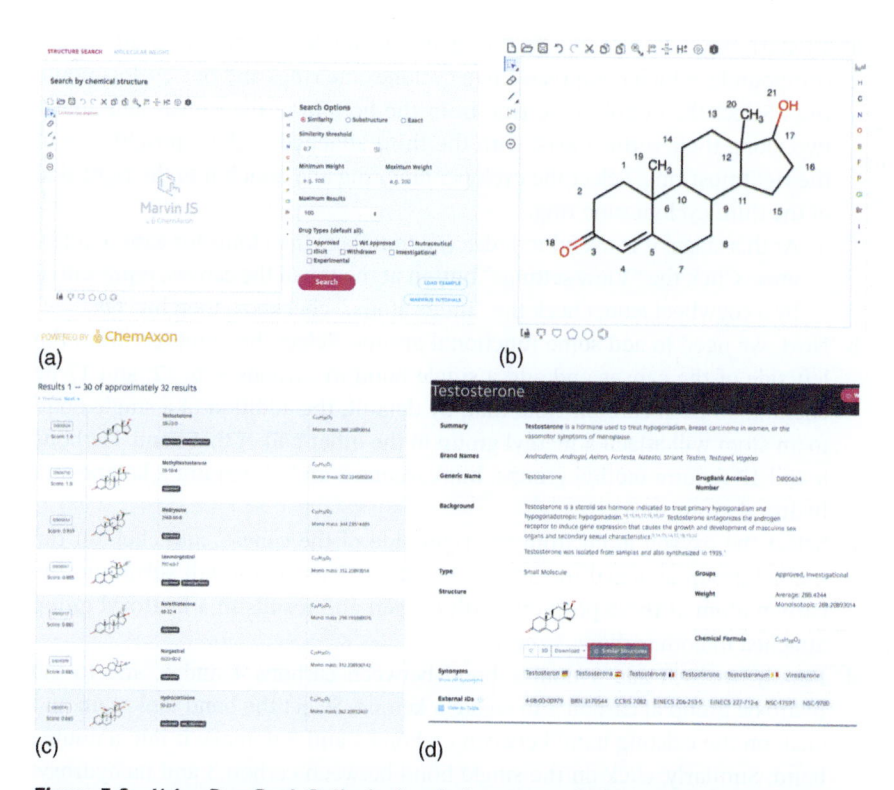

Figure 3.8 Using DrugBank Online's chemical structure similarity search. This figure illustrates the process of conducting a chemical structure similarity search. (a) The Marvin JS drawing canvas for drawing and inputting chemical structures to query. All search options shown are in their default state. (b) The chemical structure of testosterone is drawn on the canvas. Note the indexed atoms, which can aid in drawing and communicating more complex structures – atoms indices are not displayed by default but can be turned on in the settings menu indicated by the cogwheel icon at the top of the canvas. (c) Chemical structure similarity search results using testosterone (b) as the queried structure. Results are displayed in descending order of similarity to the queried structure, evident here by the inclusion of testosterone itself as the first result. (d) A screenshot of DrugBank's drug card for testosterone, with the Similar Structures button below the structure image, highlighted.

metric between the queried structure and other structures in the database is calculated. A more technical explanation of similarity scores is available via ChemAxon's documentation [25]. Note that the minimum allowable similarity threshold is 0.3 – attempting to set it any lower will instead run the search using the default value of 0.7.

3. For this exercise, we will assume the role of a researcher interested in developing a novel anabolic steroid. We will draw the structure of testosterone, a simple anabolic steroid, directly in the MarvinJS canvas in order to examine previously synthesized testosterone derivatives and identify potential novel derivatives that have yet to be tested. We will leave the stereochemistry of our molecule unspecified – when the queried structure does not contain stereo information, the search results will include molecules both with and without stereo information.

a. To start, we will draw the four-ring steroid nucleus common to all steroid compounds, which comprises three cyclohexane rings and one cyclopentane ring. Select the cyclohexane ring from the bottom of the canvas and attach two along their vertical axis, with the third attached to the top-right face of the rightmost ring. Select the cyclopentane ring and attach it to the right side of the third cyclohexane ring.
   i. At this stage, it is useful to index (i.e. number) the atoms for ease of reference. Click the "View settings" button at the top of the canvas, represented by a cogwheel icon, check the "Index atoms" checkbox, then hit "Ok."
b. Next, we need to add some functional groups. Select the bond tool from the left side of the canvas and add a single bond to carbons 3, 6, 12, and 17 by clicking on each carbon. Note that, by default, the addition of a single bond to an atom will attach a methyl group to the other end of that bond. Carbons 6 and 12 require methyl groups, but carbons 3 and 17 require a ketone and hydroxyl group, respectively.
c. Select the oxygen atom from the right side of the canvas, and click on the methyl group attached to carbons 3 and 17. This action will substitute the carbon atom at these positions with oxygen and results in a hydroxyl group attached to both carbons 3 and 17.
d. Finally, we will add a double bond between carbons 4 and 5, and to the hydroxyl group at carbon 3 to create a ketone. Select the bond tool again and click on the existing bond between carbons 4 and 5 to make it into a double bond. Similarly, click on the single bond between carbon 3 and its hydroxyl group to convert it into a double bond and the hydroxyl group into a ketone.
   i) The complete structure should look identical to the one shown in Figure 3.8b.
4. Prior to executing the search, click the "Approved" checkbox to limit the results to only compounds, which have been approved for use in humans. The remainder of the search options can stay in their default setting. After confirming your structure and search options, click the "Search" button to run the search.
5. The list of search results will appear below the MarvinJS structure editor and will be organized in descending order of similarity to the queried structure (Figure 3.8c). Each result will display along with a number of data points, including the DrugBank ID, a similarity score (with higher scores indicating better matches), a vector image of the matched structure, the name and CAS number of the matched drug, its approval status, and its formula and molecular weight.
   a. Clicking the DrugBank ID will direct you to the DrugBank drug card entry for that compound.
   b. Clicking the vector image of the returned structure will open a new window with a larger image.
6. The abovementioned protocol has described the steps involved in drawing a structure for which to search in MarvinJS. As mentioned previously, the structure search can also generate structures to query based on certain chemical notation formats like SMILES or InChI. If a compound already has a known SMILES or

InChI string, copying and pasting this string directly into the canvas is generally much easier and faster than drawing a structure from scratch.

7. A structure similarity search can also be performed from directly within a DrugBank drug card. In the "Identification" section of the drug card, next to the "Structure" heading, is an image of the drug's structure (Figure 3.8d). Clicking the button labeled "Similar Structures" directly below will immediately run a structure similarity search using all of the default search options and return a list of similar structures and their similarity scores.

This kind of chemical structure-based searching has a number of potential applications in regard to drug discovery. In the example above, our search returned a list of approved drug molecules with a structure similar to testosterone. One potential next step might be to examine structural differences in these testosterone derivatives as compared to their relative potencies in order to determine the importance of certain functional groups and their position within the molecule. Even this relatively simple approach can provide the context required to guide further research and narrow the focus of future drug discovery efforts.

When the structure is determined for a newly discovered or synthesized bioactive compound, it can often provide clues as to the compound's potential actions – in other words, structural similarity to an existing compound might imply a similar mechanism. Taking our admittedly simplified example from above, suppose we were unaware that our starting compound was testosterone. By running a structure similarity search and looking at the results, we could immediately identify our mystery compound as some type of steroid, and could then make inferences about things like its MoA and pharmacokinetics based on known properties of similar compounds. This search can also be used to identify potential protein targets (viewable by clicking the hyperlinked DrugBank ID), predict side effects, and predict unexpected interactions with unintended protein targets.

3.3.2.2 Using Sequence Search to Find Similar Targets

It is possible to search DrugBank for similar protein sequences to a known sequence, including targets, enzymes, carriers, and transporters. This can be useful to understand the types of molecules that are known to interact with your sequence (in cases of an exact match) or sequences similar to your sequence. The similarity search is powered by BLAST [26].

As an example, assume you have identified a putative target sequence based on *in silico* or *in vitro* means, and wish to understand the chemical nature of drugs that may bind to it. Navigate to the search page (https://go.drugbank.com/structures/search/bonds/sequence), either by selecting *Search -> Target Sequences* from the main navigation bar or manually entering the URL; you should see an input form (Figure 3.9a). Next:

1. Enter one or more DNA or protein sequences to search in the main text input box at the top of the form. These sequences should be in FASTA format (hovering over the small question mark icon at the top right provides a full explanation of this input format).

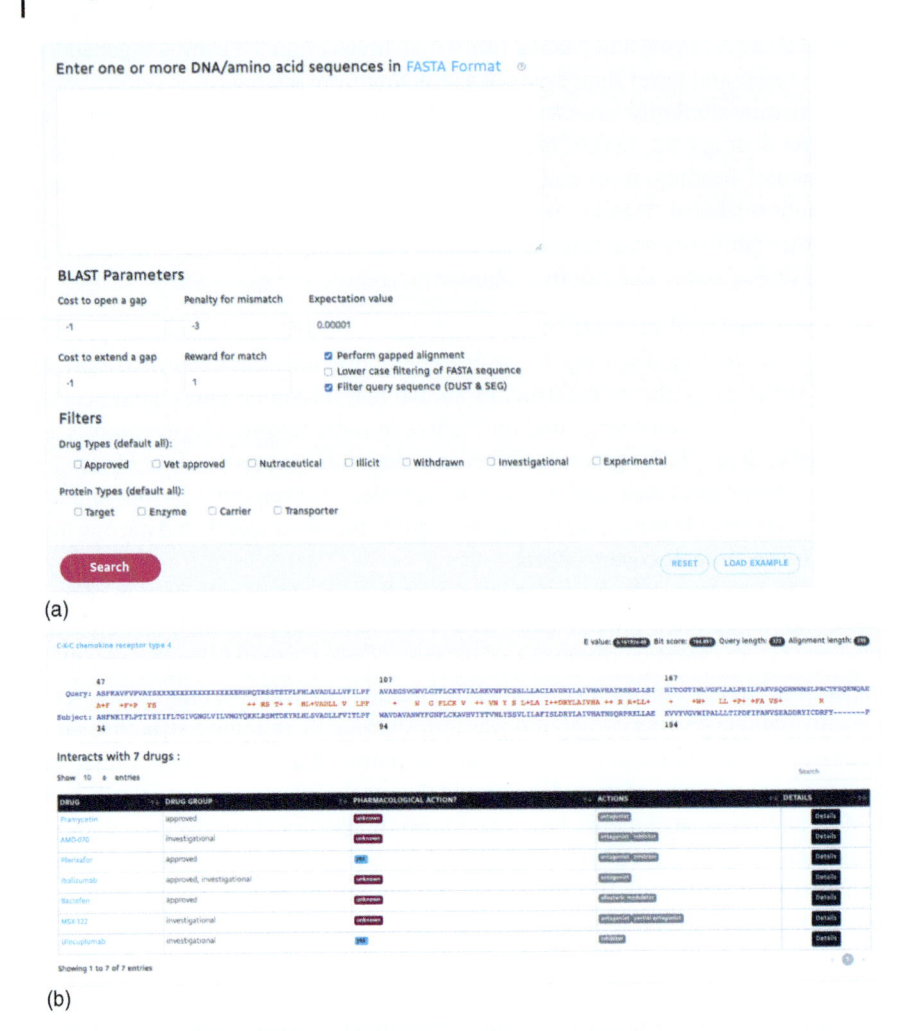

Figure 3.9 Using the DrugBank Online sequence search. This figure provides an overview of using the DrugBank Online sequence searching tool. (a) The sequence input form, which accepts one or more FASTA-formatted nucleic acid or protein sequences. Users can adjust a subset of BLAST parameters using the entry fields and radio buttons. The filters allow users to restrict the search to sequences associated with subsets of drugs based on approval status and to specific types of sequences (target, enzyme, carrier, or transporter; see Section 3.2.2.6). (b) The first result displayed after searching using the human C-X-C chemokine receptor type 5. Note the hit metrics in the top right and the BLAST output alignment present below; exact matches are denoted by the one-letter code between sequences, while similar residues are denoted with a plus symbol ("+"). The bottom table lists the drugs with which the identified sequence has known interactions in DrugBank.

2. Adjust the BLAST parameters, if desired. Note that not all parameters available in BLAST, such as the choice of substitution matrix, are available to change. The "Expectation value" controls the cutoff for returning hits; increasing this value will result in more hits but many more will be only slightly similar to the target sequence. The default gap opening cost is set at one (as opposed to the normal BLAST default of 11); this may result in hits with more gaps than otherwise

expected. For a full explanation of BLAST parameters, see the official manual (https://www.ncbi.nlm.nih.gov/books/NBK279690/).
3. Adjust the "Drug Types" filter. Only sequences associated with drugs of the selected type will be considered when searching. This is useful if, for example, you wish to consider only approved drugs, whose protein binding and MoA are more likely to be known in considerable detail. Alternatively, filtering to all but approved drugs provides insight on scaffolds currently under investigation.
4. Adjust the "Protein Types" filter. Setting this can narrow the search to the most relevant type of sequence, given the starting query (see Section 3.2.2.6 for a full explanation of each protein type).
5. Run the search (press the "Search" button).

Continuing the scenario from above, you run a search with your unknown sequence using the default BLAST parameters, including approved, withdrawn, investigational, and experimental drugs, and limiting the protein types to targets. BLAST returns 73 matches, the first of which is shown in Figure 3.9b. Each hit contains the name of the hit, together with the hit E value, bit score, and alignment length. Briefly, BLAST identifies small local matches between query and target sequence, which it attempts to extend in either direction while obeying set cutoff parameters. The longest such alignment is used to score the hit, and is also provided as part of the hit itself; in the view here, the alignment is shown on a single line and may be scrolled to the left or right if it does not fully fit within the hit table. Lastly, all relevant drug–protein interactions that fit the protein types filter are included.

Inspecting the hits for the unknown sequence, it is clear that the top hits all belong to the CXC and CC chemokine receptor families, with E values ranging from e^{-48} to e^{-33}. Indeed, the unknown query is the human C-X-C chemokine receptor type 5 (UniProt ID P32302). Although the next hit, the type 1 angiotensin II receptor, has a good E value (e^{-27}), it represents a clear departure from the cluster of top hits and will not be considered.

To get a sense of what kinds of chemical scaffolds can effectively target CXC/CC chemokine receptors, we can more closely investigate the hits. There are nine small molecules in the top hits, which are listed as either antagonist or inhibitor and for which a full structure complete with chemical classification (provided in the **Chemical Taxonomy** field of the Categories section in the relevant drug card) is present in DrugBank (Figure 3.10a). Although some similarities are apparent across scaffolds, such as a generally extended conformation and the presence of phenyl groups and amines, the scaffolds appear diverse.

It is possible to conduct a rudimentary chemical similarity analysis using data extracted directly from DrugBank. For all nine structures identified, the "Substituents" provided as part of the chemical taxonomy were extracted and used to produce a 9×94 matrix of one-hot encoded features. The most common chemical features across all molecules (present in at least three drugs) are shown in Figure 3.10b. Confirming the visual inspection of the compounds, the various nitrogen-containing functional groups make up a large proportion of the results, together with heteroaromatics, various oxygen-containing groups, and alkyl fluorides.

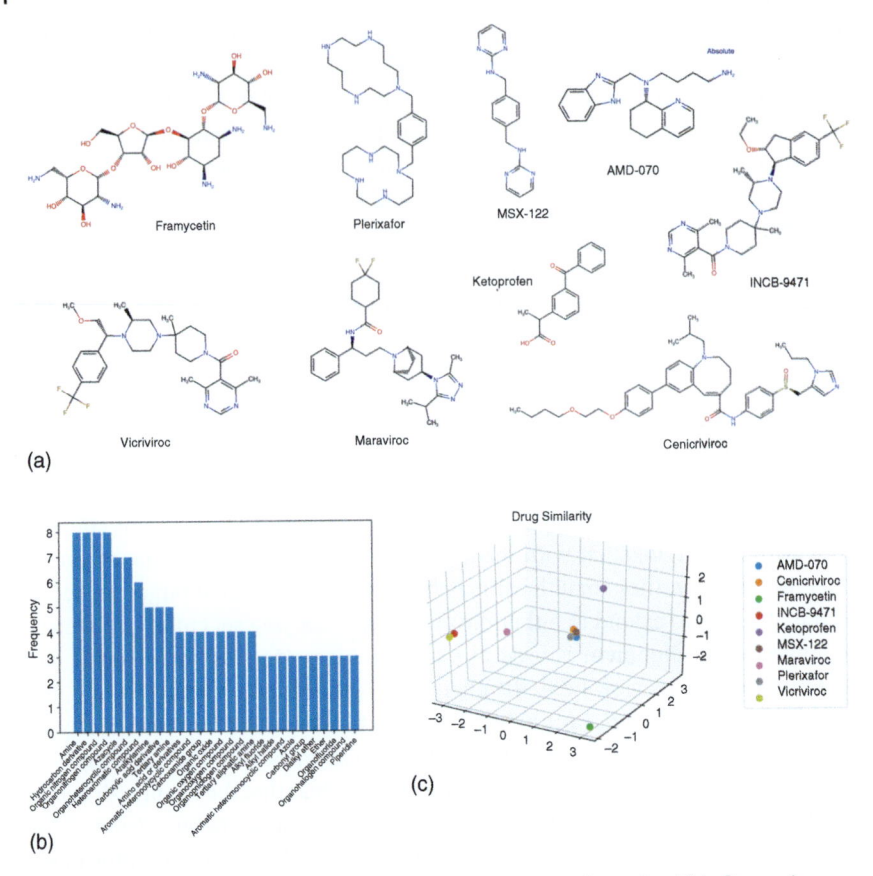

Figure 3.10 A simple structural analysis of sequence search results. This figure shows an example of how searching for similar sequences to a putative target can help to inform compound design. (a) Molecules identified within DrugBank to interact with top hits in a resulting search (see text for more details). (b) A histogram showing the prevalence of chemical features in the molecules identified in (A). For ease of visualization, features present in two or fewer molecules are not included. (c) 3D visualization of the full constituent feature matrix following PCA projection onto three components. It is clear that there are two clusters, which may serve as starting points for further analysis.

Furthermore, by using principal component analysis to project the full chemical feature matrix onto three components, it is possible to visualize the relationships between these drugs (Figure 3.10c). The resulting image reveals separation between most drugs, though INCB-9471 and vicriviroc are similar, as anticipated based on their structures. There is a single larger cluster of cenicriviroc, plerixafor, AMD-070, and MSX-122, which is not immediately apparent from a visual inspection of their structures. Furthermore, all but cenicriviroc interact with the most similar hit in the original BLAST search, C-X-C chemokine receptor type 4. This suggests that focusing on these structures, and similar ones to them, might be a reasonable place to start when identifying a new bioactive compound.

Although small-scale and highly simplistic, this example provides insight into how sequence searching may assist in the discovery of targets and the prioritization of potential scaffolds for downstream discovery work.

3.3.3 Extracting DrugBank Datasets for ML

Machine learning (ML) is increasingly applied across healthcare, from the analysis of imaging data to a myriad of applications within drug discovery pipelines [10, 27]. Although model development in these relatively new and exciting areas remains an important consideration, we argue that data quality is crucial, as health informatics represents a high-stakes domain [28]. Combined with the generally recognized "unreasonable effectiveness of data" [29], assuming a data-centric approach [30] to model training and continuous deployment practices may reap significant benefits to organizations and patients alike.

Although we do not aim to provide a comprehensive overview of relevant ML techniques here, we do highlight several ways in which public users may obtain large, focused datasets for use in building and evaluating their models. These may be used in model training, in validation of models trained on experimental or in-house datasets, or in some combination of training and testing. The datasets discussed below require a free account to access, which academic users may request using a simple form (available at: https://go.drugbank.com/public_users/sign_up; account requests require approval, which may take up to two business days to process).

The Advanced Search functionality discussed in Section 3.3.1.2 provides a powerful mechanism for querying and filtering the complete sets of drugs and targets within DrugBank. The results of a search may be exported as a CSV file, by clicking on the "Export" button at the top of the search results list (Figure 3.6b). By combining search filtering with a number of display field selections it is possible to create a focused custom dataset that can easily be loaded into an ML system or relational database system as tabular data.

Whole datasets may also be accessed under the "Downloads" tab of the main menu bar (or by navigating to https://go.drugbank.com/releases/latest). The "Complete Database" provides a wealth of information for all current DrugBank drugs in XML format with an associated schema. Relevant attributes for drug discovery include drug approval status, structural information including classifications, experimental and predicted properties, and detailed target and metabolism information; other information is also provided, which may be useful depending on the desired use case.

Simplified scientific data extracts are available through the headings at the top of the download page in SDF, CSV, and FASTA formats. These datasets have the advantage of being presorted into various categories, such as those based on the drug type and approval status. In addition to their potential use in ML applications, these other formats provide additional compatibility with existing software. Drug structures in SDF format may serve as the basis for cheminformatic studies or for *in silico* structural work. Sequences in FASTA format are easily used in comparative methods to find similar sequences (e.g. Section 3.3.2.2) or to study target relationships using phylogenetics.

A key advantage of the DrugBank datasets is the combination of breadth, depth, and accuracy, made possible by the combination of automated and curated data intake within DrugBank (Sections 3.2.1 and 3.2.2.7, Figure 3.1). Studies have consistently demonstrated the importance of data completeness and accuracy in the performance of a wide variety of ML models (e.g. see [31]). The highly structured nature of these datasets allows users to easily experiment with the addition of new features to their models, while our commitment to depth (completeness) and accuracy of data, and the inclusion of valid scientific references (Section 3.2.2.7) ensures data quality and transparency (accuracy).

3.4 Research Using DrugBank

As the pace of data and studies being released continues to grow at a breakneck rate, researchers are struggling with time-consuming work and an increasingly competitive environment. In order to stay ahead of the competition, many are turning to DrugBank for reliable, high-quality data.

Recently, a large team of researchers from Wuhan, Beijing, and Shenzhen developed a virtual screening tool using DrugBank's database to help accelerate the drug discovery process relating to COVID-19 [32]. The team used DrugBank to filter out FDA-approved drugs as well as stage 3 clinical trial drugs. Several active sites of viral proteins were then chosen to use as ligand targets for a screening process. Compounds with high binding affinities to these viral proteins were identified through *in silico* molecular docking experiments. The results included a number of drugs that were already being studied as treatments for COVID-19, but also identified a number of new possible candidates. The list included drugs that are used to treat HIV, HCV, cancer, and asthma, as well as influenza virus antagonists. Through *in silico* screening such as this, researchers can quickly identify candidate treatments for emerging diseases such as COVID-19.

Turning to Sweden, a research team there has identified lead drug compounds using DrugBank to screen against viral targets responsible for COVID-19 [33]. They compiled lists of approved, investigational, and experimental drugs to screen against four COVID-19 targets: 3C-like protease (3CLpro), papain-like protease (PLpro), RNA-dependent RNA polymerase (RdRp), and the spike (S) protein. For this study, structures of drugs identified as having high binding affinities were retrieved from DrugBank and were computationally docked to these four protein targets. The compounds were validated through a double-scoring approach using molecular dynamics and a molecular mechanics-generalized Born surface area (MM-GBSA) strategy. They found drugs that were already under review in COVID-19 clinical trials, confirming their methodology. To widen the pool of candidates, they also screened for compounds that could potentially act on multiple targets. DrugBank captures many different categorizations of drugs (such as approved, investigational, and experimental; see Section 3.2.2.2) allowing the user to filter down to those most important to their research. This is an optimal way to repurpose drugs given a vast database and known targets; researchers can readily identify leading compounds to accelerate the drug discovery process.

Another instance where DrugBank helped to speedup drug repurposing strategies involved gene networking and bioinformatic analysis. Researchers from Taiwan and Indonesia uncovered potential treatments for atopic dermatitis (AD) by integrating genetic and drug information using open data sources [34]. They gathered and mapped drug target genes to DrugBank and used parameters to filter out potential candidates based on pharmacological activity, approval status, as well as the presence of clinical and experimental drugs. After running the data, the results showed dupilumab as an effective treatment for AD. As dupilumab is already approved for this indication, this finding provided evidence for the accuracy of their methodology. The researchers found 10 more potential candidates that had preclinical and clinical trial evidence linking them through genetic interactions with AD.

Another important step in discovery and repurposing studies is the experimental validation of predicted drugs, however, it is not always performed due to resource constraints or a variety of other factors. In one illustrative example, researchers from Argentina trained 1000 linear classifiers on random subsets of independent variables (molecular descriptors) to discriminate between known active and inactive inhibitors of the *Plasmodium falciparum* protease falcipain-2 [35]. Ensemble learning was used to improve the predictive power over individual models, which was subsequently applied to the DrugBank and SWEETLEAD [36] databases to identify putative falcipain-2 inhibitors based on their positive predictive value (PPV). Of the 157 hits, four were tested for *in vitro* activity against purified falcipain-2. Methacycline, a tetracycline antibiotic, and odanacatib, an abandoned cathepsin K inhibitor investigated for use in osteoporosis, both inhibited the ability of falcipain-2 to cleave the peptidic substrate Z-LR-AMC and inhibited *P. falciparum* growth in culture. Interestingly, only odanacatib was able to inhibit proteolysis of the physiological substrate hemoglobin, highlighting the nuance of drug MoA vs. therapeutic effect.

As highlighted in this section, the accessibility of DrugBank's extensive database can offer different solutions to accelerate the drug discovery pipeline. Researchers are able to use it for *in silico* research by identifying potential drug candidates as well as for repurposing molecules. Our vast range of interconnected information creates an ideal environment for streamlined drug discovery and continues to be a strong resource for researchers to use and validate drug prediction strategies. These examples represent just a few use cases, where DrugBank provided reliable data to help find treatments for a particular disease, some of which can be emerging.

3.5 Discussion and Conclusions

The increasing importance of *in silico* methodology across healthcare, and specifically within the domain of drug discovery, has the potential to revolutionize the manner in which we deliver care. To fully realize these benefits it is necessary to have complete, well-structured, and accurate data. In this chapter, we have discussed the DrugBank database, highlighting several key datasets, providing workflows to accomplish common tasks, and discussed several research studies that demonstrate the value of this data.

The datasets discussed herein represent useful resources for drug discovery work, but do not represent an exhaustive set of those within DrugBank. Clinical trial data, as an example, can be used effectively to interrogate drug repurposing opportunities and identify underserved areas within the scope of druggable targets. Though these data are available as part of DrugBank Online (Table 3.1), expansion of this dataset and the construction of tools to assist with its interrogation are current focus areas for improvement. Similarly, although the pharmacology (and specifically pharmacokinetic) information provided in drug cards (see Section 3.2.2.3), is exceptionally detailed, it is largely in the form of unstructured text. Future efforts to create structured entries from this dataset may assist in the use of these parameters as input to various algorithms and ML models.

As mentioned in the introduction section, drug target identification is often conducted through the use of genetic associations, or is strengthened by such findings [37]. In general, the integration of genetic information in clinical diagnosis and care, though challenging, remains a source of great interest [38, 39]. The association of genomic changes with an alteration in the safety, efficacy, or other properties of a drug with respect to the individual is usually referred to as pharmacogenomics/pharmacogenetics (PGx) [40]. Although the utility of PGx data in a clinical setting has been demonstrated, the exploration of its use in other fields, such as drug discovery [41], remains to be fully evaluated. In keeping with this exciting potential, DrugBank will be investing in expanding our PGx dataset to empower new discoveries in the area of genomic medicine (see Section 3.2.2.3).

The importance of evolutionary context in drug discovery is largely limited to the use of homology searching and phylogenetic methods to ensure orthologues of putative targets are present within an animal model of choice [42]. With the recent breakthrough in *in silico* protein structural prediction [43, 44], increasing power of *in silico* structural analysis methods, and a firm emphasis on validated drug–target interactions, it is likely that this conversation will expand from a purely sequence-focused view to include important structural elements. Assisting users with analytic workflows centered around sequence and structural homology represents a fascinating possibility for future work.

Critically, though there are numerous avenues currently under development to expand DrugBank's offering, our existing data and infrastructure already represent an invaluable resource for the drug discovery community. Although commercial licensing is available, we provide many important datasets for drug discovery free of charge; by making these data freely available to researchers, we aim to empower health informatics research and democratize the research process such that an individual's ability to discover novel insights is not tied to resourcing. Future efforts to expand on these data and tools will continue this motivation, and ensure the continued success of health informatics research.

References

1 Eder, J. and Herrling, P.L. (2015). Trends in modern drug discovery. In: *New Approaches to Drug Discovery*, vol. 232, 3–22. Cham: Springer International Publishing.

2 Blay, V., Tolani, B., Ho, S.P., and Arkin, M.R. (2020). High-throughput screening: today's biochemical and cell-based approaches. *Drug Discovery Today* 25 (10): 1807–1821.

3 Dowden, H. and Munro, J. (2019). Trends in clinical success rates and therapeutic focus. *Nature Reviews. Drug Discovery* 18 (7): 495–496.

4 Lewis, K. (2020). The science of antibiotic discovery. *Cell* 181 (1): 29–45.

5 Hughes, J., Rees, S., Kalindjian, S., and Philpott, K. (2011). Principles of early drug discovery: principles of early drug discovery. *British Journal of Pharmacology* 162 (6): 1239–1249.

6 Heifetz, A., Southey, M., Morao, I. et al. (2018). Computational methods used in hit-to-lead and lead optimization stages of structure-based drug discovery. In: *Computational Methods for GPCR Drug Discovery*, vol. 1705 (ed. A. Heifetz), 375–394. New York, NY: Springer, New York.

7 Fourches, D. and Ash, J. (2019). 4D- quantitative structure–activity relationship modeling: making a comeback. *Expert Opinion on Drug Discovery* 14 (12): 1227–1235.

8 Kubota, K., Funabashi, M., and Ogura, Y. (2019). Target deconvolution from phenotype-based drug discovery by using chemical proteomics approaches. *Biochimica et Biophysica Acta, Proteins and Proteomics* 1867 (1): 22–27.

9 Batool, M., Ahmad, B., and Choi, S. (2019). A structure-based drug discovery paradigm. *International Journal of Molecular Sciences* 20 (11): 2783.

10 Chan, H.C.S., Shan, H., Dahoun, T. et al. (2019). Advancing drug discovery via artificial intelligence. *Trends in Pharmacological Sciences* 40 (8): 592–604.

11 Sanchez-Lengeling, B. and Aspuru-Guzik, A. (2018). Inverse molecular design using machine learning: generative models for matter engineering. *Science* 361 (6400): 360–365.

12 WHO Collaborating Centre for Drug Statistics Methodology (2022). ATC classification index with DDDs.

13 National Center for Biotechnology Information (2022). MeSH (Medical Subject Headings). *National Library of Medicine*. Available at www.ncbi.nlm.nih.gov/mesh.

14 CDER Manual of Policies and Procedures (2018). MAPP 7400.13: Determining the Established Pharmacologic Class for Use in the Highlights of Prescribing Information. *US FDA Center for Drug Evaluation and Research*.

15 Djoumbou Feunang, Y., Eisner, R., Knox, C. et al. (2016). ClassyFire: automated chemical classification with a comprehensive, computable taxonomy. *Journal of Cheminformatics* 8 (1): 61.

16 Tetko, I.V. and Tanchuk, V.Y. (2002). Application of associative neural networks for prediction of lipophilicity in ALOGPS 2.1 program. *Journal of Chemical Information and Computer Sciences* 42 (5): 1136–1145.

17 Cheng, F., Li, W., Zhou, Y. et al. (2012). admetSAR: a comprehensive source and free tool for assessment of chemical ADMET properties. *Journal of Chemical Information and Modeling* 52 (11): 3099–3105.

18 The UniProt Consortium, Bateman, A., Martin, M.-J. et al. (2021). UniProt: the universal protein knowledgebase in 2021. *Nucleic Acids Research* 49 (D1): D480–D489.

19 Berman, H.M. (2000). The protein data bank. *Nucleic Acids Research* 28 (1): 235–242.
20 Burley, S.K., Bhikadiya, C., Bi, C. et al. (2021). RCSB Protein Data Bank: powerful new tools for exploring 3D structures of biological macromolecules for basic and applied research and education in fundamental biology, biomedicine, biotechnology, bioengineering and energy sciences. *Nucleic Acids Research* 49 (D1): D437–D451.
21 Frolkis, A., Knox, C., Lim, E. et al. (2010). SMPDB: the small molecule pathway database. *Nucleic Acids Research* 38 (Database issue): D480–D487.
22 Wishart Research Group (2010). Small Molecule Pathway Database.
23 (2018). *The use of stems in the selection of International Nonproprietary Names (INN) for pharmaceutical substances*, World Health Organization, Geneva.
24 Chemaxon Marvin JS User's Guide. *Chemaxon Docs*.
25 Chemaxon JChem Base Query Guide: Similarity search. *Chemaxon Docs*.
26 Altschul, S. (1997). Gapped BLAST and PSI-BLAST: a new generation of protein database search programs. *Nucleic Acids Research* 25 (17): 3389–3402.
27 Freedman, D.H. (2019). Hunting for new drugs with AI. *Nature* 576 (7787): S49–S53.
28 Sambasivan, N., Kapania, S., Highfill, H. et al. (2021). "Everyone wants to do the model work, not the data work": data cascades in high-stakes AI. In: *Proceedings of the 2021 CHI Conference on Human Factors in Computing Systems*, 1–15.
29 Halevy, A., Norvig, P., and Pereira, F. (2009). The unreasonable effectiveness of data. *IEEE Intelligent Systems* 24 (2): 8–12.
30 Miranda, L. (2021). "Towards data-centric machine learning: a short review". ljvmiranda921.github.io.
31 Budach, L., Feuerpfeil, M., Ihde, N., Nathansen, A., Noack, N., Patzlaff, H., Harmouch, H., and Naumann, F. (2022). *The Effects of Data Quality on Machine Learning Performance*.
32 Xu, C., Ke, Z., Liu, C. et al. (2020). Systemic *In Silico* screening in drug discovery for coronavirus disease (COVID-19) with an online interactive web server. *Journal of Chemical Information and Modeling* 60 (12): 5735–5745.
33 Murugan, N.A., Kumar, S., Jeyakanthan, J., and Srivastava, V. (2020). Searching for target-specific and multi-targeting organics for Covid-19 in the Drugbank database with a double scoring approach. *Scientific Reports* 10 (1): 19125.
34 Adikusuma, W., Irham, L.M., Chou, W.-H. et al. (2021). Drug repurposing for atopic dermatitis by integration of gene networking and genomic information. *Frontiers in Immunology* 12: 724277.
35 Alberca, L.N., Chuguransky, S.R., Álvarez, C.L. et al. (2019). In silico guided drug repurposing: discovery of new competitive and non-competitive inhibitors of falcipain-2. *Frontiers in Chemistry* 7: 534.
36 Novick, P.A., Ortiz, O.F., Poelman, J. et al. (2013). SWEETLEAD: an in Silico database of approved drugs, regulated chemicals, and herbal isolates for computer-aided drug discovery. *PLoS One* 8 (11): e79568.

37 Schmidt, A.F., Finan, C., Gordillo-Marañón, M. et al. (2020). Genetic drug target validation using Mendelian randomisation. *Nature Communications* 11 (1): 3255.

38 Jordan, D.M. and Do, R. (2018). Using full genomic information to predict disease: breaking down the barriers between complex and mendelian diseases. *Annual Review of Genomics and Human Genetics* 19 (1): 289–301.

39 Burke, W. (2021). Utility and diversity: challenges for genomic medicine. *Annual Review of Genomics and Human Genetics* 22 (1): 1–24.

40 Roden, D.M., McLeod, H.L., Relling, M.V. et al. (2019). Pharmacogenomics. *The Lancet* 394 (10197): 521–532.

41 Roses, A.D. (2008). Pharmacogenetics in drug discovery and development: a translational perspective. *Nature Reviews. Drug Discovery* 7 (10): 807–817.

42 Holbrook, J.D. and Sanseau, P. (2007). Drug discovery and computational evolutionary analysis. *Drug Discovery Today* 12 (19–20): 826–832.

43 Jumper, J., Evans, R., Pritzel, A. et al. (2021). Highly accurate protein structure prediction with AlphaFold. *Nature* 596 (7873): 583–589.

44 Baek, M., DiMaio, F., Anishchenko, I. et al. (2021). Accurate prediction of protein structures and interactions using a three-track neural network. *Science* 373 (6557): 871–876.

4

Bioisosteric Replacement for Drug Discovery Supported by the SwissBioisostere Database

Antoine Daina[1], Alessandro Cuozzo[2], Marta A.S. Perez[1], and Vincent Zoete[1,2]

[1] SIB Swiss Institute of Bioinformatics, Molecular Modeling Group, Quartier UNIL-Sorge, Bâtiment Amphipôle, 1015 Lausanne, Switzerland
[2] University of Lausanne, Ludwig Institute for Cancer Research, Department of Oncology UNIL-CHUV, Route de la Corniche 9A, 1066 Epalinges, Switzerland

4.1 Introduction

4.1.1 Concept of Isosterism and Bioisosterism

Isosterism is one of the oldest and most established concepts in medicinal chemistry but is also a trusted, powerful, and efficient practice to foster successful drug discovery to this day. The history of bioisosterism is long, and detailed presentations can be found in the book of the same series dedicated to the subject [1] and in other substantial reviews [2–4].

However, here is a swift journey of milestones and definitions around the important notions. Origins are certainly to be found in 1919 with the work of Irving Langmuir [5], who studied the similarities of various properties between atoms, groups, radicals, and molecules. The "isosteres" were strictly defined as chemical entities that have the same number of atoms and arrangement of electrons. This definition was then broadened in 1925 by applying Grimm's "Hydride Displacement Law" and the pseudoatom notion. In the 1930s, the experiments of Erlenmeyer brought crucial inputs by (i) relaxing the isosteric classification to chemical entities sharing identical peripheral layers of electrons and thus including those having different numbers of atoms and (ii) relating isosterism to biology through experiments showing antigens bearing isosteric fragments binding equally to antibodies [6].

The term "bioisostere" appeared in 1951 and is attributed to Friedmann, who pioneered very important aspects for future application in drug research [7]. In particular, he emphasized that bioisosteric chemical entities must show similar biological activity and comply with the *broadest* definition of isosteres. In other words, isosteres are not necessarily bioisosteres if they do not share the same bioactivity. Reversely, bioisosteres are not always isosteres if restricted to the strict classical definition. Later definitions are going even further in practical sense, such as the one of Thornber, who defined a form of *non-classical* isosterism characterized by chemical and physical similarity and *roughly* similar biological effects [8].

4.1.2 Classical vs. Non-classical Bioisostere and Further Molecular Replacements

The most recent definitions of bioisosterism relate to drug discovery in a pragmatic sense, with the idea that all depend on the biological and chemical contexts of the field explored. Regarding biological context, the same pair of similar compounds can display comparable pharmacological properties on a given protein target or assay while showing divergent bioactivities on other targets or in other experimental setups.

In addition, the effect produced by exchanging a molecular fragment in a molecule is very dependent on the chemical context. For instance, replacing a methyl group with a halogen atom can have different impacts on molecular and physicochemical properties if it takes place as an aromatic substitution or at the end of a long alkyl chain.

Echoing such ordinary problems of daily medicinal chemistry routine, experts in the field have clearly softened the criteria for alikeness in terms of both biological and chemical contexts. Among the refined vocabulary employed, the distinction between *classical* and *non-classical* bioisosteres is noteworthy.

As the name suggests, *classical bioisosteres* come from the initial definitions of isosterism focusing on strict comparison at the atomic and electronic levels. Atoms or groups are typically classified as monovalent, divalent, or trivalent bioisosteres. Medicinal chemists apply such classical bioisosteric replacements routinely. Typically, this definition applies, for example, between fluorine and hydrogen; amino and hydroxyl; thiol and hydroxyl; hydroxyl, amino, and methyl groups (comply with Grimm's Hydride Displacement Law); chloro, bromo, thiol, and hydroxyl groups (relaxed criteria according to Erlenmeyer) [3]. Some modest extensions of the concept can reasonably be seen as classical bioisosteres like tetrasubstituted atoms (tetravalent carbon, tetrasubstituted silane, ammonium exchanges) or very similar ring replacements (e.g. pyridine for phenyl).

Further extensions of the concept enter the territory of *non-classical bioisosteres*, which can differ in molecular structures and properties, for instance in terms of the number of atoms, or steric or electronic considerations. Well-known examples include the replacement of carboxylic acid by tetrazole, as successfully applied for designing nonpeptide oral angiotensin receptor antagonists and resulting in the antihypertensive drug Losartan (Figure 4.1a). In general, the tetrazole moiety shows an acidity similar to carboxylic acid while improving other properties important for a drug [13, 14]. In this biological and chemical context, the bioisosteric exchange also produced stronger *in vitro* and *in vivo* activities due to better pharmacokinetics and pharmacodynamics [9].

Although less strict than *classical bioisoteres*, such *non-classical* bioisosteric transformations still aim at mimicking some properties of a molecular fragment to be

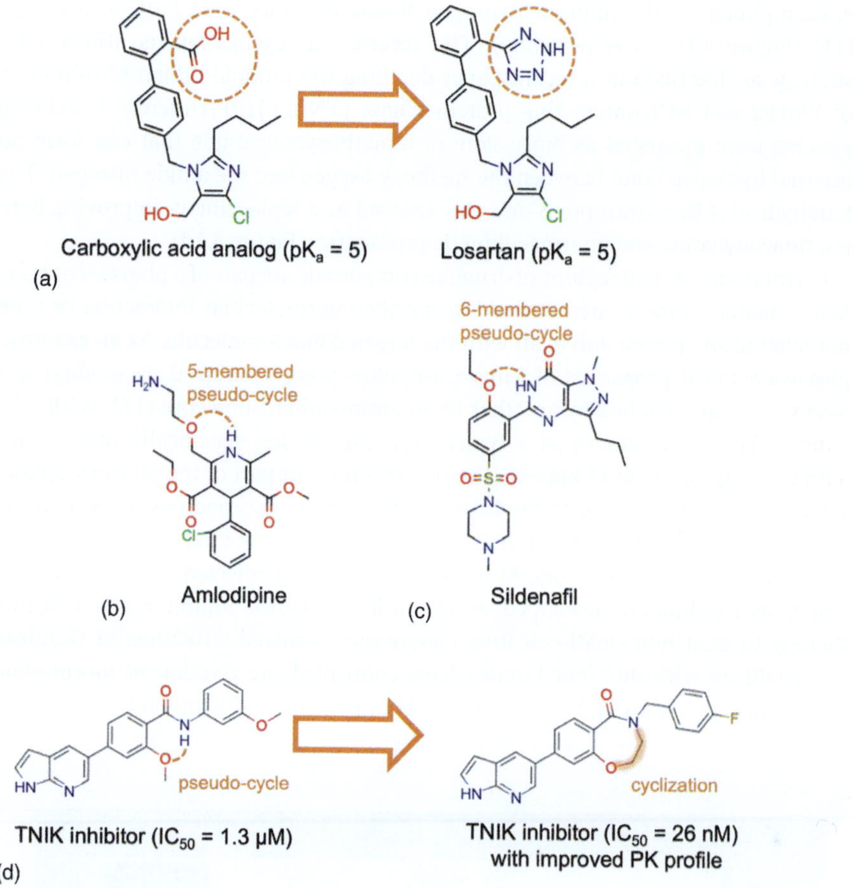

Figure 4.1 Drug-related *non-classical* bioisosteres. (a) Both the bioactivity and the bioavailability of angiotensin receptor antagonists were improved by switching from carboxylic acid to tetrazole [9]; (b) and (c) examples of FDA-approved drugs involving internal hydrogen bonds forming pseudo-cycles, possibly ring bioisosteres. Source: Adapted from Refs. [10, 11]; (d) example of bioisosteric replacement of the central core of TNIK inhibitor by cyclization [12].

replaced, even by a different means than sticking to an identical number of atoms and electrons.

Conceptually, it is possible to go even further and apply molecular replacements of fragments without necessarily trying to mimic any property *a priori*. The objective of retaining bioactivity is perforce linked to molecular recognition at the target, and hence, any modification of small molecule ligand should be meant not to alter the position in space of chemical features essential for the recognition, a.k.a. the pharmacophore. Keeping the pharmacophoric points at the correct location can be achieved by more subtle and sophisticated means than exchanges of similar moieties as described previously. For instance, taking advantage of intramolecular interactions to mimic a ring with a noncyclic moiety is exemplified by the internal hydrogen bonds in amlodipine [10] or sildenafil [11] (Figure 4.1b, c, respectively). The reverse, i.e. cyclization, is also a valid strategy, as described in a recent paper detailing the rational design of inhibitors of TRAF2 and NCK-interacting protein kinase (TNIK) [12]. Different fused ring systems were evaluated as bioisostere of o-methoxybenzamide that can form an internal hydrogen bond between the methoxy oxygen and the amide nitrogen. The tetrahydro-1,4-benzoxazepin-5-one was selected as a replacement, improving both pharmacodynamic and pharmacokinetic profiles (see Figure 4.1d).

Furthermore, not all regions of druglike compounds are part of a pharmacophore. Some chemical groups are not making specific intermolecular interaction or even not making any interaction at all with the targeted macromolecule. As an example, physicochemical properties of kinase inhibitors were optimized by modifying a long side chain attached by an ether to an aminoquinazoline core [15]. While the latter is known nowadays as a typical scaffold making specifically interactions with the hinge domain of kinases, the side chain is not part of the pharmacophore *stricto sensu* and was used to modulate physicochemical properties while keeping bioactivity. Terminal polar heterocycles were particularly effective in increasing the solubility of the inhibitors. Morpholine was finally selected for the molecule, which was ultimately developed as Gefitinib, an EGFR inhibitor and first-line therapy to treat non-small cell lung carcinoma. Resolved structures of Gefitinib cocrystallized with different kinases have confirmed the position of morpholine in the solvent (Figure 4.2, e.g. Gefitinib bound to an EGFR mutant, PDB entry:

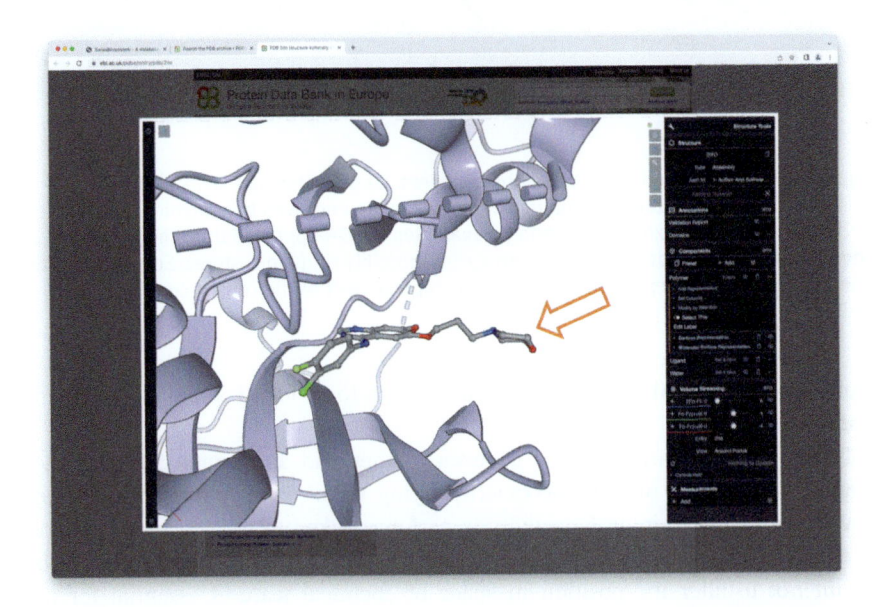

Figure 4.2 Crystallized complex of EGFR with inhibitor Gefitinib. Screenshot of Mol* Viewer [16] as embedded on Protein Data Bank in Europe portal (PDB ID: 2ITO, https://www .ebi.ac.uk/pdbe/). EGFR is displayed as mauve cartoon and Gefitinib ligand in ball-and-stick with carbon atoms in grey. The orange arrow points to the morpholine in the solvent.

2ITO). Grippingly, morpholine is the second most queried fragment inputted by SwissBioisostere users (refer to Section 4.4.2).

Regardless of the medicinal chemistry strategy followed (if any), the fact remains that replacing one part of a molecule only, while keeping the rest unchanged generates a couple of compounds. In case of similar biological activity, we consider the compounds as *bioisosteres* and the exchange of fragments as a *bioisosteric replacement*.

To support medicinal chemists in choosing effective bioisosteric replacements, this very pragmatic generalization of the concept stresses the need for tools not limited to molecular or physicochemical descriptions but based on bioactivity knowledge. Nowadays, the wealth of bioactivity data is sufficient, both in quality and quantity, to enable such knowledge-based tools. The SwissBioisostere database and its web interface are the examples we want to describe in this chapter.

4.1.3 Bioisosteric Replacement in Drug Discovery

Drug discovery can be defined as all the strategies and techniques aimed at finding small molecules active on a defined biological target (i.e. hit compounds), selecting leads with most appropriate properties for chemical modifications enabling optimization, and ultimately promoting the drug candidates with the best chance of success into the development phases. It is a long and costly workflow involving trial-and-error paths and empirical feedback loops – in fact, much more complex than the idealized scheme often presented. For decades, substantial efforts have been put to lower the attrition rate and accelerate the generation of hypotheses, knowledge, or evidences to support decisions and finally to reduce the risks associated with the even more time-consuming and expensive drug development phases.

Such decision-making support can be successfully achieved by a bioisosteric replacement strategy, routinely followed by medicinal chemists. The approach consists in defining and applying the chemical modifications that improve one or several sub-optimal properties while keeping the bioactivity at least at the same level [17]. Drug discovery is highly multi-objective, hence the large variety of properties to be potentially corrected: toxicity or lack of specificity for the target, synthesis or intellectual property issues, improper Absorption, Distribution, Metabolism, and Excretion (ADME) or pharmacokinetic profiles, to name the most obvious ones [18].

In this section, we propose to describe and exemplify bioisosterism practices applied to *hit finding* and *lead optimization*.

When a pharmacologically relevant target has been selected, chemical entities showing activity must be identified with procedures grouped under the term *hit finding*. In usual workflows, high-throughput screening as well as literature and patent analysis are the primary sources for hits. The most promising hits have to be clearly detected, unambiguously defined chemically, biochemically validated in diverse assays, and further evaluated as suitable or not for promotion as lead compounds. These activities are of utmost importance to promote the best possible start of demanding medicinal chemistry programs. During hit finding, experts must obviously address technical points, such as synthetic accessibility of a given scaffold, for instance, but also, more broadly, questions regarding the freedom to operate. Intellectual property to avoid conflict with already protected fields is critical.

The objective is to escape a given chemotype to overcome the specific issues of a given chemical series. Consequently, one can expect the chemical space to be vast and distant from the first molecular hits. An efficient approach to explore new areas of this broad space consists in exchanging the whole central core of a hit compound but keeping the pharmacophoric points at the periphery of the molecule to retain bioactivity [19]. In this methodology conceptualized and called *scaffold hopping* by Gisbert Schneider [20], bioisosteric replacements concern "linker" or "scaffold" fragments, including multiple connection points to the constant part of bioisostere compounds (for technical aspects, see Section 4.2.3 and Figure 4.4).

Upon successful completion of all the hit-related processes described above, the chemical entities are termed "lead compounds" and enter optimization, for which bioisosteric replacements are also routinely and efficiently conducted. During *lead optimization*, a validated chemotype is subject to numerous modest structural modifications [21]. The exploration of the chemical space allows to consider the relationship between the structure and the properties that need to be optimized to design a drug candidate. Compared to the hit-finding step, the exploration of the space remains within the vicinity of the lead compound. Structural modifications are principally made at the periphery of the molecules, such as at the end of a chain or at a substituent position. The bioisosteric replacement is mainly applied on "side chains," with exchanged fragments having a single connection point with the rest of the molecule (for technical aspects, see Section 4.2.3, and Figure 4.4).

The motivation for proposing SwissBioisostere and the way it has been designed was to meet the needs of medicinal chemists' practice. This is exposed in detail in Section 4.2.

4.2 Construction and Dissemination of SwissBioisostere

4.2.1 Intention and Requirements

As introduced in Section 4.1, bioisosterism is routinely used for drug discovery. This intuitive approach cannot follow a generalized logical path since it depends on the biological and chemical contexts of the explored domain. There are neither universally applicable rules nor guidelines to support the important and daily task of replacing parts of a template molecule with new chemical moieties. Often, the practice of bioisosteric replacement relies solely on the expertise of medicinal chemists.

The likelihood of success of bioisosteric replacement approaches increases when applied in a systematic and rational manner [2, 3]. Medicinal chemists can benefit from computational support for bioisosteric drug design. However, the usefulness of such tools depends on some requirements. First, the bioisosteric knowledge should

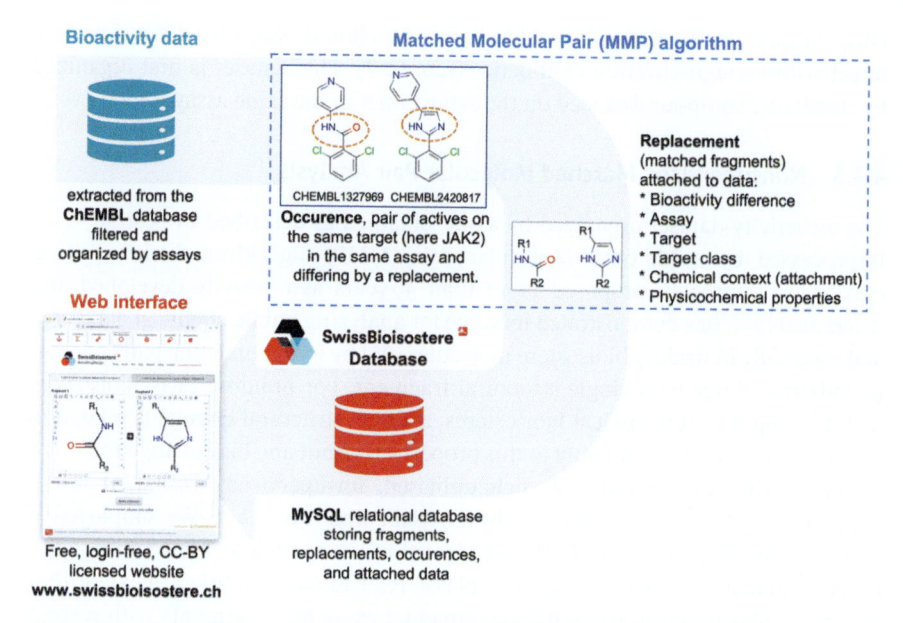

Figure 4.3 Construction of the SwissBioisostere database and web interface.

be primarily rooted in bioactivity data linked to the structure of compounds and processed with an unbiased technique, without considering other molecular parameters like physicochemical properties, for instance (refer to Section 4.2.3). Second, the bioactivity data itself should be of high quality and broad in terms of chemical and biological spaces (refer to Section 4.2.2).

The physicochemical and molecular descriptors are not included in the definition of molecular replacements, but, reversely, they are of great importance for the users to estimate the impact of these replacements on such properties. This, together with the difference in bioactivity, should be organized for easy access to enable a global assessment of the consequences of selected molecular replacements (refer to Section 4.2.4 and Section 2.5).

The general workflow for the construction of SwissBioisostere is displayed in Figure 4.3.

4.2.2 Bioactivity Data

The major data source for building SwissBioisostere is ChEMBL (https://www.ebi.ac.uk/chembl/), a manually curated high-quality bioactivity database relying mainly on medicinal chemistry literature and secondarily other sources, like publicly available screening campaigns [22, 23]. It provides the possibility to download the entire database in different formats. This allows to efficiently link the chemical context (molecular structure and descriptors) and the biological context (bioactivity, target, and target class) to assays and publications, for a large set of bioactive compounds. For the needs of SwissBioisostere, ChEMBL data were filtered to keep only small molecules (molecular weight <800 g/mol), active *in vitro*

(IC_{50}, EC_{50}, K_i, or K_d < 10 µM) in a binding or functional assay on a defined protein target with enough curation confidence (score >7). This dataset is first organized by classifying compounds tested on the same target in the same assay.

4.2.3 Nonsupervised Matched Molecular Pair Analysis

The bioactivity dataset organized by assay, obtained as described in Section 4.2.2, is processed by a Matched Molecular Pair (MMP) algorithm. Such intuitive, easy-to-use approach, proposed more than 40 years ago, heavily developed and diversified [24], has demonstrated its value for analyzing public chemical databases and especially in finding bioisostere molecules [25] by individualizing pairs of compounds that differ by a single structural fragment. For building SwissBioisostere and defining truly unclassical bioisosteres, a single structural change is related to variation in bioactivity and only to this property, without any bias of any kind.

One well-known example of such unbiased, unsupervised MMP [26] is the fragment-based method described by Hussain and Rea [27]. We employed a custom-made implementation of this algorithm, in particular by defining additional fragmentation rules (for details, please refer to [28]). In brief, the algorithm cuts molecules tested in the same experimental assay into fragments with respect to their bond types. Only single bonds may be cut if linking at least one carbon, no hydrogen, and not being part of any cycle, chemical function, or simple sugar pattern (e.g. glucose or fructose). To generate fragments, no more than three bonds can be cut at the same time. As such, three kinds of fragments are considered: *side chain* fragments with one attachment point; *linker* fragments with two attachment points; and *scaffold* fragments with three attachment points (Figure 4.4a). All remaining (one, two, or three) moieties are tagged "R-groups" and correspond to the constant part of the molecule (Figure 4.4b). This allows finally to define an *occurrence* as two molecules tested on the same assay (and thus on the same target) differing only by one fragmental exchange with the rest of the structure constant (R-groups). This fragmental exchange is defined as the *replacement* (Figure 4.3).

4.2.4 Database

The MMP analysis on bioactivity data as described above enables the user to find possible bioisosteric replacements, for instance, if the majority of occurrences (pairs of molecules) for a given replacement are showing similar bioactivity when tested in the same assay. The analysis can be further refined thanks to attached data, such as physicochemical properties, or biological and chemical contexts not employed to guide the MMP but important for design actions to be applied in lead optimization or hit finding. A relational database was built using MySQL (https://www.mysql.com) with the aim of structuring the extensive wealth of knowledge and making it straightforwardly searchable through a large variety of languages, including web-oriented programs. As an example, the main and largest table contains more than 65 million data points, corresponding to all replacement occurrences. These base data are linked to all additional knowledge, like molecular and physicochemical properties or target classes, through several other interconnected tables.

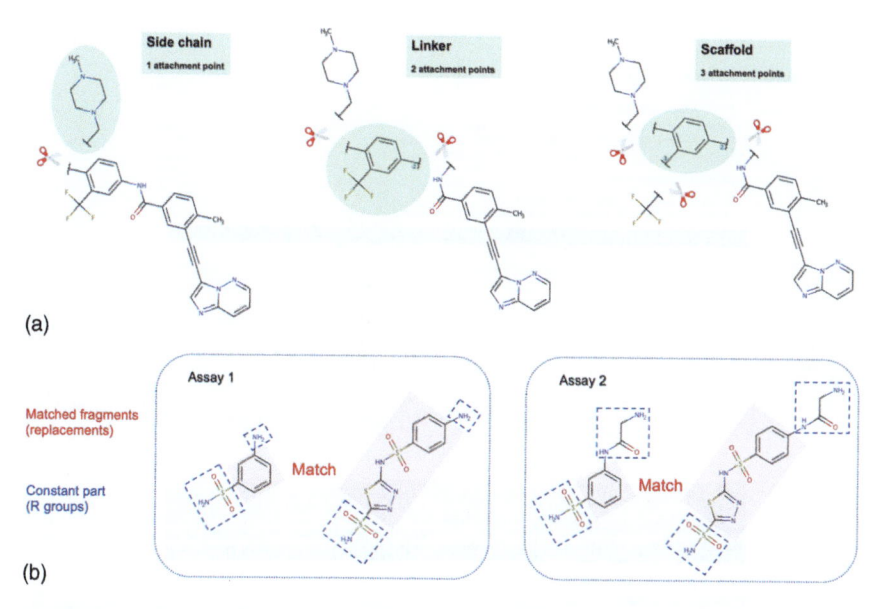

Figure 4.4 Unsupervised Matched Molecular Pair (MMP) algorithm for building SwissBioisostere. (a) Example of some fragmentations of Ponatinib (other cuts are possible); our implementation of MMP can consider three kinds of fragments: *side chain*, *linker*, and *scaffold* fragments with one, two, and three attachment points, respectively. This allows (b) to define matched fragments (here *replacements* of linkers boxed in red) among pairs of molecules tested on the same target in the same assay (here, two *occurrences* for the same replacement from two different assays); all remaining (one, two, or three) chemical moieties correspond to the *constant part* of the molecule (blue dashed boxes).

4.2.5 Web Interface

The SwissBioisostere database is openly accessible on the Web, freely browsable and searchable by reaching www.swissbioisostere.ch. This login-free website has been online since 2012 [29] and has undergone a major update (both frontend and backend) in 2021 [28]. Users can perform their own requests and analyses within the graphical web interface; they can also export results, access to related ChEMBL and PubMed entries, and interoperate with other CADD web tools. Use cases and examples are given in Section 4.4.3. Please refer to the reference [28] for the details on how to take full advantage of all capabilities.

Importantly, like for our CADD web tools, the results generated by Swiss-Bioisostere are under CC-BY license. This extends the freedom to operate, including for commercial and for-profit usages. The current website is optimized for Firefox (www.mozilla.org) or Google Chrome (www.google.com/chrome/). The best user experience is obtained by using a recent version of either browser.

Detailed support to the user on all options regarding input, output, visualization, analysis, filtering, export, access to databases of origin, and interoperability with other CADD tools is obtained directly on the website through the main menu. Apart from frequently asked questions (FAQ), the items "Tutorials" and "Help" give access

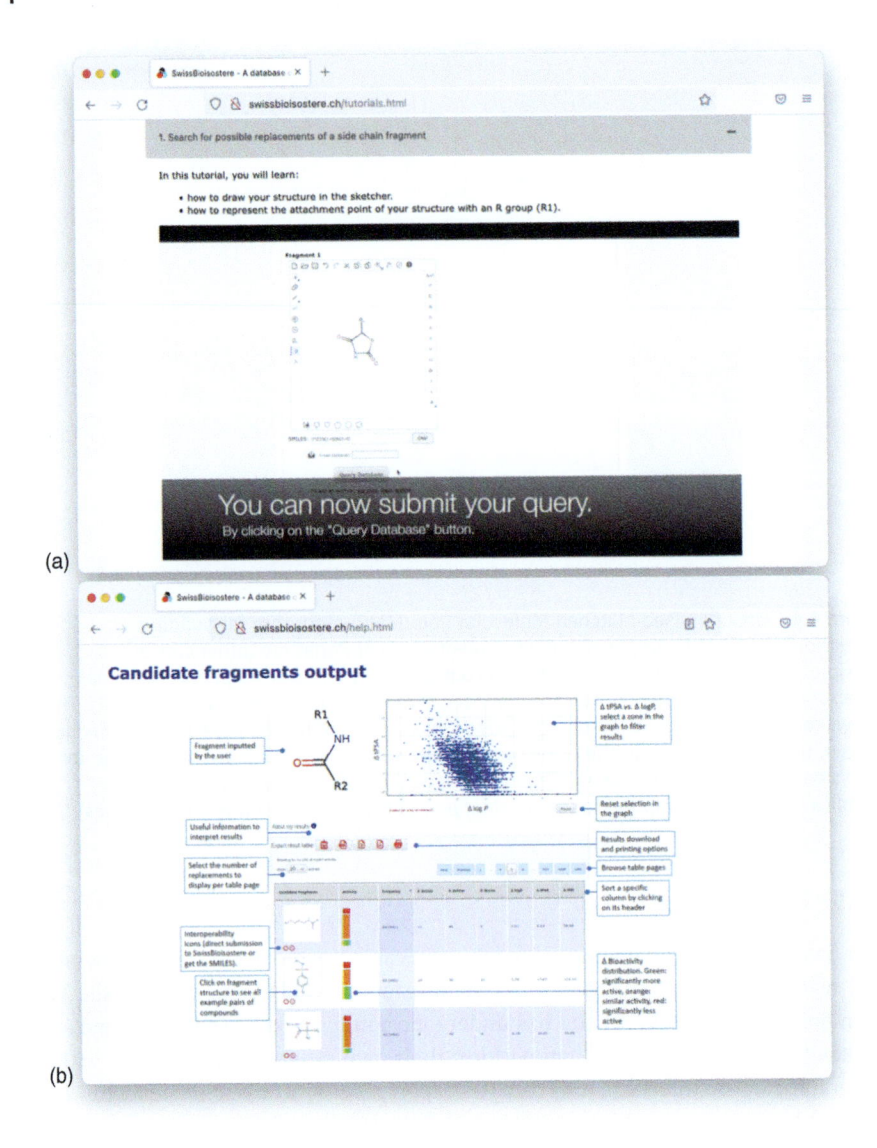

Figure 4.5 User support on SwissBioisostere website. Short video tutorials (a) and static help page (b) are available to assist the user through all technical aspects of the graphical interface.

to video tutorials and static help pages (see Figure 4.5). Particularly useful are the short screen capture videos of about 1 to 2 minutes, which cover comprehensively the most technical aspects of the graphical interface. As of today, the tutorials show how to: (i) input a side chain fragment; (ii) analyze results of possible replacements of a fragment; (iii) analyze results of specific replacement occurrences; (iv) input linker and scaffold fragments; and (v) input a specific replacement. The last two tutorials show users how they can benefit from SwissDrugDesign environment interoperability: (vi) send any compound from SwissBioisostere to other SwissDrugDesign tools in order to perform additional analyses (vii) send any molecule from another SwissDrugDesign tool to SwissBioisostere. The static help page acts as a checklist summarizing the input/output requirements and available options. If a user has other concerns or a specific question, a contact form is also provided.

The following few basic points are noteworthy. Users can input molecular fragments directly from the input page using either one or both molecular sketchers. Two types of requests are available: (option 1) requests for possible replacements of a molecular fragment with input in the left-hand sketchers; (option 2) requests for occurrences of a specific replacement with input in both left- and right-hand sketchers. Request options and display/undisplay of the right-hand sketcher are available by clicking on the corresponding grey tabs above sketchers. When a query of possible replacements (request type 1, see Figure 4.10a) is completed, results are returned in a new browser tab as a first output page containing the list of candidate fragments sorted by default according to the difference of bioactivity (see Figure 4.10b). If the user clicks on a given candidate fragment, a second request is performed for occurrences of the specific replacement. Upon completion, a new browser tab displays a second output page, listing all occurrences for the specific replacement (i.e. all pairs of molecules differing by this replacement and tested in the same assay, see Figure 4.10c). As mentioned before, such a request for occurrences can also be performed directly from the input page with an input in both sketchers (request type 2).

4.3 Content of SwissBioisostere

4.3.1 Global Content

At the time of writing this chapter (early 2022), the chemoinformatic pipeline described in Section 4.2 was applied to data extracted and filtered from ChEMBL version 28 to analyze a total of 1,124,168 datapoints representing 483,927 compounds tested for bioactivity on 2036 protein targets of 35 classes through 61,199 assays. The workflow that generated the database behind the production website www.swissbioisostere.ch was able to describe 25,305,017 unique replacements, implying 1,216,118 unique fragments [28]. Overall, the browsable *replacement space* of SwissBioisostere is as vast as 65 million datapoints, of which more than 36 million are directly linked to a publication and straightforwardly accessible in one click through a PubMed link (see Figures 4.10 and 4.11). The rest of the replacement information originates from assays not published but curated by ChEMBL, as well. Most are part of large high-throughput screening (HTS) public campaigns, targeting neglected diseases or COVID-19, for instance. It is important to understand that addition of new data in SwissBioisostere depends on ChEMBL releases and SwissBioisostere updates. As such, SwissBioisostere must be seen as a CADD tool to support drug discovery and certainly not as a means to track the very latest communications in medicinal chemistry.

4.3.2 Biological and Chemical Contexts

An important asset of SwissBioisostere is to support the user by providing both the biological and chemical contexts for the replacements under investigation. The underlying idea is that if a replacement has already been successfully applied to many similar molecules active on the same target or on similar targets from the same class, confidence in the bioisosteric nature of the replacement is higher.

The number of unique fragments and of unique replacements broken down by the target classes are shown in Figure 4.6. Please note that the replacements are more numerous than the fragments because a given fragment can be replaced by several ones. The most populated target classes are by far the G-protein coupled receptors, especially the GPCR of family A, with 6,400,517 replacements involving 385,018 fragments; the kinases with 6,960,300 replacements involving 237,918

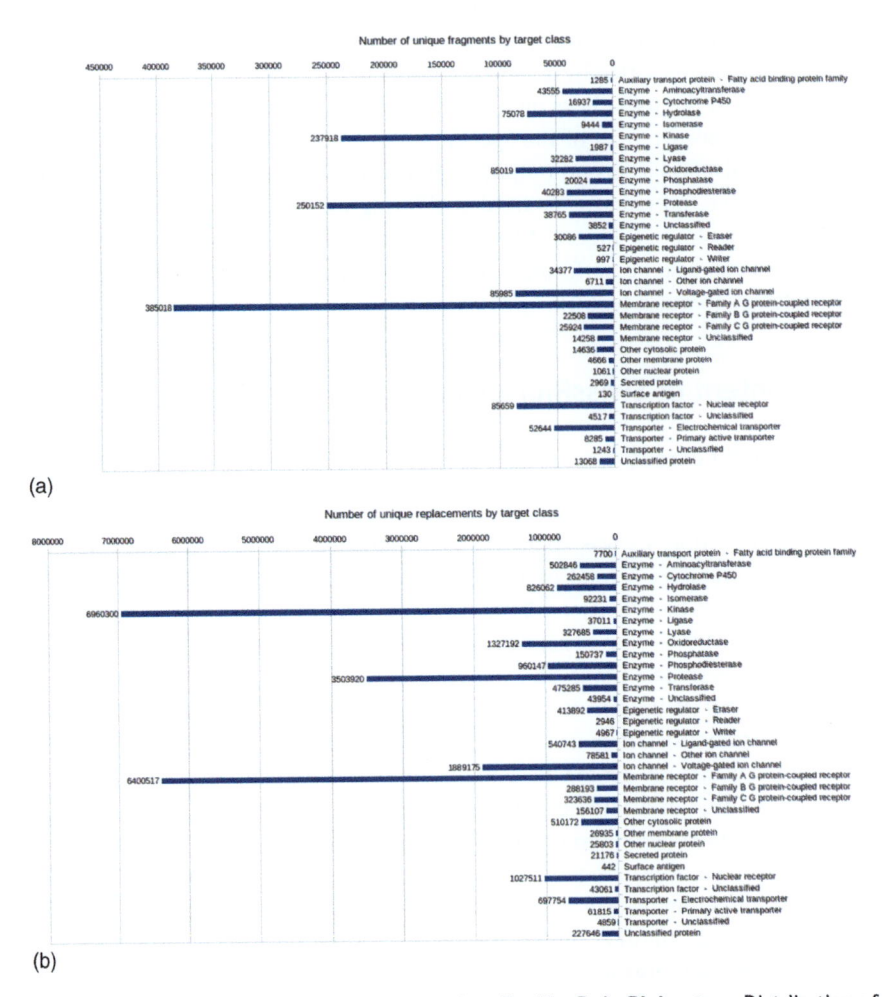

Figure 4.6 A picture of the biological space described by SwissBioisostere. Distribution of unique fragments (a) and unique replacements (b) as a function of the 35 target classes.

fragments; and the proteases with 3'503'920 replacements involving 250,152 fragments. This appears intuitively to be a true picture of the recent history of medicinal chemistry. Obviously, the likelihood of finding relevant and accurate information on molecular replacements is particularly high among the massive data accumulated on these extensively studied drug targets. However, a strength of SwissBioisostere is that it also contains data on much less popular niches with the same level of confidence. Finding validated examples of bioisosteric small molecules active on target classes like, for instance, surface antigens or transcription factors can impact very positively speculative early-phase drug discovery projects. This is even more true if the chemical context of the molecular replacement is similar.

For the chemical context, the output pages of the SwissBioisostere web interface provide analyses and selection tools to estimate which replacements are most relevant for specific needs. As described in Figure 4.12, the user can interactively select the physicochemical space of interest or refine the chemical context as properties of the attachment points.

As quantified in detail in Section 4.4.3.4.1, aromatic groups have a tremendous influence on organic chemistry and in particular on medicinal chemistry [37]. This trend is clearly observable in Figure 4.7a, where it can be seen that about 75% of all fragments in SwissBioisostere contain at least one aromatic ring. The rest excludes any aromatic moieties, with 14% involving nonaromatic cycles and 11% being linear moieties. Similarly, the relative proportion of side chains decreases according to the order: aromatic, nonaromatic cycles, and linear fragments. Both the scaffolds and the linkers follow the reverse trend.

Moreover, when looking at the composition of fragments, one can appreciate that only 0.7% are purely carbon moieties, whereas more than 76% contain heteroatoms, excluding halogens (Figure 4.7b). This is an important wealth of information for efficient drug design, both allowing optimization of physicochemical and pharmacokinetic properties of the desired compounds (please refer to Section 4.4.3.3) as well as exploration of pharmacophores for better molecular recognition by the targeted binding sites. The proportion of fragments containing at least one halogen atom, more than 22%, is also significant and reflects the importance of these elements in medicinal chemistry. Indeed, many halogenated molecules have reached the clinical phases and the market as a result of a long-time strategy to exploit the special nature of fluorine, chlorine, bromine, and to a lower extent, iodine [38]. While originally used primarily to optimize physicochemistry and stabilize metabolism, halogen atoms are nowadays known for their subtle but very specific intermolecular interactions, which enable refined strategies for structure-based design [39].

4.3.3 Fragment Shape Diversity

Closely related to aromaticity and molecular "flatness," it has been observed that increasing the tridimensional nature of the molecules improves the chance of drug candidates to successfully progress through development phases [37]. Besides, it has long been shown that molecular shape is strongly associated with bioactivity and

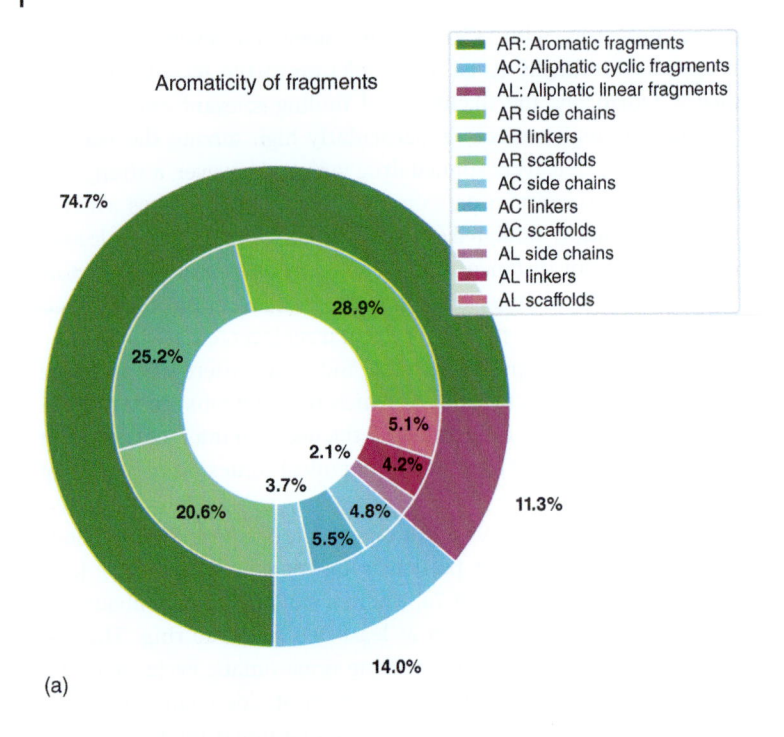

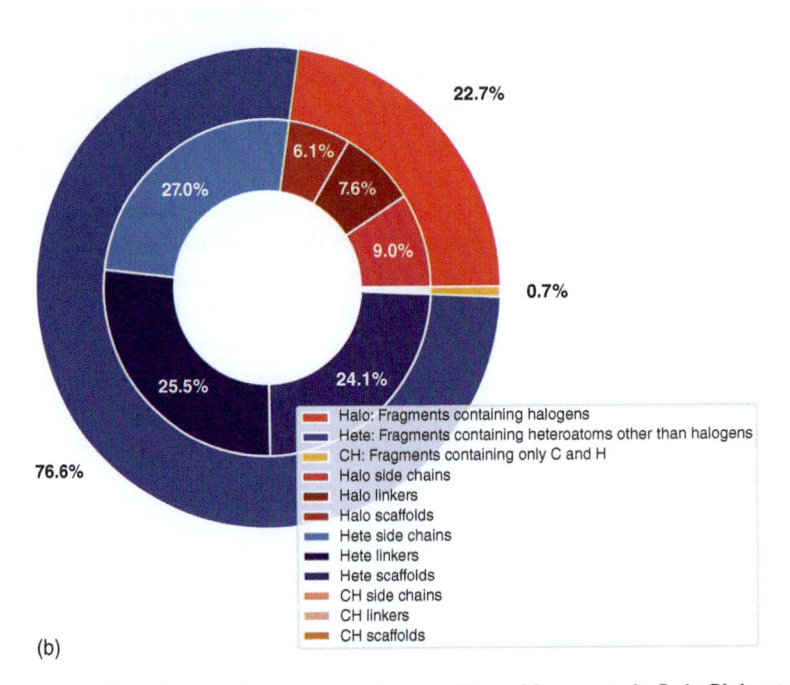

Figure 4.7 The chemical nature and composition of fragments in SwissBioisostere. The proportion of aromatic, cyclic, and linear moieties (a) and the proportion of heteroatoms and halogens (b).

that diversity in shape will increase the ability of chemical collections to address multiple protein targets in HTS [40]. We analyzed the content of SwissBioisostere using the method based on normalized ratios of principal moments of inertia (NPR) developed by Sauer and Schwartz [41]. It allows visualization of distinct shapes in a triangular space defined by the two principal components, as on the scheme in Figure 4.8a, where purely rod-shaped molecules are at the top left corner, the purely spherical molecules are at the top right corner and the purely disc-shaped molecules are at the bottom corner. Classification as "rod," "sphere," or "disc" is possible when dividing geometrically the triangular space into three zones of equal surface defined by connecting the three midpoints of each side to the geometric center of the triangle, as depicted in Figure 4.8b. The same picture shows the result of the NPR analysis of 1.2 million fragments included in SwissBioisostere, spread over the space, with the majority of them being rods, then discs. Essentially spherical fragments are much rarer.

Remarkably, the global molecular shape distribution for fragments is very comparable to that of full small molecules. The reader may refer to the respective articles for the NPR analysis of bioactive compound collections (e.g. MDDR or GOLD-set [41]) or of vendor catalogs recorded in the ZINC database [42].

The NPR analysis stratified by side chains, linkers, and scaffolds (Figure 4.8c) indicates small differences in the shape repartition, among which the most significant is certainly the overrepresentation of rod-like shaped side chains compared to linkers and scaffolds.

Overall, as seen in Figure 4.8d, the fragments queried by users via the SwissBioisostere Web interface follow a very similar trend, demonstrating a good match between user demands and the content of our knowledgebase.

Using the triangle space divided into three zones allowed to inspect the replacements as switching between or staying in the same shape class. Interestingly, whereas the "sphere" fragments are less numerous in SwissBioisostere, the replacements involving spherical moieties (either staying in the same class or moving from/to "rod" or "disc") are overrepresented (data not shown). This might indicate that medicinal chemistry habits have included the importance of synthesizing and assaying more tridimensional compounds.

4.4 Usage of SwissBioisostere

4.4.1 Website Usage

In 2021, SwissBioisostere received about 11,200 unique users, showing an increase of 35% since 2020 and 79% since 2019. These users, who came from 163 different countries, opened 18,500 web sessions (+42% since 2020 and +87% since 2019) totalizing 50,400 page views (+32% since 2020 and +65% since 2019) and submitted 18,400 requests (+7% since 2020 and +13% since 2019).

Figure 4.8 Molecular shape distribution of fragments. (a) Schematic representation of the output, purely rod-shaped fragments are in top-left corner; perfectly spherical fragments are in top-right corner, and disc-shaped fragments are in the bottom corner. (b) Distribution of all 1.2 million fragments in the divided shape space for classification (red dashed lines). (c) Distribution of SwissBioisostere fragments stratified by side chain, linker, and scaffold fragments. (d) Distribution of fragments inputted by users on the web interface.

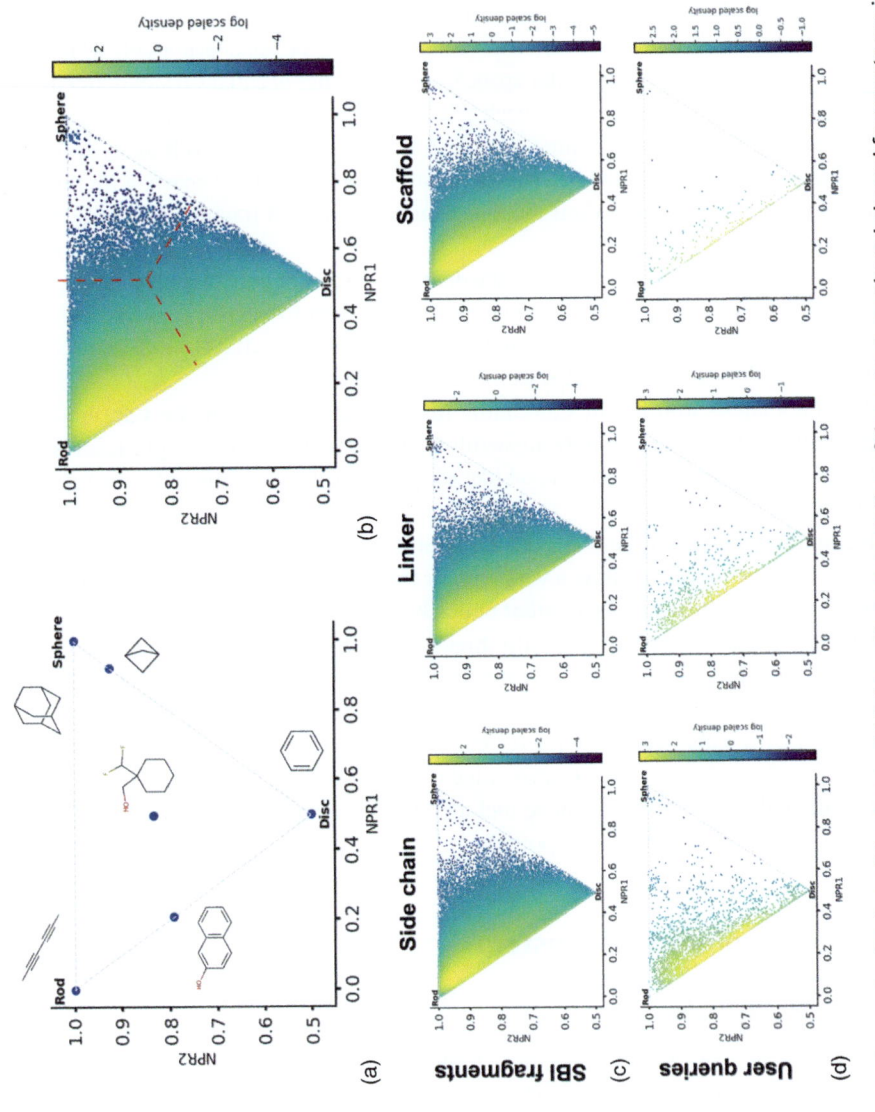

4.4 Usage of SwissBioisostere | 117

4.4.2 Most Frequent Requests

The requests of users through the web interface were briefly discussed in Section 4.3.3, to indicate the match with the content of the database. In addition, we analyzed the most frequent users' inputs on the website. In Figure 4.9, the most frequent fragments when searching for all possible replacements of a molecular fragment are represented (option 1 in Section 2.5). Strikingly, all fragments are side chains (with only one attachment point), except the amide linker (with two attachment points) ranked #7. While this chemical group is massively studied [43], the fact that it is one of the examples provided in the input page of SwissBioisostere probably artificially increases the number of submissions. Intuitively, all other fragments most frequently queried for replacement make total sense. These moieties are very common in druglike molecules (e.g. pyridine and phenyl), represent well-known medicinal chemistry options to fine-tune a property (e.g. morpholine to increase solubility, refer to Figure 4.2), or belong to a group of problematic fragments (e.g. nitro substituents toxified by metabolism).

4.4.3 Examples Related to Drug Discovery

4.4.3.1 Use Cases

Several cases of typical search and analysis with SwissBioisostere are provided in the methodological article [28] describing the database and the interface, in particular, hit-finding examples, carboxylic acid bioisosteres, and amide bioisosteres thorough investigations. Whereas replacements and occurrences are numerous for side chains and linkers, less data regards fragments with three attachment points. By scanning the literature, it becomes clear that the three-attachment moiety exchanges, certainly more synthetically complicated, are less frequently attempted and that scaffold hopping is often limited to modification of linkers. Consequently, only 16.7% of SwissBioisostere data involve scaffolds [28]. Nevertheless, remarkable information about scaffolds is just a few clicks away. We can take the example of the small molecule drug that generated the biggest revenue in 2021, Apixaban, an inhibitor of factor Xa administered as anticoagulant (Figure 4.10a). Searching in SwissBioisostere for replacements of its pyrazolopyridinone central core, four possible scaffold fragments relying on six datapoints of pairs of molecules can be found (user can perform this request through the scaffold example found at the bottom of the submission page, see Figure 4.10b). All compounds were experimentally evaluated on coagulation factor X and published in two research articles [30, 44],

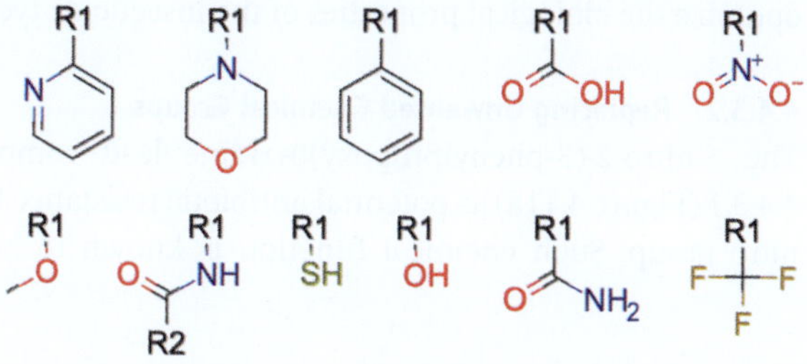

Figure 4.9 Most frequent fragments inputted by users on www.swissbioisostere.ch.

which describe the medicinal chemistry milestones leading to the discovery and optimization of what will become a blockbuster medicine. Figure 4.10b shows the submission web page of the SwissBiosisostere interface (including links to input examples). Upon request completion, all possible candidate fragments to replace the inputted moiety are provided in a tabular fashion in a first result page, together with analysis, filtering, and export options (Figure 4.10c). Clicking on the chemical structure of a fragment makes another tab open in the web browser to display all occurrences of molecule pairs (Figure 4.10d). This page enables further analyses, including compound and assay descriptions, by accessing directly related entries in ChEMBL [22] as well as the publication of origin (if any) through PubMed (https://pubmed.ncbi.nlm.nih.gov). Importantly, interoperability icons (below all molecules) allow to submit any molecule to other CADD web tools developed by us at the SIB Swiss Institute of Bioinformatics. In one click, SwissBioisostere users can execute ligand-based virtual screening through SwissSimilarity [31], estimate the most probable protein targets with SwissTargetPrediction [45], evaluate physico-chemical, pharmacokinetic, and other related parameters with SwissADME [33], or submit as another SwissBioisostere query. Conversely, any molecule generated by these tools can be submitted equally to SwissBioisostere [46]. Simple web searches of chemical knowledge bases such as SwissBioisostere can not only provide global pictures and figures on decades of drug discovery but also allow to observe significant focused successful moves in the history of medicinal chemistry.

A recent article describes the successful usage of SwissBioisostere to design inhibitors of the NorA efflux pump, a protein responsible for antibiotic resistance in *Staphylococcus aureus* [34]. The study started with a known inhibitory boronic chemotype as a template. The bioisosteric strategy was conducted to generate more druglike, equipotent inhibitors. Among the 77 candidate fragments to replace boronic acid provided by SwissBioisostere, 42 were selected to be further evaluated in silico through molecular docking and ADME predictions. Finally, a nitro analog was synthesized and evaluated *in vitro*. It exhibited improved bactericide potentialization of antibiotic ciprofloxacin by higher efflux inhibition. This result together with reduced cytotoxicity on host cells, qualified 5-nitro-2-(3-phenylpropoxy)pyridine as a lead compound for resistance breaker to resensitize *S. aureus* (Figure 4.11a). This fruitful example confirmed that, although SwissBioisostere does not contain many bioactivity data on antibiotics, because of some filtering criteria, the method can be applied to other species targets such as for antibacterial drug discovery. This extends to agrochemistry, as for instance reported in a recent article [35] describing how SwissBioisostere supported efficiently heterocyclic replacements to further optimize the biological properties of the insecticide tyclopyrazoflor (Figure 4.11b).

4.4.3.2 Replacing Unwanted Chemical Groups

The 5-nitro-2-(3-phenylpropoxy)pyridine lead compound described in Section 4.4.3.1 (Figure 4.11a) as potential antibiotic resistance breaker contains an aromatic nitro group. Such chemical function is known to be toxified by metabolism to

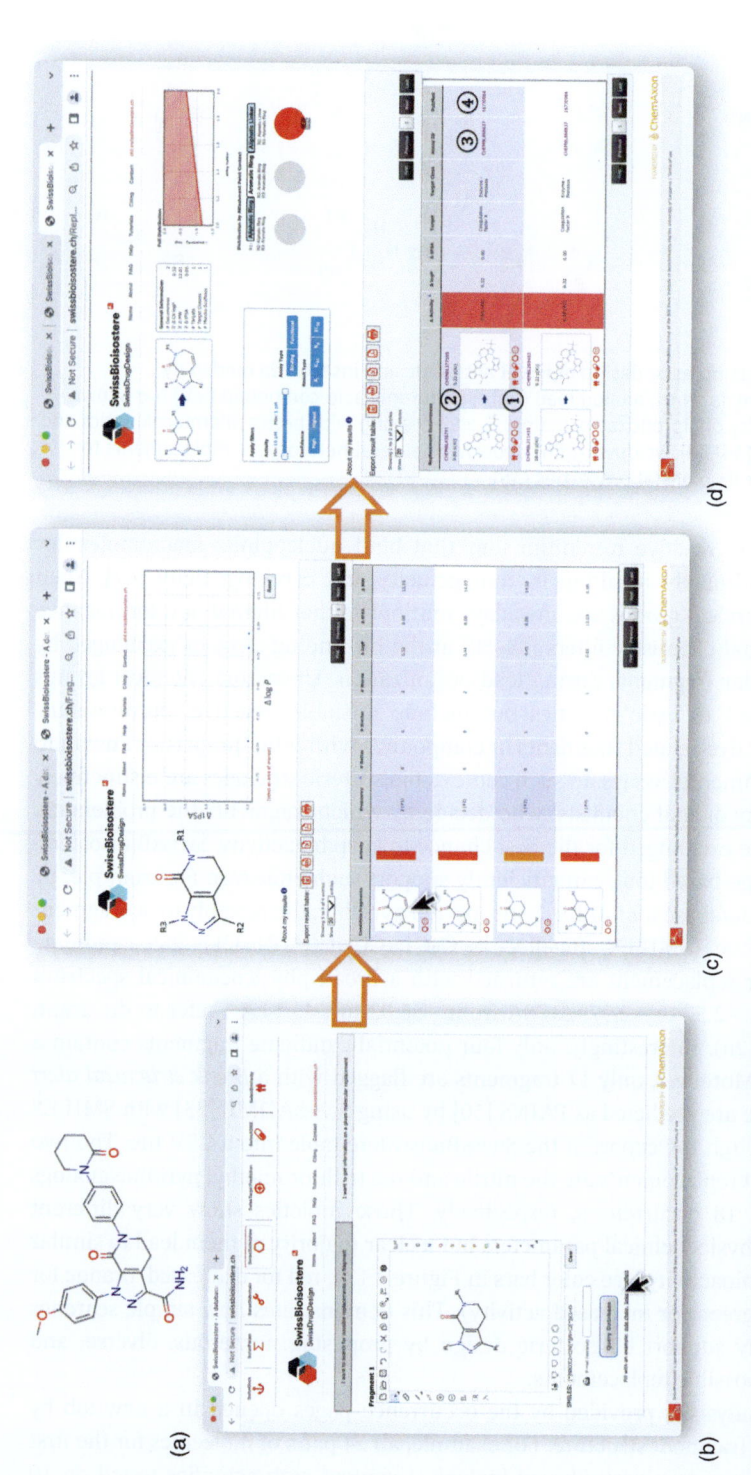

Figure 4.10 Examples of scaffold replacement request, analysis, and interoperability. (a) Chemical structure of Apixaban, inhibitor of the coagulation factor X and best-selling small molecule drug in 2021. The submission page (b) includes some examples; by clicking on "scaffold," the user can input the pyrazolopyridinone fragment typical of coagulation factor X inhibitors [30]. By clicking the "Query Database" button, another tab opens with the first result panel (c) tabulating the candidate replacing fragments. By clicking on the structure of a fragment, a third tab opens with the occurrences of pairs of molecules (d). Each occurrence (row) allows further analysis by ① submitting any molecule to another SwissDrugDesign tool by clicking on the corresponding interoperability button ("twins" for SwissSimilarity [31], "target" for SwissTargetPrediction [32], "pill" for SwissADME [33], or "hexagon" for resubmitting to SwissBioisostere; the "face" displays the SMILES of the molecule); or by accessing external databases: ChEMBL [22] for the ② compounds or the ③ assay, and PubMed (https://pubmed.ncbi.nlm.nih.gov) for the publication ④ (if any).

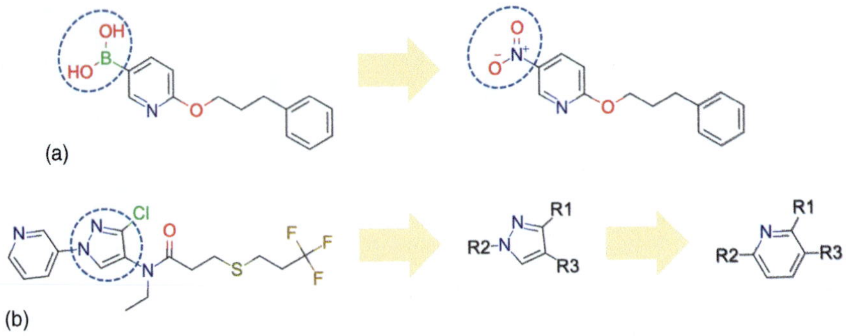

Figure 4.11 Examples or design of novel antibiotic and insecticide guided by SwissBiosiostere. (a) Nitro analog lead (right) of boronic acid compound (left) has shown increased activity of ciprofloxacin against *S. aureus* along with better pharmacokinetics and toxicity profile [34]. (b) Tyclopyrazoflor underwent several heterocyclic replacements to improve further its biocidal properties [35].

generate highly reactive nitrenium ions that bind nucleophilic macromolecules covalently, ultimately resulting in mutagenicity and carcinogenicity [47]. Such unwanted chemical groups are nowadays routinely either filtered out, for instance using medicinal chemistry filters [48–50] at the hit-finding steps or exchanged by other molecular fragments during lead optimization. Unwanted chemical groups are not limited to toxic moieties but include unstable, reactive, promiscuous, aggregator, or dye-related fragments or compounds with other properties known to perturb experimental assays. In such context, bioisosteric strategies are instinctively followed by medicinal chemists, who decide by which fragments the problematic group must be exchanged for the best chance to keep bioactivity. SwissBioisostere, as a knowledge-based tool, can efficiently support such endeavor. For example, by querying the database for 5-nitro-2-substituted pyridine, the possibly toxic fragment described above (SMILES: [O−][N+](=O)C1=CC=C([*])N=C1), 285 candidate fragments for replacement are returned with a broad physicochemical spectrum ($\Delta \log P$ from −2.57 to +2.97; ΔtPSA from −56.03 to +43.14 Å^2, refer to the graph on Figure 4.12a). Interestingly, only four potential candidate fragments contain a nitro group. Moreover, only 17 fragments are flagged with a *Brenk structural alert* [48] and none are predicted as PAINS [50] by using SwissADME [33] with SMILES obtained through the export of the SwissBioisostere table into a CSV file. The two most frequent replacements are the nitrile and the trifluoromethyl pyridine analogs with 24 and 18 occurrences, respectively. Those moieties show very different impacts on physiochemical parameters but a clear majority of them lead to similar or increased bioactivity (see color bars in Figure 4.12a, red for decreased, orange for similar, and green for increased activity). This demonstrates how simple searches can efficiently support bioisosteric design by proposing numerous, diverse, and meaningful possible replacements.

Further analysis is provided by the occurrence pages opened in a new tab by clicking on a fragment structure. For example, all 24 pairs of molecules for the first replacements are in a pretty broad biological context with activities tested on 10

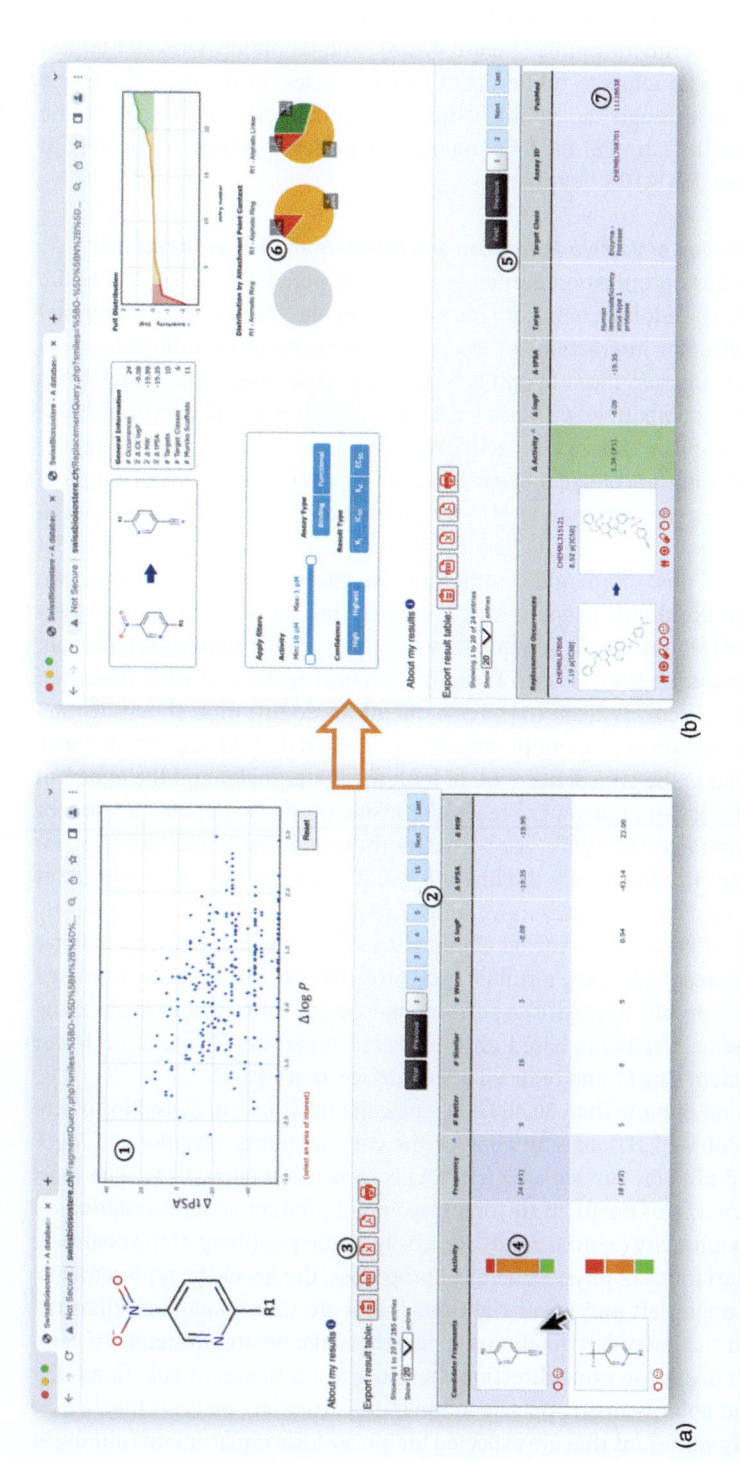

Figure 4.12 Searching for aromatic nitro bioisosteres. (a) 285 candidate fragments to replace the possibly toxic 5-nitro-2-substituted pyridine group, with a broad physicochemical spectrum as displayed in the lipophilicity vs. apparent polarity graph ①) or in the sortable columns ②; the export options ③ expand the possibility of further analysis, for example, the CSV format includes the SMILES of all fragments, useful inputs for other tools; the activity color bar ④ allows a quick evaluation of the impact of the replacement on experimental bioactivities (red for decreased, orange for similar, and green for increased activity). (b) A closer look at the most frequent replacement, i.e. the nitrile analog, with each row corresponding to distinct occurrences; the biological context is given in the "target" and "target class" sortable columns ⑤; the chemical context as deconvolution of attachment points is given as pie-charts ⑥; both molecules are bioisostere of Tipranavir (CF$_3$ analog) and tested on the same target in the same assay as published in [36] directly accessible through the PubMed link ⑦.

targets of 6 different classes, whereas the chemical context is limited to aliphatic ring and linker attachment points (Figure 4.12b). The datapoint with the largest increase in bioactivity refers to inhibitors of HIV proteases. In the research article directly accessible through the PubMed link [36], both molecules belong to the final series for optimization of the CF_3 analog, further developed as Tipranavir, an approved drug used in AIDS treatment.

4.4.3.3 Optimization of Passive Absorption and Blood–Brain Barrier Diffusion

Pharmacodynamics optimization aiming at increasing potency or selectivity at the target often involves adding chemical groups to molecules, e.g. to make additional specific intermolecular interactions or to open a side cavity of a binding site. This typically generates larger, more lipophilic, and polar molecules. Such compounds are in general not compatible with proper ADME, which is mandatory to achieve sufficient bioavailability and for a bioactive molecule to reach its target, and finally for the expected pharmacological event to occur. Several studies linked physico-chemical properties with optimal ADME, for comprehensive reviews please refer to [51, 52]. For example, the BOILED-Egg is a simple predictive classification model for gastrointestinal absorption and central nervous system (CNS) distribution, two important pharmacokinetic properties to control during the steps of discovery for an oral drug [53]. Figure 4.13a schematizes the main steps of optimization from a BCR–ABL kinase inhibitor lead to Ponatinib, an oral anticancer drug described elsewhere by the discovery team [54]. Each chemical modification shows distinct variations (dashed arrows) of both descriptors (WLOGP [55] and tPSA [56]). The general trend is the typical decrease of both the lipophilicity and the apparent polarity (semi-transparent arrow) to reach the inside of the "egg;" the "white" for passive absorption and the "yolk" for permeation through the blood-brain barrier (BBB). Lowering simultaneously the lipophilic and polar natures of a molecule is not an obvious medical chemistry move, since lipophilicity and polarity are mostly anti-correlated. This can however be obtained by removing non-pharmacophoric regions of the molecule, like the terminal cyclopropylbenzene-1,4-diamine, crossed in Figure 4.13b. Another strategy is to perform bioisosteric replacement by selecting potential candidate fragments based on the desired properties, in our case lower partition coefficient (log P) and reduced polar surface area (tPSA).

The distribution of more than 36,400,000 replacements (those of SwissBioisostere linked with a PubMed ID) as a function of the corresponding variations of log P (ΔWLOGP) and of polar surface area (ΔtPSA) is shown in Figure 4.13c. The most populated regions of this heatmap are for replacements producing small variations of polarity and lipophilicity (central zone). Reversely, at the periphery of the heatmap, the larger the variations of physicochemical properties, the fewer the replacements. Moreover, the upper-left and lower-right quadrants are more populated than the upper-right and the lower-left quadrants. This echoes the greater difficulty of varying log P and tPSA in the same direction than to select a fragment able to modify lipophilicity and polarity in an opposite manner. In particular, the dash-lined circle indicates grossly variations that are expected for bioisosteric replacements aiming at increasing passive absorption and CNS penetration by lowering log P and tPSA at

Figure 4.13 Optimization of ADME properties. (a) optimization from a BCR–ABL kinase inhibitor lead to Ponatinib, an anticancer oral drug [54] into the BOILED-Egg [53]. Source: Adapted from Ref. [53]. (b) Chemical modifications of the lead to generate Ponatinib. (c) Heatmap of distribution of SwissBioisostere replacement and the impact on apparent polarity (ΔtPSA) and lipophilicity (ΔWLOGP); dash-lined circle approximates replacements aiming at increasing passive absorption and CNS penetration by lowering log P and tPSA at the same time. (d) The 644 possible replacing fragments of methylimidazole found in SwissBioisostere web interface, allowing the selection of the region of interest (here ΔtPSA < 0 and ΔWLOGP < 0). This analysis pointed out only 11 fragments able to decrease lipophilicity and apparent polarity at the same time, including Ponatinib dimethylpiperazine.

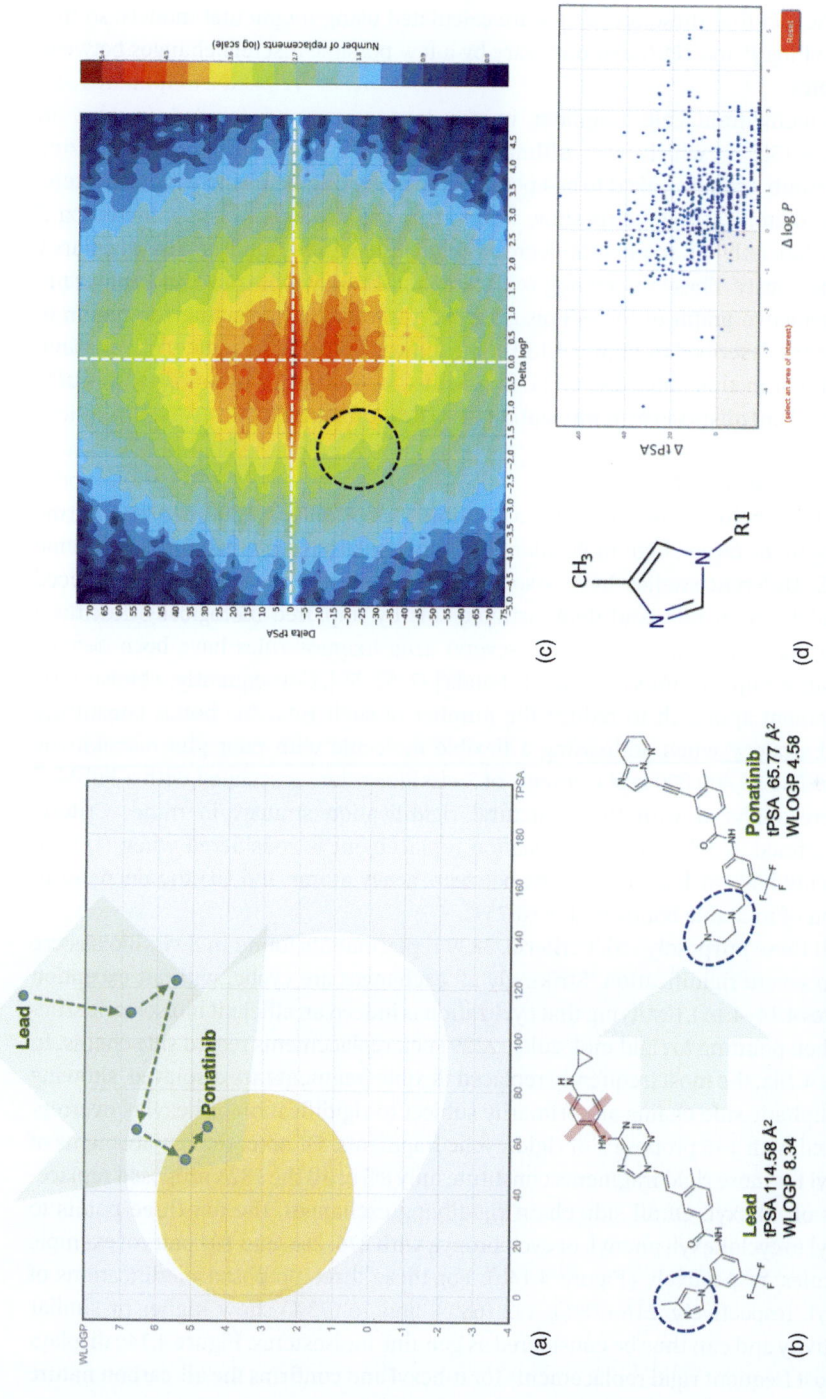

the same time. This zone is clearly less populated than its symmetric counterparts in other quadrants. Of note, the discontinuities in the heatmap simply originate from the fact that these properties are calculated using fragmental models, so that values of log P and tPSA can only vary by a few possible discrete changes between molecules.

The methylimidazole fragment in the lead compound (circled in blue in Figure 4.13b) – which was ultimately exchanged by the dimethylpiperazine in Ponatinib – can be linked to 644 possible replacing fragments in SwissBioisostere. Among them, 223 fragments show lower tPSA values, and 148 show lower log P values, but only 11 fragments decrease both lipophilicity and apparent polarity simultaneously. These interesting replacements are easy to retrieve and analyze in the interactive graph of SwissBioisostere web interface by selecting the region of interest (as described in Figure 4.13d). The dimethylpiperazine moiety of Ponatinib is included in this short list of 11 fragments, as well as 10 other ideas to guide medicinal chemists in the optimization of ADME properties.

4.4.3.4 Reduction of Flexibility

Apart from being associated with a possible loss of entropy that can impact the binding to the target, high molecular flexibility is also strongly linked to suboptimal ADME. Different studies have associated flexible small molecules with reduced bioavailability in rats, and demonstrated this by impaired biological or artificial membrane permeation. Therefore, several drug likeness rules have been defined with various upper limits of rotatable bonds [37, 57–59]. Consequently, a bioisosteric replacement approach to reduce the number of such rotatable bonds constitutes a valid strategy when addressing a flexible molecule with poor pharmacokinetic profile. The 36,400,000 replacements of SwissBioisostere associated with a PubMed ID were analyzed with this structural rigidification strategy in mind. Criteria were defined as follows: a rigidification replacement is considered when (i) both fragments have at least five bonds between heavy atoms and (ii) the decrease in fraction of rotatable bonds is at least 75%.

With these purposely strict criteria, 3839 replacements found in SwissBioisostere lead to severe rigidification. Strikingly all exchanges are cyclic, without exception (Figures 4.14–4.16), testifying that cyclization is indeed an efficient bioisosteric strategy when pointing to rigid molecules. 2229 such replacements regard side chains. In Figure 4.14a, the most frequently replaced flexible fragments are displayed, showing that aliphatic side chains are primarily subject to rigidification. n-hexyl is overrepresented with 145 proposals of rigid/cyclic fragments. Of note, the replacements of n-hexyl for more rigid fragments constitute only 8% of all the 1823 proposed replacements of n-hexyl. Of all side chain rigidifying exchanges, the top three points to n-hexyl to cyclohexyl, phenyl, or cyclopropyl, with 276, 266, and 104 pairs of example molecules, respectively (Figure 4.14b). For those three proposed modifications of n-hexyl, respectively, 216 (78%), 182 (68%), and 76 (73%) show higher or similar bioactivity and can thus be considered as genuine bioisosteres. Figure 4.14c displays the most frequent rigid replacements for n-hexyl and confirms the all-carbon nature

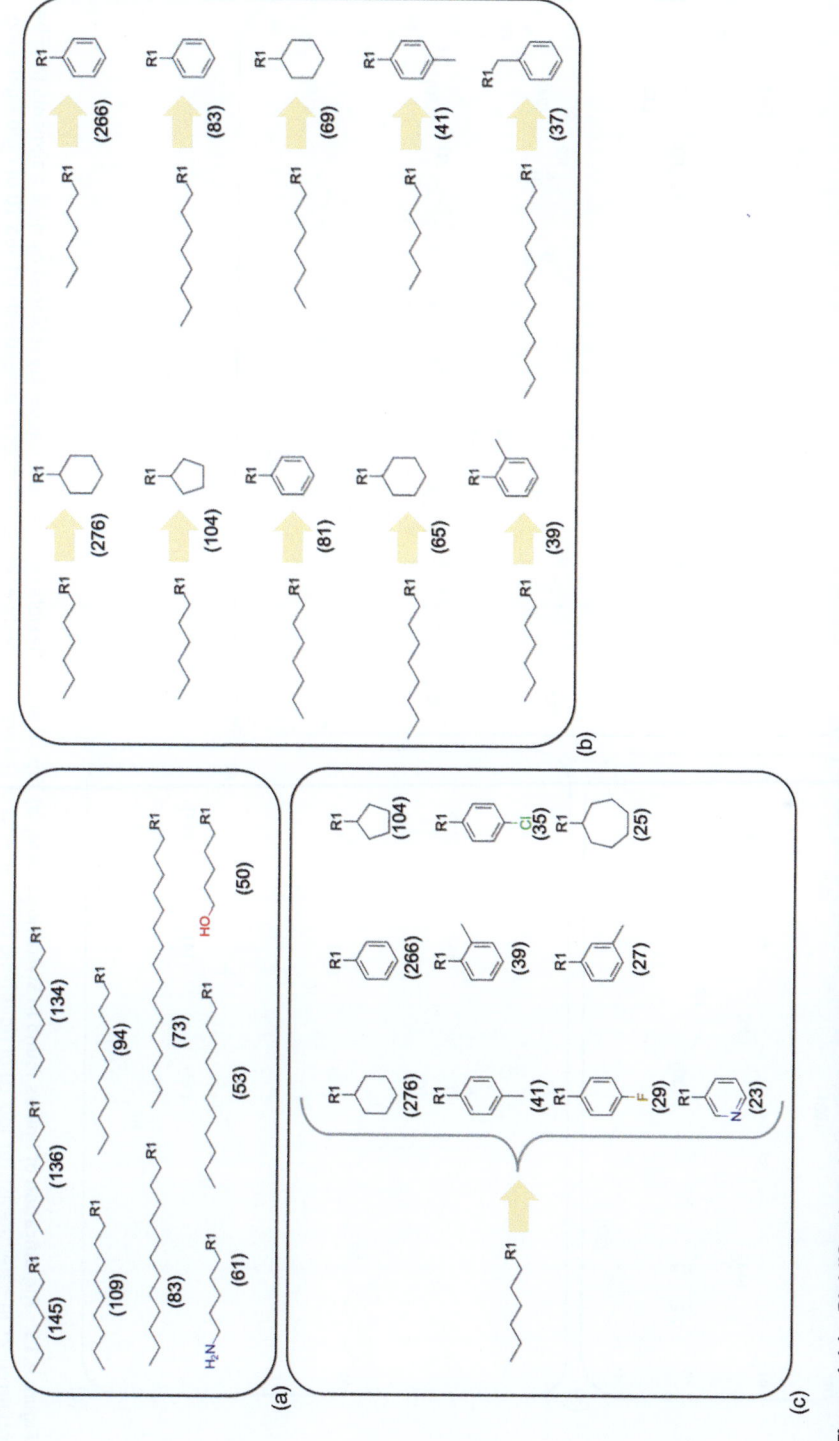

Figure 4.14 Rigidification of side chains as found in SwissBioisostere. (a) Top 10 of the flexible side chains as found in SwissBioisostere. (a) Top 10 of the flexible side chains most frequently replaced by rigid fragments (number of occurrences, i.e. pairs of example molecules, in parenthesis). (b) Top 10 rigidifying replacements of side chains, with number of occurrences in parenthesis (c) Top 10 of rigidifying replacements for *n*-hexyl, with number of occurrences in parenthesis.

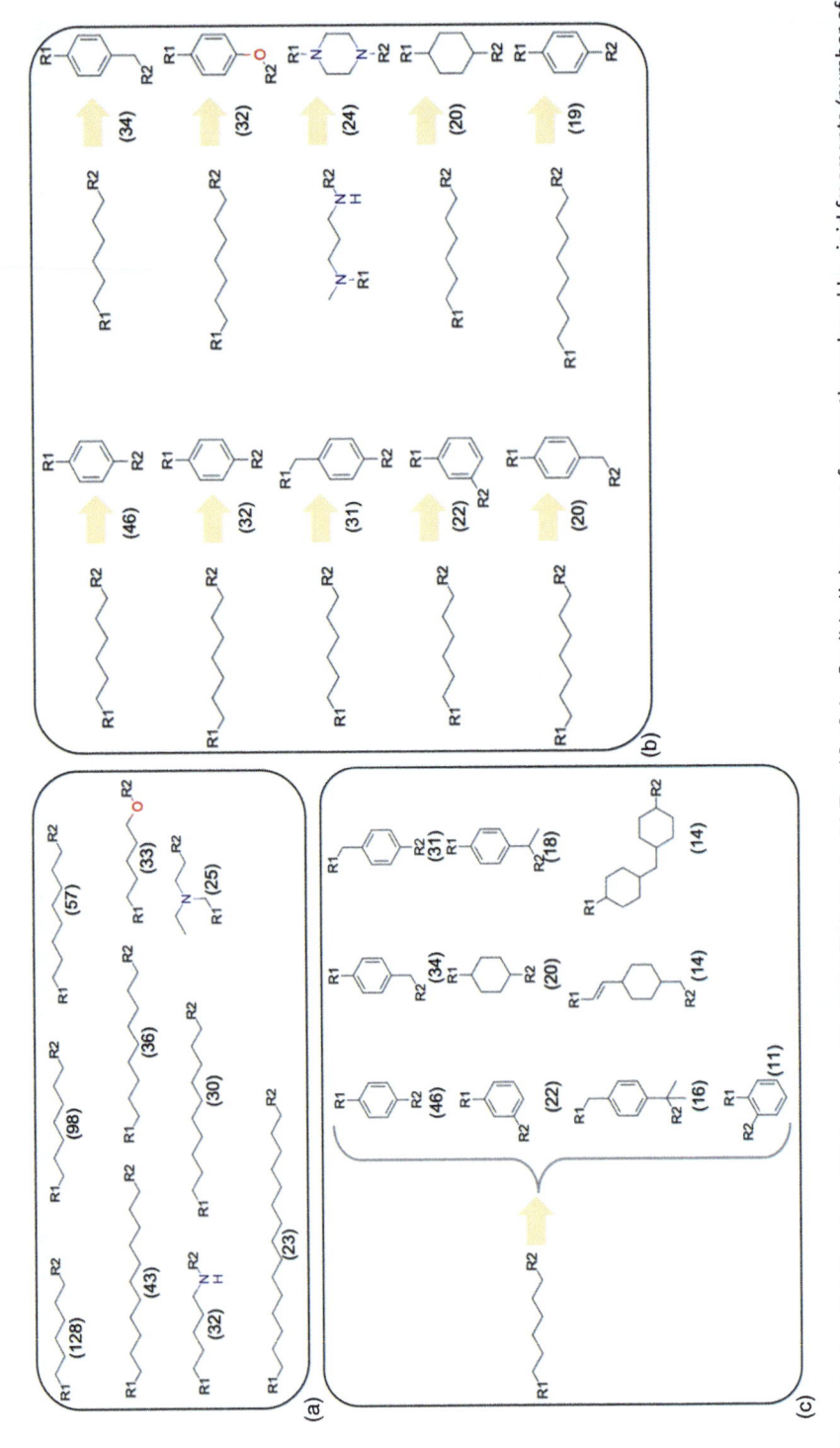

Figure 4.15 Rigidification of linkers found in SwissBioisostere. (a) Top 10 of the flexible linkers most frequently replaced by rigid fragments (number of occurrences in parenthesis). (b) Top 10 of rigidifying replacements of linkers, with number of occurrences in parenthesis (c) Top 10 of rigid rigidifying replacements for 1,6-hexyl with occurrences in parenthesis.

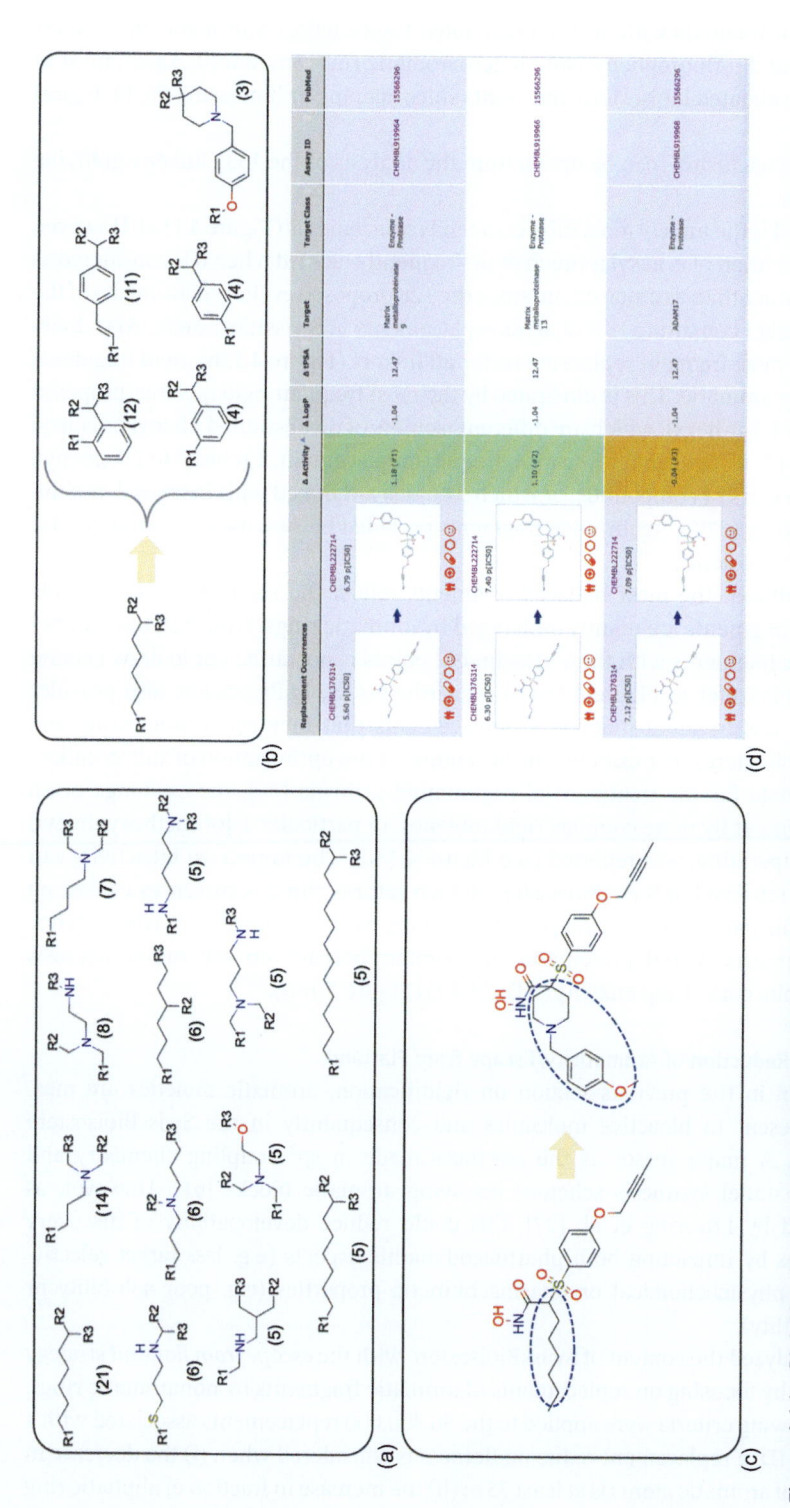

Figure 4.16 Rigidification of scaffolds found in SwissBioisostere. (a) Top 13 of the flexible scaffolds most frequently replaced by rigid fragments (number of occurrences in parenthesis). (b) Top 5 of rigid replacements for 1,1,6-hexyl, with number of occurrences in parenthesis. (c) Example of rigid bioisosteric replacement for 1,1,6-hexyl for the discovery of tumor necrosis factor-alpha converting enzyme (ADAM-17) and matrix metalloproteinase inhibitors [60]. (d) Retrieval and analysis of occurrences with increasing activity on both metalloproteinases and similar activity on ADAM-17.

of the cyclic fragment with the few exceptions of some halogen aromatic substituents (p-chloro and p-fluorophenyl) and heteroaromatic rings (pyridine). Again, most of those are validated bioisosteric fragments since keeping or increasing the biological activity.

Similar conclusions can be drawn from the analysis of the 1331 linker-rigidifying exchanges.

1,6-hexyl is the moiety most subject to rigid replacements (Figure 4.15a). However, the rigidification of n-hexyl is much more frequently tackled when it is considered as a linker rather than as a side chain, since the 128 proposed cyclic replacements of the n-hexyl linker constitute 15% of all its replacements in SwissBioisostere. Also, looking at the most frequent replacements for all linkers (Figure 4.15b), rigid fragments are mainly aromatic. This is illustrated by the most frequent rigid moieties proposed to replace 1,6-n-hexyl, which are different isomers of disubstituted phenyl or benzyl (Figure 4.15c). For example, the most frequent replacement, 1,6-hexyl to 1,4-phenyl, counts 46 pairs of compounds, of which 31 cases are linked with increased or similar bioactivity (67%). Again, such fragments provided by SwissBioisostere are useful bioisosteric moieties.

For scaffolds, the most replaced fragments follow the same trend, i.e. flexible aliphatic fragments are mainly exchanged by aromatic rings. However, the number of flexible fragments with three attachment points is not sufficient to draw general conclusions (refer to Figure 4.16a,b). Nevertheless, SwissBioisostere also provides access to less frequent fragmental replacements that may reveal interesting and useful bioisosteres. For example, in the course of the optimization of sulfonylalkyl-hydroxamate for the treatment of rheumatoid arthritis [60], the exchange of an alkyl fragment by more complex rigid moieties, in particular 1-[(4-methoxyphenyl)methyl]piperidine, was reported (see Figure 4.16c). The impact on bioactivity can be easily retrieved in SwissBioisostere, which returns three occurrences consisting of the same pair of bioisosteric potent inhibitors with an increased *in vitro* potency on two matrix metalloproteinases and similar potency on the tumor necrosis factor-alpha converting enzyme (ADAM-17) (Figure 4.16d).

4.4.3.5 Reduction of Aromaticity/Escape from Flatland

As shown in the previous section on rigidification, aromatic moieties are massively present in bioactive molecules and consequently in the SwissBioisostere database. A major reason is the advances made in sp^2 coupling chemistry and related parallel synthesis schemes involving aromatic blocks [61]. However, as suggested by Lovering et al. [37], this could reduce developability of discovery molecules by impacting both pharmacodynamic aspects (e.g. less target selectivity) and physicochemical or pharmacokinetic properties (e.g. poor solubility or permeability).

We analyzed the content of SwissBioisostere with the *escape from flatland* strategy in mind, by focusing on replacements of aromatic fragments by nonaromatic rings. The following criteria were applied to the 36,400,000 replacements associated with a PubMed ID: a replacement reducing flatness is considered when (i) the decrease in fraction of aromatic atoms is at least 75%; (ii) the increase in fraction of aliphatic ring atoms is at least 75%; and (iii) the fraction of double bond in the replacing atom is less than 10%. These strict criteria allowed to spot 9967 ring replacements with substantially increased tridimensionality, the vast majority (8345) are side chains with 1392 aromatic cycles possible to be exchanged by 535 nonaromatic rings. Expectedly, the most replaced aromatic moieties are phenyl (substituted or not), benzyl, and isomers of pyridine (Figure 4.17a). The most frequent replacements, as described in Figure 4.17b, point to purely carbon cycles. Interestingly, the second most frequent aliphatic ring exchange to phenyl is cyclopropyl (1291 occurrences, Figure 4.17c), a ring system of unique nature that makes carbons resemble to sp^2 hybrids and orbitals to π-cloud. 75% of the occurrences of the phenyl-to-cyclopropyl exchange led to molecules with similar or even better activity than the initial ones, which makes this replacement a bioisostere of interest. The first nonaromatic heterocycle replacing phenyl is morpholine (291 occurrences, Figure 4.17c), a medicinal chemistry classic to increase solubility of druglike compounds that can be found in different FDA-approved drugs, e.g. Gefitinib (refer to Figure 4.2). Another remarkable example is given by the presence of adamantyl among the most frequent phenyl replacements (255 occurrences, Figure 4.17c). Such very lipophilic and tridimensional bioisosteres have been heavily studied in medicinal chemistry for their ability to improve metabolic stability and access to CNS targets in different therapeutic areas. [62–64].

1502 replacements of aromatic linkers to less flat nonaromatic rings can be found in SwissBioisostere. These exchanges happen between 373 aromatic fragments and 310 nonaromatic rings. As for side chains, the most replaced aromatic moieties involve phenyl or pyridine (Figure 4.18a). Again, the most frequent replacements in Figure 4.18b illustrate that the majority of replacing fragments are purely carbon linkers, apart from 1,4-phenyl replaced by 1,4-piperidine, with 64% of the 57 occurrences showing similar or higher bioactivity. The other most frequent replacements of 1,4-phenyl involve cyclohexyl and other piperidines (Figure 4.18c). The ability to easily browse less recurrent replacements through the SwissBioisostere interface allows to spot real nuggets, such as small bicyclic bridged compounds. Nowadays, bicyclo[1.1.1]pentane is a known useful phenyl mimic [66]. For example, the bicyclo[1.1.1]pentane analog of Darapladib, a lipoprotein-associated phospholipase A2 (LpPLA2) inhibitor developed against atherosclerosis, resulted in slightly lower *in vitro* potency – yet still at a subnanomolar level – but also allowed to reduced lipophilicity and aromaticity, leading to enhanced permeability and solubility (see Figure 4.18d) [65]. Another recent example reported an improvement of physicochemical properties and a great improvement of the metabolic stability of indoleamine-2,3-dioxygenase 1 (IDO1) inhibitors, useful for cancer immunotherapy, by replacing the 1,4-phenyl linker of the lead compound (see Figure 4.19) [67]. The bicyclo[1.1.1]pentane analogs were experimentally found to have excellent potency, selectivity, and much-improved pharmacokinetics due to lower metabolic hydrolysis of the amide moiety. As well, the three-dimensional overlap of both bioisosteres in the IDO1 binding pocket was confirmed by X-ray crystallography. Of note, the most recent literature is included in the next version of ChEMBL and consequently in further updates of SwissBioisostere (see Section 4.3.1).

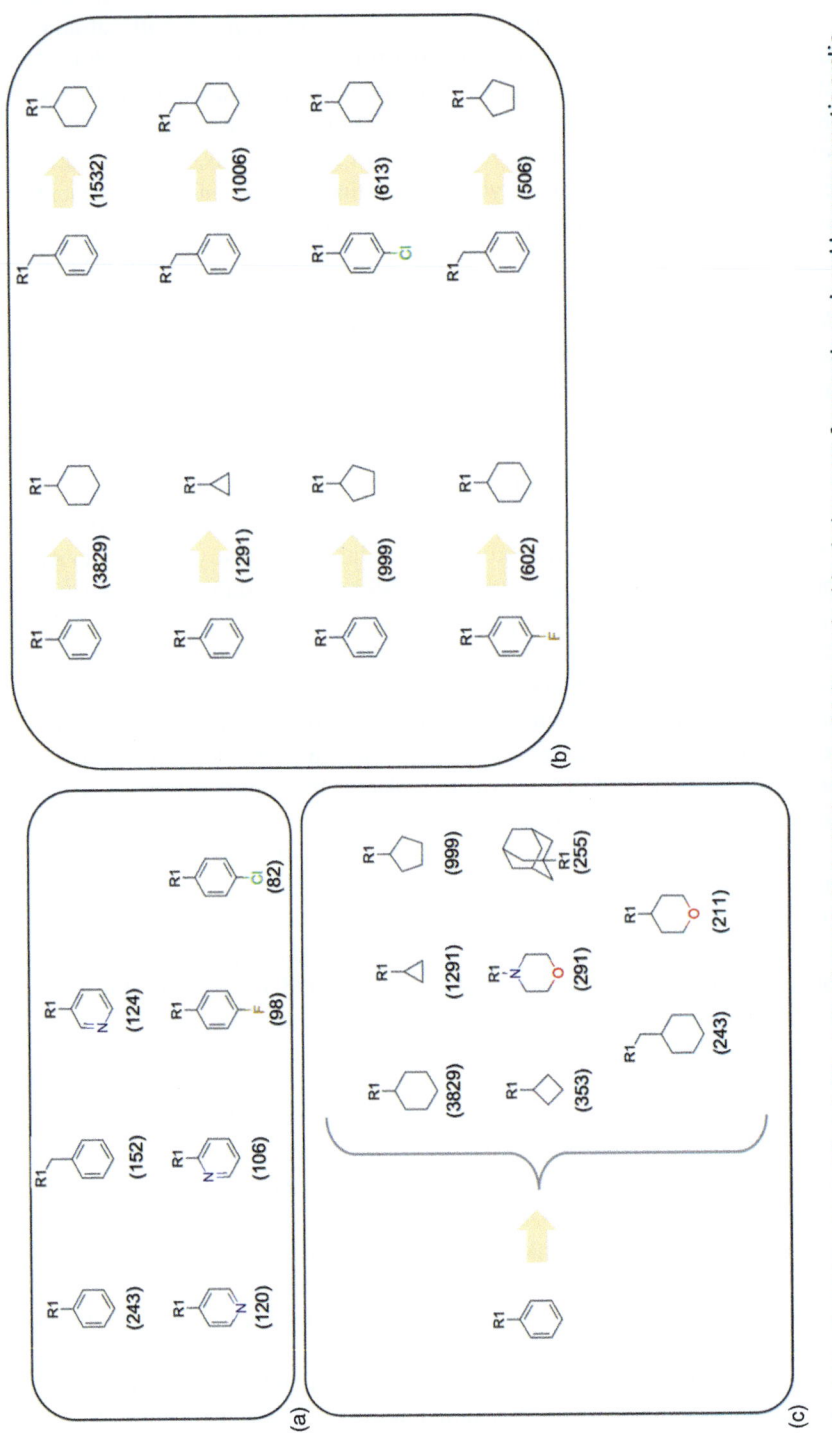

Figure 4.17 Reducing aromaticity of side chains found in SwissBioisostere. (a) Aromatic side chains most frequently replaced by nonaromatic cyclic fragments (number of occurrences in parenthesis). (b) Most frequent replacements reducing aromaticity for side chains, with number of occurrences in parenthesis. (c) Most frequent replacements reducing aromaticity for phenyl, with number of occurrences in parenthesis.

Figure 4.18 Reducing aromaticity of linkers found in SwissBioisostere. (a) Aromatic linkers most frequently replaced by nonaromatic cyclic fragments (number of occurrences in parenthesis). (b) Most frequent replacements reducing linker aromaticity with number of occurrences in parenthesis. (c) Most frequent replacements reducing aromaticity for 1,4-phenyl with occurrences in parenthesis. (d) SwissBioisostere entry of bicyclo[1.1.1]pentane analog of Darapladib, showing subnanomolar LpPLA2 inhibitor, with improved solubility and permeability [65].

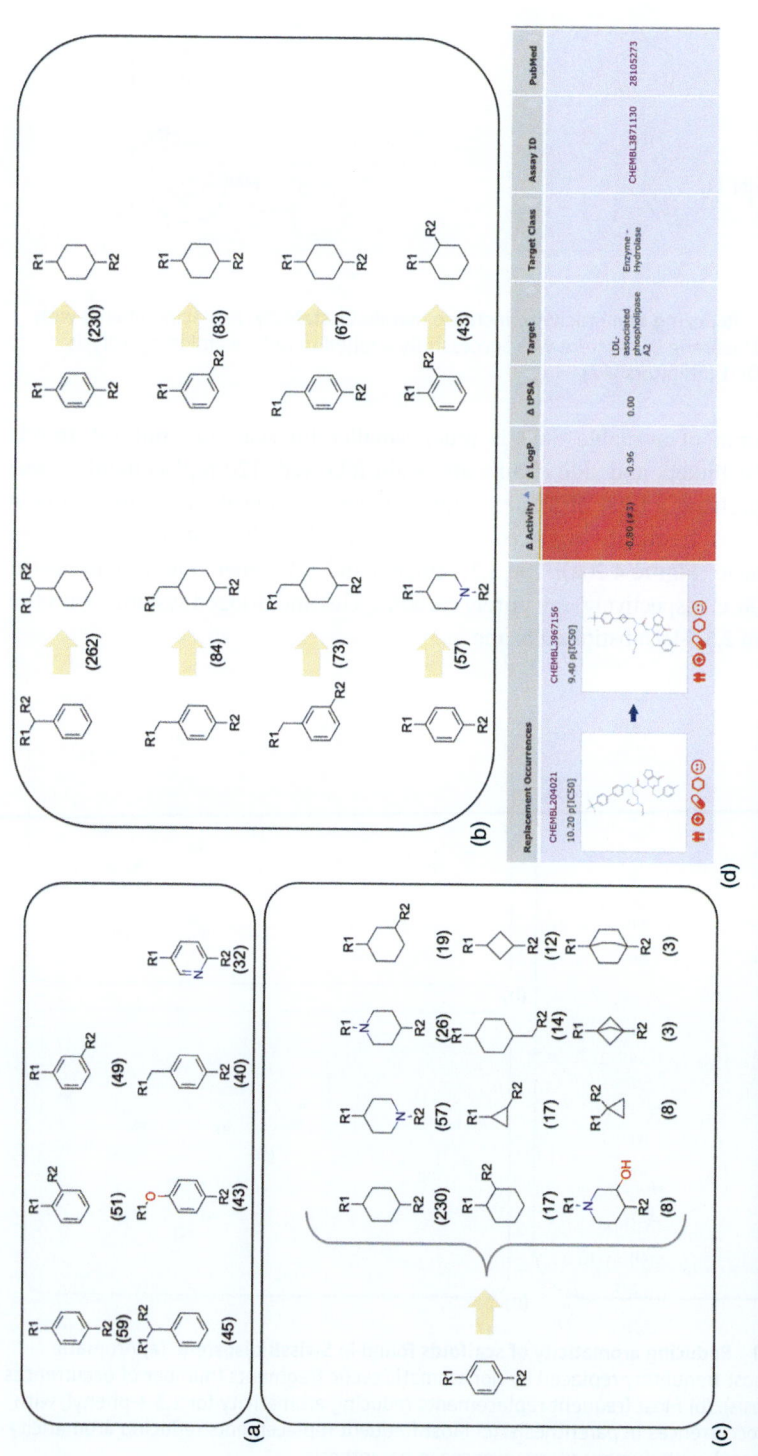

Figure 4.19 Reducing aromaticity to increase metabolic stability. Replacing phenyl with bicyclo[1.1.1]pentane bioisostere was successfully applied to reduce amide hydrolysis liability of IDO1 inhibitors [67].

The amount of available data is much smaller for scaffolds, but the trends observed for linkers and side chains are again followed. 120 replacements lower flatness, involving a total of 51 aromatic moieties exchanged by 58 nonaromatic rings. The most frequently replaced aromatic scaffolds include phenyls, pyridines, and thiophene (Figure 4.20a). The 1,3,4-phenyl and 1,3,5-phenyl replacements (in Figure 4.20b, c, respectively) are purely carbon cycles and bridged systems, with the exception of 2,5,5-trisubstituted oxane.

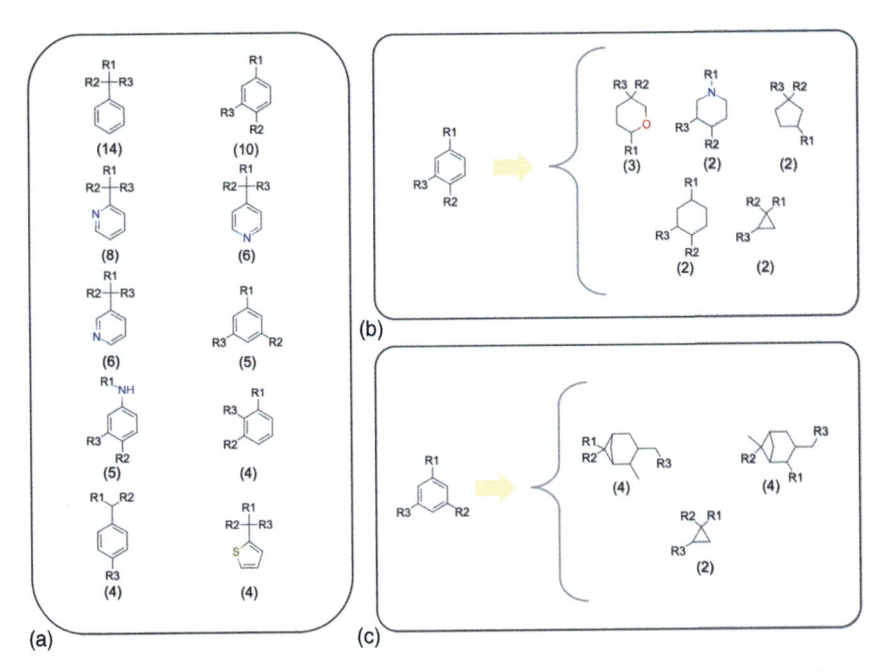

Figure 4.20 Reducing aromaticity of scaffolds found in SwissBioisostere. (a) Aromatic scaffolds most frequently replaced by nonaromatic cyclic fragments (number of occurrences in parenthesis). (b) Most frequent replacements reducing aromaticity for 1,3,4-phenyl, with number of occurrences in parenthesis. (c) Most frequent replacements reducing aromaticity for 1,3,5-phenyl, with number of occurrences in parenthesis.

4.5 Conclusive Remarks

SwissBioisostere consists in a knowledge and structural database of molecular replacements built on highly curated data extracted from ChEMBL. The MMP engine was used to define molecular replacements in pairs of relevant small molecules based on chemical structure and bioactivity only. Although not part of the definition of replacements, other related informations have been stored in the database, like molecular and physicochemical properties, which are important to assist medicinal chemists and other drug discovery experts in their hit finding and lead optimization endeavors. Because universal rules cannot be applied to guarantee a replacement to be bioisosteric, well-defined chemical and biological contexts of the replacement are critical to selecting the most appropriate molecular exchanges for a distinct objective in each setting. With these practical considerations in mind, a user-friendly web interface was developed and made accessible at www.swissbioisostere.ch. This free website does not require any login information, and the output is provided under CC-BY license to ensure anyone can benefit from this broad wealth of accurate information and to enable freedom to operate in various environments, including for for-profit or commercial applications.

The examples and use cases described in this chapter illustrate how Swiss-Bioisostere can support drug discovery complementarily to other web tools developed under the umbrella of the SwissDrugDesign project (https://www.molecular-modelling.ch/swiss-drug-design.html).

Acknowledgment

The authors are deeply grateful to SIB, Swiss Institute of Bioinformatics (www.sib.swiss) for supporting the SwissDrugDesign project. We would like to thank Prof. Olivier Michielin for the useful discussions as well as Wiley-VCH for the kind invitation to present our work. Chemaxon is acknowledged for the licensing agreement. The backend of the SwissBioisostere website (www.swissbioisostere.ch) involves MarvinJS and JChem microservices for some calculations (www.chemaxon.com).

References

1 Brown, N. (2012). *Bioisosteres in Medicinal Chemistry*. Wiley.
2 Meanwell, N.A. (2011). Synopsis of some recent tactical application of bioisosteres in drug design. *Journal of Medicinal Chemistry* 54 (8): 2529–2591.
3 Patani, G.A. and LaVoie, E.J. (1996). Bioisosterism: a rational approach in drug design. *Chemical Reviews* 96 (8): 3147–3176.
4 Lipinski, C.A. (1986). Chapter 27. bioisosterism in drug design. *Annual Reports in Medicinal Chemistry* 21: 283–291.
5 Langmuir, I. (1919). The structure of atoms and the octet theory of valence. *PNAS* 5 (7): 252–259.

6 Erlenmeyer, H. and Leo, M. (1932). Über pseudoatome. *Helvetica Chimica Acta* 15 (1): 1171–1186.
7 Friedman, H. (1951). Influence of isosteric replacements upon biological activity. *NASNRS* 206: 295–358.
8 Thornber, C.W. (1979). Isosterism and molecular modification in drug design. *Chemical Society Reviews* 8 (4): 563.
9 Carini, D.J., Duncia, J.V., Aldrich, P.E. et al. (1991). Nonpeptide angiotensin II receptor antagonists: the discovery of a series of N-(biphenylylmethyl)imidazoles as potent, orally active antihypertensives. *Journal of Medicinal Chemistry* 34 (8): 2525–2547.
10 Arrowsmith, J.E., Campbell, S.F., Cross, P.E. et al. (1986). Long-acting dihydropyridine calcium antagonists. 1. 2-Alkoxymethyl derivatives incorporating basic substituents. *Journal of Medicinal Chemistry* 29 (9): 1696–1702.
11 Stepanovs, D. and Mishnev, A. (2012). Molecular and crystal structure of sildenafil base. *Zeitschrift für Naturforschung Part B* 67 (5): 491–494.
12 Li, Y., Zhang, L., Yang, R. et al. (2022). Discovery of 3,4-dihydrobenzo[f][1,4] oxazepin-5(2H)-one derivatives as a new class of selective TNIK inhibitors and evaluation of their anti-colorectal cancer effects. *Journal of Medicinal Chemistry* 65 (3): 1786–1807.
13 Ballatore, C., Huryn, D.M., and Smith, A.B. (2013). Carboxylic acid (bio)isosteres in drug design. *ChemMedChem* 8 (3): 385–395.
14 Lassalas, P., Gay, B., Lasfargeas, C. et al. (2016). Structure property relationships of carboxylic acid isosteres. *Journal of Medicinal Chemistry* 59 (7): 3183–3203.
15 Plé, P.A., Green, T.P., Hennequin, L.F. et al. (2004). Discovery of a new class of anilinoquinazoline inhibitors with high affinity and specificity for the tyrosine kinase domain of c-Src. *Journal of Medicinal Chemistry* 47 (4): 871–887.
16 Sehnal, D., Bittrich, S., Deshpande, M. et al. (2021). Mol* Viewer: modern web app for 3D visualization and analysis of large biomolecular structures. *Nucleic Acids Research* 49 (W1): W431–W437.
17 Bunch, L. (2013). Bioisosteres in medicinal chemistry. Edited by Nathan Brown. *ChemMedChem* 8 (6): 1012–1012.
18 Langdon, S.R., Ertl, P., and Brown, N. (2010). Bioisosteric replacement and scaffold hopping in lead generation and optimization. *Molecular Informatics* 29 (5): 366–385.
19 Hu, Y., Stumpfe, D., and Bajorath, J. (2017). Recent advances in scaffold hopping. *Journal of Medicinal Chemistry* 60 (4): 1238–1246.
20 Schneider, G., Neidhart, W., Giller, T., and Schmid, G. (1999). "Scaffold-Hopping" by topological pharmacophore search: a contribution to virtual screening. *Angewandte Chemie (International Ed. in English)* 38 (19): 2894–2896.
21 Hughes, J.P., Rees, S., Kalindjian, S.B., and Philpott, K.L. (2011). Principles of early drug discovery. *British Journal of Pharmacology* 162 (6): 1239–1249.
22 Mendez, D., Gaulton, A., Bento, A.P. et al. (2019). ChEMBL: towards direct deposition of bioassay data. *Nucleic Acids Research* 47 (D1): D930–D940.

23 Gaulton, A., Hersey, A., Nowotka, M. et al. (2017). The ChEMBL database in 2017. *Nucleic Acids Research* 45 (D1): D945–D954.

24 Kenny, P.W. and Sadowski, J. (2005). Chemoinformatics in drug discovery. In: *Methods and Principles in Medicinal*, 271–285. Weinheim: Wiley-VCH.

25 Dossetter, A.G., Griffen, E.J., and Leach, A.G. (2013). Matched molecular pair analysis in drug discovery. *Drug Discovery Today* 18 (15–16): 724–731.

26 Tyrchan, C. and Evertsson, E. (2017). Matched molecular pair analysis in short: algorithms, applications and limitations. *Computational and Structural Biotechnology Journal* 15: 86–90.

27 Hussain, J. and Rea, C. (2010). Computationally efficient algorithm to identify matched molecular pairs (MMPs) in large data sets. *Journal of Chemical Information and Computer Sciences* 50 (3): 339–348.

28 Cuozzo, A., Daina, A., Perez, M.A.S. et al. (2021). SwissBioisostere 2021: updated structural, bioactivityand physicochemical data delivered by a reshapedweb interface. *Nucleic Acids Research* 50 (D1): D1382–D1390.

29 Wirth, M., Zoete, V., Michielin, O., and Sauer, W.H.B. (2013). SwissBioisostere: a database of molecular replacements for ligand design. *Nucleic Acids Research* 41 (D1): D1137–D1143.

30 Pinto, D.J.P., Orwat, M.J., Quan, M.L. et al. (2006). 1-[3-Aminobenzisoxazol-5′-yl]-3-trifluoromethyl-6-[2′-(3-(R)-hydroxy-*N*-pyrrolidinyl)methyl-[1,1′]-biphen-4-yl]-1,4,5,6-tetrahydropyrazolo-[3,4-c]-pyridin-7-one (BMS-740808) a highly potent, selective, efficacious, and orally bioavailable inhibitor of blood coagulation factor Xa. *Bioorganic & Medicinal Chemistry Letters* 16 (15): 4141–4147.

31 Bragina, M.E., Daina, A., Perez, M.A.S. et al. (2022). The SwissSimilarity 2021 web tool: novel chemical libraries and additional methods for an enhanced ligand-based virtual screening experience. *International Journal of Molecular Sciences* 23 (2): 811.

32 Daina, A., Michielin, O., and Zoete, V. (2019). SwissTargetPrediction: updated data and new features for efficient prediction of protein targets of small molecules. *Nucleic Acids Research* 47 (W1): W357–W364.

33 Daina, A., Michielin, O., and Zoete, V. (2017). SwissADME: a free web tool to evaluate pharmacokinetics, drug-likeness and medicinal chemistry friendliness of small molecules. *Scientific Reports* 7: 42717.

34 Thamilselvan, G., Sarveswari, H.B., Vasudevan, S. et al. (2021). Development of an antibiotic resistance breaker to resensitize drug-resistant *Staphylococcus aureus*: in silico and in vitro approach. *Frontiers in Cellular and Infection Microbiology* 11: 700198.

35 Chen, M., Li, Z., Shao, X., and Maienfisch, P. (2022). Bioisosteric-replacement-driven lead optimization of tyclopyrazoflor. *Journal of Agricultural and Food Chemistry* https://doi.org/10.1002/cbdv.200790032.

36 Turner, S.R., Strohbach, J.W., Tommasi, R.A. et al. (1998). Tipranavir (PNU-140690): a potent, orally bioavailable nonpeptidic HIV protease inhibitor of the 5,6-Dihydro-4-hydroxy-2-pyrone sulfonamide class. *Journal of Medicinal Chemistry* 41 (18): 3467–3476.

37 Lovering, F., Bikker, J., and Humblet, C. (2009). Escape from flatland: increasing saturation as an approach to improving clinical success. *Journal of Medicinal Chemistry* 52 (21): 6752–6756.

38 Hernandes, M.Z., Cavalcanti, S.M.T., Moreira, D.R.M. et al. (2010). Halogen atoms in the modern medicinal chemistry: hints for the drug design. *Current Drug Targets* 11 (3): 303–314.

39 Meanwell, N.A. (2018). Fluorine and fluorinated motifs in the design and application of bioisosteres for drug design. *Journal of Medicinal Chemistry* 61 (14): 5822–5880.

40 Sauer, W.H.B. and Schwarz, M.K. (2003). Size doesn't matter: scaffold diversity, shape diversity and biological activity of combinatorial libraries. *Chimia* 57 (5): 276.

41 Sauer, W.H.B. and Schwarz, M.K. (2003). Molecular shape diversity of combinatorial libraries: a prerequisite for broad bioactivity †. *Journal of Chemical Information and Computer Sciences* 43 (3): 987–1003.

42 Irwin, J.J., Tang, K.G., Young, J. et al. (2020). ZINC20-A free ultralarge-scale chemical database for ligand discovery. *Journal of Chemical Information and Modeling* 60 (12): 6065–6073.

43 Kumari, S., Carmona, A.V., Tiwari, A.K., and Trippier, P.C. (2020). Amide bond bioisosteres: strategies, synthesis, and successes. *Journal of Medicinal Chemistry* 63 (21): 12290–12358.

44 Pinto, D.J.P., Orwat, M.J., Koch, S. et al. (2007). Discovery of 1-(4-methoxyphenyl)-7-oxo-6-(4-(2-oxopiperidin-1-yl)phenyl)-4,5,6,7-tetrahydro-1H-pyrazolo[3,4-c]pyridine-3-carboxamide (apixaban, BMS-562247), a highly potent, selective, efficacious, and orally bioavailable inhibitor of blood coagulation factor Xa. *Journal of Medicinal Chemistry* 50 (22): 5339–5356.

45 Zoete, V., Daina, A., Bovigny, C., and Michielin, O. (2016). SwissSimilarity: a web tool for low to ultra high throughput ligand-based virtual screening. *Journal of Chemical Information and Computer Sciences* 56 (8): 1399–1404.

46 Daina, A. and Zoete, V. (2019). Application of the SwissDrugDesign online resources in virtual screening. *International Journal of Molecular Sciences*, Vol. 13, Pages 1805-1831 20 (18): 4612.

47 Testa, B. and Krämer, S.D. (2007). The biochemistry of drug metabolism – an introduction. *Chemistry & Biodiversity* 4 (3): 257–405.

48 Brenk, R., Schipani, A., James, D. et al. (2008). Lessons learnt from assembling screening libraries for drug discovery for neglected diseases. *ChemMedChem* 3 (3): 435–444.

49 Bruns, R.F. and Watson, I.A. (2012). Rules for identifying potentially reactive or promiscuous compounds. *Journal of Medicinal Chemistry* 55 (22): 9763–9772.

50 Baell, J.B. and Holloway, G.A. (2010). New substructure filters for removal of pan assay interference compounds (PAINS) from screening libraries and for their exclusion in bioassays. *Journal of Medicinal Chemistry* 53 (7): 2719–2740.

51 Wan, H. and Holmen, A. (2009). High throughput screening of physicochemical properties and in vitro ADME profiling in drug discovery. *Combinatorial Chemistry and High Throughput Screening* 12 (3): 315–329.

52 Hop, C.E.C.A. (2011) Encyclopedia of Drug Metabolism and Interactions. 1–43. https://doi.org/10.1002/9780470921920.edm049

53 Daina, A. and Zoete, V. (2016). A BOILED-Egg to predict gastrointestinal absorption and brain penetration of small molecules. *ChemMedChem* 11 (11): 1117–1121.

54 Huang, W.-S., Metcalf, C.A., Sundaramoorthi, R. et al. (2010). Discovery of 3-[2-(imidazo[1,2-b]pyridazin-3-yl)ethynyl]-4-methyl-*N*-{4-[(4-methylpiperazin-1-yl)methyl]-3-(trifluoromethyl)phenyl}benzamide (AP24534), a potent, orally active pan-inhibitor of breakpoint cluster region-abelson (BCR-ABL) kinase including the T315I gatekeeper mutant. *Journal of Medicinal Chemistry* 53 (12): 4701–4719.

55 Wildman, S.A. and Crippen, G.M. (1999). Prediction of physicochemical parameters by atomic contributions. *Journal of Chemical Information and Computer Sciences* 39 (5): 868–873.

56 Ertl, P., Rohde, B., and Selzer, P. (2000). Fast calculation of molecular polar surface area as a sum of fragment-based contributions and its application to the prediction of drug transport properties. *Journal of Medicinal Chemistry* 43 (20): 3714–3717.

57 Veber, D.F., Johnson, S.R., Cheng, H.-Y. et al. (2002). Molecular properties that influence the oral bioavailability of drug candidates. *Journal of Medicinal Chemistry* 45 (12): 2615–2623.

58 Muegge, I., Heald, S.L., and Brittelli, D. (2001). Simple selection criteria for drug-like chemical matter. *Journal of Medicinal Chemistry* 44 (12): 1841–1846.

59 Ritchie, T.J., Ertl, P., and Lewis, R. (2011). The graphical representation of ADME-related molecule properties for medicinal chemists. *Drug Discovery Today* 16 (1–2): 65–72.

60 Venkatesan, A.M., Davis, J.M., Grosu, G.T. et al. (2004). Synthesis and structure–activity relationships of 4-alkynyloxy phenyl sulfanyl, sulfinyl, and sulfonyl alkyl hydroxamates as tumor necrosis factor-α converting enzyme and matrix metalloproteinase inhibitors. *Journal of Medicinal Chemistry* 47 (25): 6255–6269.

61 Ritchie, T.J. and Macdonald, S.J.F. (2009). The impact of aromatic ring count on compound developability–are too many aromatic rings a liability in drug design? *Drug Discovery Today* 14 (21–22): 1011–1020.

62 Joubert, J., Geldenhuys, W.J., Van der Schyf, C.J. et al. (2012). Polycyclic cage structures as lipophilic scaffolds for neuroactive drugs. *ChemMedChem* 7 (3): 375–384.

63 Tse, E.G., Houston, S.D., Williams, C.M. et al. (2020). Nonclassical phenyl bioisosteres as effective replacements in a series of novel open-source antimalarials. *Journal of Medicinal Chemistry* 63 (20): 11585–11601.

64 Wilkinson, S.M., Gunosewoyo, H., Barron, M.L. et al. (2014). The first CNS-Active carborane: a novel P2X 7 receptor antagonist with antidepressant activity. *ACS Chemical Neuroscience* 5 (5): 335–339.

65 Measom, N.D., Down, K.D., Hirst, D.J. et al. (2016). Investigation of a bicyclo[1.1.1]pentane as a phenyl replacement within an LpPLA 2 inhibitor. *ACS Medicinal Chemistry Letters* 8 (1): 43–48.

66 Zhao, J.-X., Chang, Y.-X., He, C. et al. (2021). 1,2-Difunctionalized bicyclo[1.1.1]pentanes: long–sought-after mimetics for ortho/meta-substituted arenes. *Proceedings of the National academy of Sciences* 118 (28): e2108881118.

67 Pu, Q., Zhang, H., Guo, L. et al. (2020). Discovery of potent and orally available Bicyclo[1.1.1]pentane-derived indoleamine-2,3-dioxygenase 1 (IDO1) inhibitors. *ACS Medicinal Chemistry Letters* 11 (8): 1548–1554.

Part II

Macromolecular Targets and Diseases

5

The Protein Data Bank (PDB) and Macromolecular Structure Data Supporting Computer-Aided Drug Design

David Armstrong[1], John Berrisford[2], Preeti Choudhary[1], Lukas Pravda[3], James Tolchard[4], Mihaly Varadi[1], and Sameer Velankar[1]

[1]*Protein Data Bank in Europe, EMBL-EBI, Wellcome Genome Campus, Hinxton, Cambridge, CB10 1SD, UK*
[2]*AstraZeneca, AstraZeneca Academy House, 136 Hills Rd, Cambridge, CB2 8PA, UK*
[3]*Exscientia, The Schrodinger Building, Oxford Science Park, Oxford, Oxfordshire, United Kingdom, OX4 4GE*
[4]*Centre de RMN à Très Hauts Champs de Lyon, Claude Bernard University Lyon 1, 5 rue de la Doua, 69100 Villeurbanne, France*

5.1 Introduction

The Protein Data Bank (PDB) [1], managed by the global Worldwide PDB (wwPDB) consortium [2], is one of the oldest scientific databases in life sciences. The PDB archives structural models of biological macromolecules, derived from experimental data. The wwPDB partners, the Research Collaboratory for Structural Bioinformatics (RCSB) [3], Protein Data Bank in Europe (PDBe) [4], Protein Data Bank Japan (PDBj) [5], Electron Microscopy Data Bank (EMDB) [6], and Bio Mag Res Bank (BMRB) [7], manage the PDB archive based on the FAIR principles [8], ensuring structural biology data are Findable, Accessible, Interoperable and Reusable.

The PDB archive contains over 200,000 structures of proteins, DNA, and RNA, and their complexes with small molecules, such as cofactors and inhibitors. This data, along with related metadata and experimental data, are stored in the PDB archive in PDBx/mmCIF formatted files [9]. Since 2019, it has been mandatory for X-ray crystallographic structures to be deposited in the PDBx/mmCIF format [10], ensuring maximum capture and validation of metadata for these structures.

The PDB is a vital resource for computer-aided drug design and contains structural information for large numbers of drugs, with 5494 unique ligands in the PDB mapped to entries in DrugBank [11]. Additionally, there are numerous potential drug targets as well as structures containing macromolecular drug targets. This data are of paramount importance in determination of key drug binding sites in macromolecules [12], and in understanding existing binding modes to support designs of novel compounds to target these binding sites.

In addition to the three-dimensional (3D) coordinate information archived in the PDB, standardization of polymer sequences and chemical identifiers in PDB entries facilitates the integration of additional metadata from external resources

[13, 14]. This additional biological and chemical information is vitally important in understanding the scientific context of the structures in the PDB, which is required to determine functional information.

As part of the European Bioinformatics Institute (EMBL-EBI), the PDBe [4] is uniquely placed to integrate macromolecular structure data from partner resources at EBI and beyond. This allows the integration of relevant biological and chemical data to better demonstrate the functional importance of structures in the PDB. The PDBe-Knowledge Base (PDBe-KB) [15] builds upon this, with partnerships extending across the structural bioinformatics community, allowing the integration of even more data related to macromolecular structure and function. This includes a large number of partners involved in cheminformatics who provide data relating to small molecules and their macromolecular binding sites, including canSAR [16], 3DLigandSite [17], P2Rank [18], and many more, detailed at pdbe-kb.org/partners.

The wwPDB, by adhering to the FAIR principles, ensures that all PDB data are provided freely, with no limits upon its use. All PDBe and PDBe-KB tools and resources are also free to use, with scripts and software pipelines made open source wherever possible. In addition to access through the PDBe [4] and PDBe-KB [15] websites, all PDBe data are made available through publicly accessible APIs [19, 20], while much of this data is also available via a distributed PDBe knowledge graph [20].

This chapter will introduce the type of data available in the PDB, how it is organized and curated, and how it can be used to support drug design. It will also give an overview of the tools and resources at PDBe and PDBe-KB, highlighting how these can support understanding of drug binding and function in PDB structures to improve research within this area.

5.2 Small Molecule Data in Protein Data Bank (PDB) Entries

5.2.1 What Data are in the PDB Archive?

The PDB is the single global archive of experimentally determined 3D structure data of biological macromolecules. Each PDB structure must contain a polymeric entity, i.e. protein or nucleic acid, however, information can also be included for all non-polymeric ligands within the structure.

The atomic coordinates of a PDB entry are built with a specific hierarchy, ensuring that each molecule and its constituent parts can be clearly identified. The smallest component of the hierarchy is at the atomic level, with each separate coordinate line in the archive file describing the specific position of an atom in 3D space. Each atom is defined as part of a larger chemical component or residue, defined by a 3-character ID code.

These chemical components can be either individual bound ligands in the structure or individual residues within a polymeric molecule, with each defined by a unique identifier (asym or chain ID) and numbering for clear identification. Beyond each specific polymeric chain ID, each unique and individual molecule in the structure is also given a specific "entity" identifier, which is used to link all the metadata

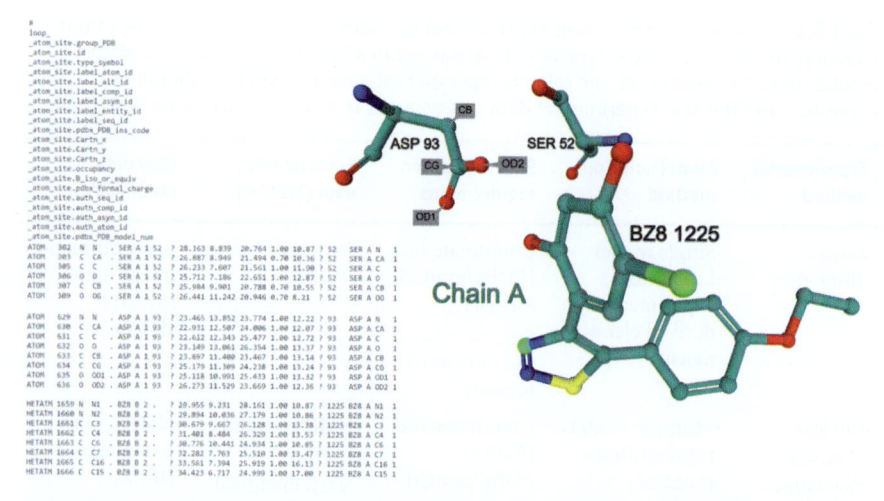

Figure 5.1 A sample of the atomic coordinates from a PDBx/mmCIF format file (PDB entry 2yi7) is shown on the left. The individual items in the "atom_site" category are listed first, highlighting the data present in each column for the subsequent data. A subset of the atomic coordinates is displayed below, with graphical representation of these coordinates, displayed on the right of the image, only selected atoms are labeled for clarity.

relating to this molecule. More information about ligand molecules in the PDB will be discussed in Section 5.3 (Figure 5.1).

As previously mentioned, the PDB is an archive of experimentally determined structures and, as such, is limited to a subset of accepted experimental structure determination techniques. Depending on the experimental method used, the archive PDB entry file will contain information specific to the technique, while additional experimental data files are also collected to allow assessment of experimental data in the context of the derived coordinate models. The three main methods accepted for PDB depositions are diffraction techniques such as X-ray crystallography, cryo-electron microscopy (cryoEM), and nuclear magnetic resonance (NMR). A summary of the PDB deposition data requirements for each of these techniques is given in Table 5.1.

The oldest and most common technique for determining structures in the PDB is X-ray crystallography, which involves the generation of crystalline structures of the biological sample. These crystals are then exposed to a high-powered X-ray beam, often at a synchrotron facility, and the specific diffraction pattern from these X-rays is collected by a detector. Before this diffraction pattern can be used for structure calculation, first the phases must be determined, using techniques such as molecular or isomorphous replacement.

Using the intensities and phases of the spots (or reflections) in the diffraction pattern, crystallographers can calculate a map of electron density for the biological specimen, into which the atomic model can be built. In addition to coordinates, since 2008, submission of PDB structures solved by X-ray crystallography must also include submission of the structure factor files defining the experimental reflections data.

Table 5.1 A summary of the main experimental methods accepted for PDB depositions, including information on the type of data deposited in a PDB entry file, the mandatory requirements for deposition, the related experimental data and where it should be deposited, and the raw experimental data and where it is recommended to be deposited.

Experimental method	Model solution method	PDB deposition requirements	Experimental data (archive)	Raw data (archive)
X-ray diffraction	Single model built into experimentally derived electron density map	Coordinate file (PDBx/mmCIF format) Structure factor file (mtz or CIF format)	Structure factors (PDB)	X-ray diffraction image data (SBGrid, IRRMC)
Nuclear Magnetic Resonance (NMR)	Multiple models representing a range of conformers that satisfy experimental restraints	Coordinate file (PDB or PDBx/mmCIF format) NMR restraints file (STAR or NEF format)	NMR restraints (BMRB) NMR chemical shifts (BMRB)	NMR spectral parameters (BMRB) NMR relaxation data (BMRB)
Cryo-electron microscopy (cryoEM)	Single model built into experimentally derived electric potential map	Coordinate file (PDB or PDBx/mmCIF format) Image for public display at EMDB EMDB map deposition (MRC or CCP4 format)	Electric potential map (EMDB)	Electron microscopy images (EMPIAR)

The first cryoEM structure in the PDB was released in 1991, however, it has taken a long time for the technique to establish itself as a routine method for high-resolution structure determination. The technique involves the imaging of biological molecules and complexes under cryogenic conditions, using a transmission electron microscope. The sample is flash-frozen in a thin layer with electrons passing through the sample to a detector, where images of each particle are captured. These images are then sorted and processed computationally to generate a 3D map of the sample, to allow fitting of a molecular model.

The use of cryoEM has allowed the determination of larger and more heterogeneous complexes than was previously possible with X-ray crystallography, however until recently, was not able to reach resolutions sufficient to interpret atomic-level details. However, recent advances in the technique, including improved software and hardware including free-electron detectors, have led to cryoEM becoming the fastest-growing experimental method for studying macromolecular structure [21]. This is due to the determination of high-resolution structures in conditions that better represent the native environment of the sample. Since 2016, submission of cryoEM structures to the PDB has also required submission of the experimental maps to the EMDB [6].

The third main technique used for solving structures in the PDB is NMR. This method involves the use of powerful magnetic fields to discern minor differences in the resonance frequencies, also known as chemical shifts, of atoms in the macromolecule. These chemical shifts are used to determine interactions among atoms in the molecule and generate atomic restraints, which can be used to build the structure of the macromolecules.

In solution-state NMR, the biological macromolecules can move freely in the solvent, allowing these experiments to capture the range of structural conformations adopted by these molecules. These structures are therefore deposited as multiple models in the PDB, highlighting an ensemble of potential structural conformations adopted by the macromolecules. An alternative technique is solid-state NMR [22], which uses similar underlying principles, however, is used to determine structures of molecular structures within solid or semisolid materials, including macromolecules within biological membranes.

Though the three experimental methods mentioned above account for the vast majority of PDB entries, there are also additional variations in diffraction methods that can be used to solve structures in the PDB. Firstly, neutron crystallography [23] is a similar technique to X-ray crystallography, however, it relies upon neutron scattering to determine the macromolecular structure. The benefit of this technique is that the neutrons interact with atomic nuclei, rather than electrons, which improves observation of hydrogen atoms in the structure. Neutron and X-ray crystallography are often used in conjunction to provide both high-resolution data and to determine positions of hydrogen atoms.

There are also methods that utilize X-ray crystallography to allow high-throughput determination of ligand binding in macromolecules. Fragment screening [24] experiments involve the "soaking" of various small molecule fragments into crystals of the sample. Determining how these different fragments bind within the protein structure can help to improve the mechanistic understanding of a protein and the identification of suitable drug candidates. Pan-Dataset Density Analysis (PanDDA) experiments [25] can be used to compare multiple fragment screening datasets to identify weak signals of bound small molecules within the noise of the data and can further improve the determination of small molecule binding sites.

5.2.2 Definition of Small Molecules in OneDep

In the PDB archive, ligands are defined as any molecule that is not part of a larger polymeric molecule, i.e. proteins, nucleic acids, or branched carbohydrates [26]. In the case of peptide-like ligands, if these contain at least two standard peptide bonds, then these are classed as polymeric entities. Small molecule ligands in the PDB can have a range of distinct functions, for example, as substrates, products, and inhibitors.

Each distinct ligand in the PDB archive is assigned its own unique 3-character ID code, to support easy identification across the full archive [26]. Each of these ligands includes a detailed chemical description, which is contained within the wwPDB Chemical Component Dictionary (CCD), and discussed in more detail in the next section.

5.3 Small Molecule Dictionaries

5.3.1 wwPDB Chemical Component Dictionary (CCD)

The wwPDB maintains a reference dictionary containing chemical descriptions of each unique chemical component present in the whole PDB archive. These components are the building blocks for PDB entries and include amino acids, nucleotides, metal ions, and other nonpeptide small molecules. These chemical component descriptions are stored in the wwPDB's CCD (https://www.wwpdb.org/data/ccd) [26].

Each component is given a unique identifier and has a CCD definition that describes the molecule. As of July 2022, there are around 37,000 unique definitions in the wwPDB CCD. The unique identifier is currently limited to a maximum of three characters. Most definitions contain a three-character unique identifier, with one- or two-character identifiers mostly used for identification of DNA and RNA bases or for components containing individual elements. Some examples of chemical components include manganese (Mn), adenosine-triphosphate (ATP), and glutamate (GLU). Previously, these identifiers were assigned with some meaning to their chemical definition, however, due to the high number of chemical components in the dictionary, these CCD identifiers are now randomly assigned for any new ligands.

If the CCD definition is defining a standard amino acid or nucleotide, the IUPAC protein one-letter code [27] is also provided, for example, Glutamate has the unique identifier GLU and the one-letter code E. Small modifications of standard amino acids or nucleotides, generally, where the modification contains fewer than 10 atoms, have their own CCD definitions, for example, phospho-serine has the identifier SEP. These modified amino acids or nucleotides have the same one-letter code as their standard amino acid parent, therefore SEP, which is a modified serine amino acid, also contains the one-letter code S.

Peptide-based chromophores provide a more complex example. In proteins, chromophores typically comprise three amino acids condensed into one molecule. In the CCD component, the one-letter code lists all amino acids that make up the chromophore. For example, the CCD definition for the chromophore CR2, which comprises the amino acids GLY-TYR-GLY and has the corresponding one-letter code GYG.

In addition to providing a unique identifier, each CCD definition describes the chemistry of the molecule. This includes the name of each atom in the molecule, the order of bonds between atoms, stereochemistry of chiral atoms, and any charges on individual atoms or the whole molecule. There are two sets of 3D coordinates included in the CCD definition: the model coordinates, extracted from the PDB entry from which the CCD was initially generated, and idealized coordinates (from the lowest energy conformation), generated using the expected geometry of the ligand from the CCD definition.

Additional metadata are also included in the CCD definition, including the name of the molecule and any synonyms. If a common name is known for the compound, then it is provided either as the name or as one of the synonyms, otherwise, systematic names are provided. The systematic name is the default name generated by the OpenEye [28] software at the time of creation of the compound. Chemical descriptors in InChI and SMILES formats are provided and are automatically generated by OpenEye during creation of the compound.

Every molecule in the PDB must have a corresponding CCD definition. During deposition and biocuration of PDB entries, each compound in the deposited file is compared to existing CCD definitions using a graph match algorithm [29]. If refinement restraints are provided in the uploaded coordinate file, then this information is used for comparing the molecule to entries in the CCD, otherwise, the coordinates are used for searching. If a molecule fails to find a match in the CCD, then depositors are asked for further details of the molecule so that a new CCD definition can be made. A new CCD definition is then defined during biocuration and added to the CCD. The name of the molecule is either defined by the depositor, if a common name is available, or a systematic name is generated based on the chemistry of the molecule.

5.3.2 The Peptide Reference Dictionary

The PDB archive also contains examples of complex ligands, which comprise combinations of amino acid and amino acid-like components. These peptide-like molecules commonly possess important biological functions, such as antibiotic or inhibitory activity, however, a description of their global chemistry does not fit within the classic PDB definitions of polymers and ligands. Therefore, to support the curation of this important class of molecules, their chemical and biological descriptions are described in a separate dictionary. The "Peptide Reference Dictionary" (PRD) resource [30] provides a standardized framework for these definitions so that each PRD entity can be described in a way that outlines both its subcomponent composition and global characteristics. These PRD definitions are stored in the wwPDB Biologically Interesting Molecule Reference Dictionary (BIRD) (https://www.wwpdb.org/data/bird).

The process of defining a new PRD molecule, or matching connected CCDs to an existing PRD, occurs during the biocuration process. Any atomistic information, such as reference coordinates, bonding, and chemical descriptors are then listed in PRD-chemical definition files, whereas subcomponent sequence, CCD-linking, and any related biological details, such as biological function, are stored in PRD-molecular definition files. By using the PRD dictionary to standardize biocuration, it allows for the precise interrogation, comparison, and retrieval of global and

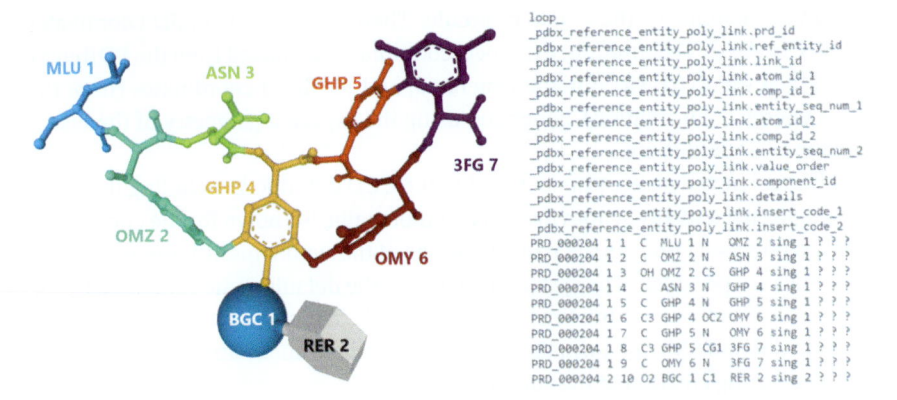

Figure 5.2 An example of PRD is the antibiotic Vancomycin (PRD_000204). Vancomycin consists of seven nonstandard amino acids (ball and stick, distinguished by color) and two sugar components (cyan and grey in a 3D representation of the SNFG notation). The PRD polymer linking section of the PRD molecular definition file is shown on the right-hand side.

subcomponent-specific data, which would otherwise not be possible. Links to PRD definition files can be found on relevant PDB entry pages and references to key PRD identifiers (ID, name, type, and function) are stored in PDB entry PDBx/mmCIF files under the pdbx_molecule_features category (Figure 5.2).

5.4 Additional Ligand Annotations in the PDB Archive

In addition to the standard chemical and biomolecular definitions already described, where possible, the PDB biocuration pipeline generates additional ligand-related information to best describe ligand complexity and intramolecular connectivity and to do so with a consistent and objective methodology [31]. Many software packages rely upon these data for purposes such as molecular refinement and accurate molecular visualization.

5.4.1 Linkage Information

The most common ligand-associated annotations found in PDB entry files refer to intermolecular bonding. These refer to all nonstandard linkages between and among polymer components and CCD ligands. This information was historically found in PDB-format *LINK*, *SSBOND*, and *CONECT* records, however, the current PDBx/mmCIF archive format provides additional data, including leaving group information, atomic descriptions, and author numbering for up to three chemical component partners per interaction [9]. At present, to ensure standardization across the whole PDB archive, all link records and bonding distances are calculated and validated during the biocuration process [31]. The PDBx/mmCIF dictionary currently supports covalent, hydrogen, covalent–metal, and disulfide-bond interaction "types" [32] (Figure 5.3).

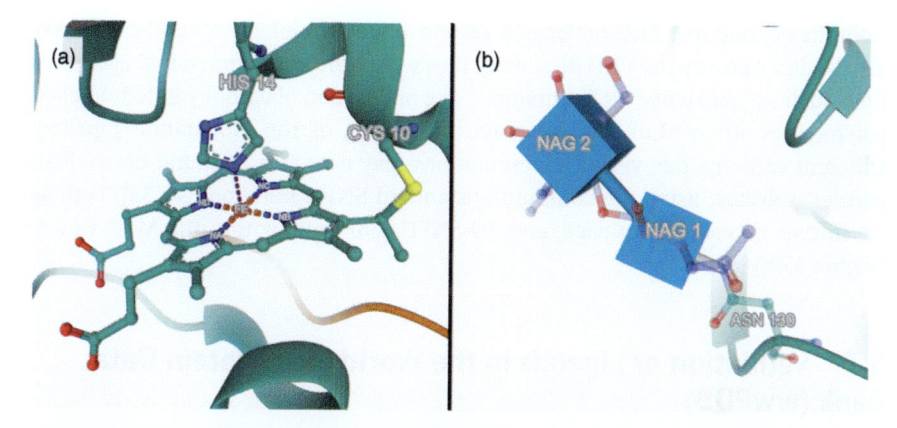

Figure 5.3 Two examples of PDB linkage information and default visualization styles in the Mol* viewer: **(LEFT: 5AUS)** covalent interaction between heme c ligand and cysteine side chain (CYS10-HEC), and metal coordination between the iron in heme c and a histidine side chain (HIS14-FE); **(RIGHT: 4TPL)** a covalent carbohydrate linkage between two N-acetyl-D-glucosamine (NAG) ligands (NAG2-NAG1) and covalent N-Glycosylation between a NAG and an asparagine side chain (NAG1-ASN207).

5.4.2 Carbohydrates

The most recent development concerning PDB ligand definitions relates to the annotation of polymeric carbohydrates [33]. These new "branched polymer" descriptions (entity_type item "branched") are composed of multiple and sequential CCD monosaccharides. The description of polymeric carbohydrates is outlined within the PDBx/mmCIF model file for a given PDB entry, under the new pdbx categories entity_branch, entity_branch_descriptor, entity_branch_link, entity_branch_list, and branch_scheme (Figure 5.4a). Whilst chemically distinct

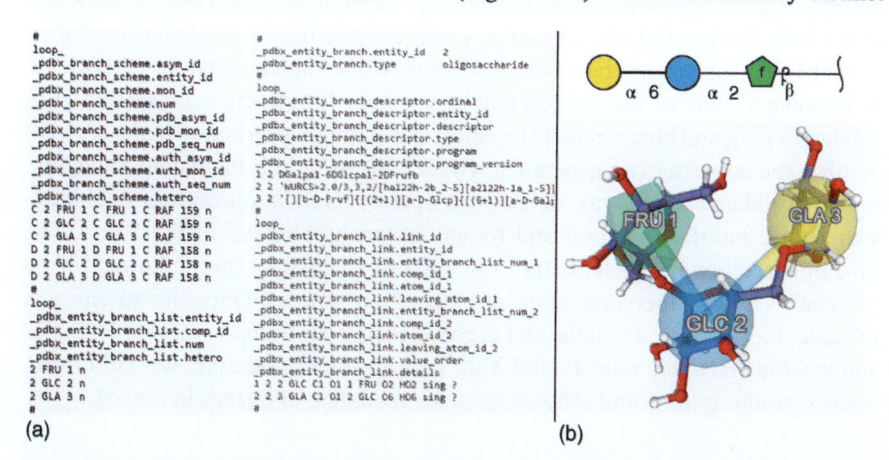

Figure 5.4 (a) Example categories from a PDBx/mmCIF PDB model file describing a branched polymer carbohydrate. The example highlights how entity 2 (raffinose (RAF), PRD_900002) is comprised of the subcomponents FRU, GLC, and GLA (fructose, glucose, and galactose) and lists the corresponding atomic linkages. (b) Examples of wwPDB carbohydrate representations by 2D and 3D symbol nomenclature for glycans (SNFG) (top and middle, respectively). Source: (b) These images were taken from the PDBe entry pages for PDB accession 5ofx; https://pdbe.org/5ofx.

from the peptide-like PRD molecules, carbohydrates of biological significance may also be described by the PRD dictionary files where they hold functional classifications such as "nutrients" or "inhibitors." The annotation of carbohydrate-branched polymers occurs within the automatic processing of the biocuration pipeline. Different carbohydrate visual representations may now also be found on wwPDB partner websites, using the community standard SNFG notation [34, 35], both as 2D images on each entry page, and 3D-SNFG [36] units within the Mol* viewer (Figure 5.4b).

5.5 Validation of Ligands in the Worldwide Protein Data Bank (wwPDB)

Currently, PDB contains over 34,000 unique small molecules bound to over 133,600 protein structures. Numerous groups have highlighted the need for standardized validation in structures in the PDB archive [37–44]. Several errors have even led to the retraction of the respective publication(s) and subsequent obsoletion of the PDB entry [43]. A Validation Task Force (VTF) was set up to centralize and standardize validation across the wwPDB archive, which included metrics to judge the reliability of the ligand-bound macromolecular structures as they play a pivotal role in many computational methods like ligand docking and structure-based drug design. This resulted in development of the wwPDB validation reports (VR), first introduced in 2012.

wwPDB validation pipeline (VP) generates detailed wwPDB VR comprising an assessment of structure quality using widely accepted standards and criteria recommended by various method-specific VTFs [45–47]. To enhance ligand validation, in 2015, wwPDB, CCDC (Cambridge Crystallographic Data Center), and D3R (Drug Design Data Resource) co-organized the ligand validation workshop (LVW) [48] whose recommendations were recently implemented in VP [14]. VP is an integral part of the unified OneDep system for structure deposition [13], validation [49], and biocuration [31]. Before depositing the structure in the wwPDB archive, the depositor can generate a wwPDB VR using the standalone validation server (validate.wwpdb.org) or API (wwpdb.org/validation/onedep-validation-web-service-interface) to find and fix any issues highlighted in the VR. At the time of deposition, a "preliminary" VR is issued to the depositor, followed by the "official" VR after the completion of biocuration process. Once the structure is released, the VR is made public and is provided as both human-readable PDF files and machine-readable mmCIF and XML files. In the next section, we will further discuss various criteria and software used for validation of ligands in the VR.

5.5.1 Various Criteria and Software Used for Validating Ligand in Validation Reports

wwPDB validation criteria for ligands can be broadly divided into two categories (I) geometric validation of the atomic coordinates, without considering the associated

Table 5.2 Summary of the software used for validating ligands in wwPDB validation reports.

Property	Detailed steps involved	Software used	Software URL
Atomic coordinates of all bound ligands	Extracts ligand of interest (LOI) reorder and rename atoms in ligands according to the Chemical Component Dictionary (CCD)	Maxit (Macromolecular Exchange and Input Tool) [50]	https://sw-tools.rcsb.org/apps/MAXIT
Geometric quality	Computes following for all ligands: • Bond-length, bond-angle, torsion angle and ring outliers	Mogul [51]	https://ccdc.cam.ac.uk/solutions/csd-core/components/mogul
	Chirality and planarity outliers	Validation-pack [50]	https://mmcif.wwpdb.org/docs/software-resources.html
2D diagrams of geometric quality	Highlights geometric analysis provided by CCDC Mogul	buster-report [43]	https://www.globalphasing.com/buster/manual/autobuster/manual/autoBUSTER9.html
3D graphical depiction of the model fit to data	Each model fit to experimental electron density is shown from different orientations to approximate a 3D view	buster-report [43]	As above

experimental data, and (II) validation of fit between the atomic coordinates of the ligand and the associated experimental data. The summary of various software used in VR is shown in Table 5.2.

5.5.2 Identification of Ligand of Interest (LOI)

Since 2017, the depositors are required to identify the ligand(s) in the structure that is either the focus of their study or is considered biologically important. This LOI information is recorded during the deposition of structure in the OneDep system [13]. All its details can be found in the "Entry composition" section of the VR. In the VP, Maxit [50] extracts the atomic coordinates of ligand(s), reorder and rename its atoms according to the CCD after which geometric quality of these is assessed further.

5.5.3 Geometric and Conformational Validation

Following the recommendation of wwPDB X-ray VTF, ligand geometry is validated against the Cambridge Structural Database (CSD) of high-quality small molecule organic structure [45]. Firstly, CSD structures with similar bond order are identified and then a distribution for the observed values for each bond length, bond angle, torsion angle, or ring in the ligand is built using the program Mogul [51]. It then computes the Z-score, which quantifies deviation from the observed values. Bond lengths and bond angles with absolute Z-score >2.0 are flagged as "outliers" in the VR. The normalized Z-scores (RMSZ) of bond lengths/angles are calculated to facilitate the overall assessment of the ligand. RMSZ scores are expected to lie between 0 and 1. For low-resolution structures, geometry should be tightly restrained and small values are expected. For very high-resolution structures, values approaching 1 may be attained. Values greater than 1 generally indicate over-fitting of the data. For acyclic torsion angles, Mogul computes the local density measure [52], which is the ratio of incidences in the CSD within 10° of the torsion angle in question, to the number of total incidences of the torsion angles in the CSD. The torsion angle is flagged as an outlier if the local density measure is <5%. For isolated rings, Mogul compares the given ring with comparable rings in small molecule structures in the CSD and calculates an RMSD value based on corresponding constituent torsion angles for each comparable ring. If both the mean and minimum of these RMSDs are >60°, the ring is flagged as an outlier. Chirality outliers are calculated by Validation-pack [14] and are assessed based on chiral volume. If the sign of the computed volume is incorrect, the handedness is wrong. If the absolute volume is less than $0.7 Å^3$, the chiral center is as a planar moiety, which is highly likely to be erroneous. All these geometric outliers are listed in the "Ligand geometry" section of the VR.

Apart from merely identifying the geometric outliers, it is also important to know the extent of distortion from the Mogul expectation. After the latest update of VP [14], this information is now clear in 2D colored images generated by Buster-report [53]. This image depicts Mogul quality analysis of bond lengths, bond angles, torsion angles, and ring geometry [43] and is added to the "Ligand geometry" section of VR. Color scheme used in these images is coded according to validation results with green indicating commonly observed values, magenta indicating unusual values, and grey indicating that there was insufficient data to derive a validation score (see Figure 5.5b). Unusual values include model quality and electron density fit. For model quality, individual bond lengths or angles with absolute Z-score >2, the torsion angle with <5% of local density measure, or RMSD >60° are considered unusual and colored in magenta. These images can be helpful for depositors to identify any putative incorrect restraint values used during refinement before depositing the structure.

5.5.4 Ligand Fit to Experimental Electron Density Validation

Apart from validating the geometric quality of the ligand, it is also crucial to inspect local agreement of a structure model with the observed electron density and

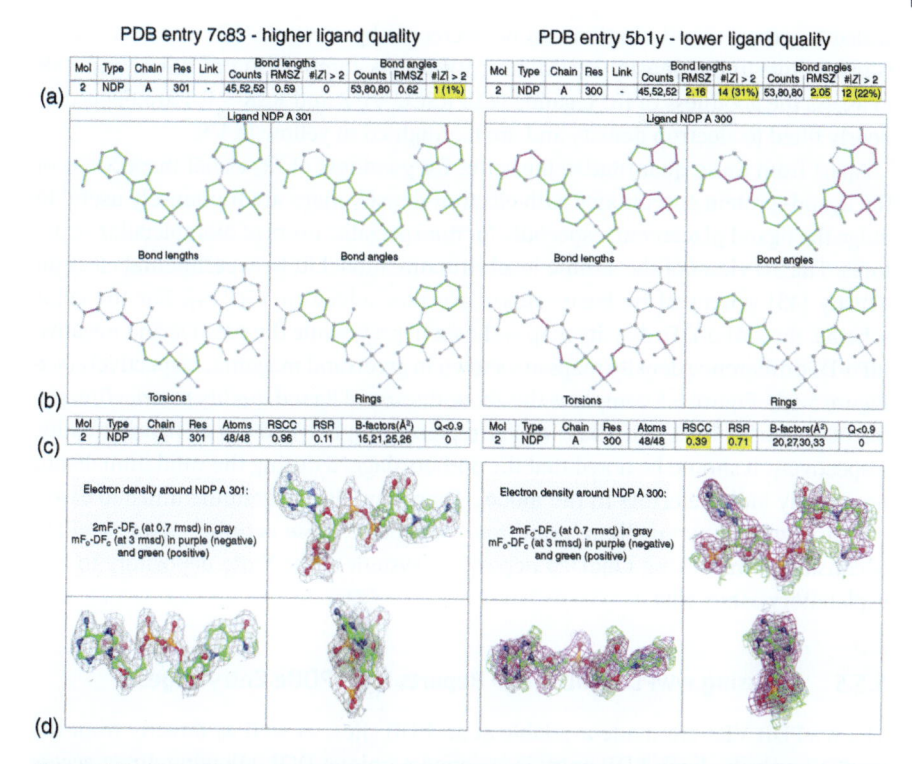

Figure 5.5 Validation assessment metric/images taken from the wwPDB validation reports for the ligand NDP in PDB ID 7c83 and 5b1y representing higher/good and lower/bad ligand geometric quality, respectively. (a) Bond lengths/angles RMSZ and Z score indicating geometric quality (b) 2D image representing ligand geometric quality. Here the commonly observed values are shown in green, while magenta color shows unusual values. Features with insufficient data to derive a validation score are highlighted in grey. (c) RSR and RSCC values indicating model fit to experimental electron density map for the ligand NDP (d) 3D view of atomic model fit to experimental electron density map (shown in grey) for the ligand NDP. Here positive and negative difference density maps are shown in green and magenta, respectively. Outliers in 1A and 1C are highlighted in yellow.

determine the accuracy of ligand placement. wwPDB validation pipeline uses the REFMAC5 program [54] from CCP4 suite to calculate electron density maps based on the coordinates in the entry and deposited experimental X-ray structure factors using a procedure adapted from EDS [55]. To quantify how well the observed and calculated electron density matches, VP computes **Real-Space R** (RSR) value for each residue/ligand in structure using the MAPMAN program [55]. Lower the value of RSR, more closely the observed and calculated electron density matches, thus the residue/ligand fits better to experimental data. RSR value of 0 indicates "perfect agreement" and RSR > 0.4 indicates poor fit or low data resolution. MAPMAN also computes another alternative to RSR, called the **Real Space Correlation Coefficient** (RSCC). RSCC ranges from 1.0 to −1.0 indicating "perfect correlation" to "perfect anticorrelation". The RSR and RSCC values can be found in the "Fit of model and data" section of VR. RSR computation requires the two density maps to be scaled together; this limitation can be overcome by using RSCC. However, RSCC is insensitive to the density level. Thus, VR uses a combination of RSCC and RSR to assess the goodness of fit. Ligands with RSCC < 0.8 and RSR > 0.4 are flagged as poorly fitted to electron density and are highlighted in yellow in VR.

Apart from these quantitative measures for goodness of fit, visual inspections of the ligand–protein coordinates with electron-density maps are immensely useful to judge the ligand placement, especially for nonspecialist users of biomolecular structures. The 3D views of the atomic-level structure model fit to experimental electron density [43] generated by buster-report are now added in VR [14]. For the color scheme, the 2mFo-DFc density map is shown in grey, while the positive and negative mFo-DFc difference density maps are shown in green and magenta, respectively (see Figure 5.5d). Figure 5.5 compares the above discussed ligand quality metrics/images for PDB entries 7c83 and 5b1y, which represent higher and lower ligand quality, respectively. It should be noted that the outliers flagged during the validation do not necessarily indicate errors in the model. These can also be genuine unusual cases, which may be functionally relevant too. To capture these genuine cases, wwPDB is constantly improving OneDep deposition system to facilitate depositors to add explanatory comments.

5.5.5 Accessing wwPDB Validation Reports from PDBe Entry Pages

The wwPDB VRs are made available at all PDB sites, as well as directly from the wwPDB website. Each PDB entry is assigned a unique DOI, allowing direct access to the coordinates and VRs at the wwPDB website. Therefore, you can access the wwPDB page for a specific PDB entry by using the following URL, where [PDB_ID] is the PDB entry ID: https://doi.org/10.2210/pdb[PDB_ID]/pdb. This page contains minimal information about the entry and download links, which includes the VR in either PDF or XML format.

You can also access the VRs from the PDBe entry pages, either by navigating to the specific entry page or directly from the PDBe search results. On the PDBe entry pages, there are options to "view" or "download" files relating to that specific entry. These options include the option to view or download the VR in either PDF or XML format. Furthermore, there is the option to "download files" for an entry in the PDBe search results and this includes download of VR files (Figure 5.6).

5.5.6 Other Planned Improvements to Enhance Ligand Validation

wwPDB validation is being improved continuously with the help of valuable feedback from wwPDB VTFs, depositors, and our diverse community of users. As per the recommendations for LVW, percentile scores for the overall ligand quality will soon be incorporated into the VR [14]. The wwPDB OneDep system was recently modified to record the restraints for ligands used by depositors during the refinement process. Furthermore, these restraint values will be included in VR, where these will be compared with Mogul target values helping users to identify the outliers that do not accord with Mogul assessment. Additionally, the EDS program of VP is being

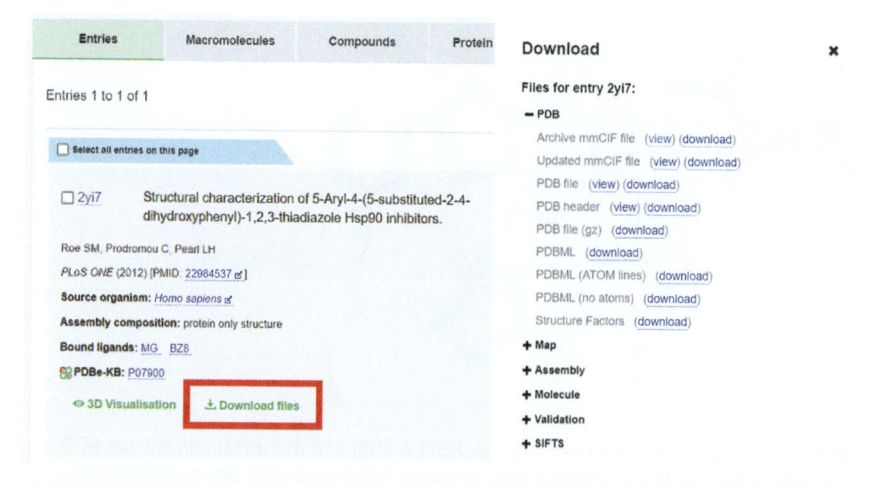

Figure 5.6 Image displaying the download options from the search results on the PDBe pages (PDBe.org).

refactored to use the latest software and as a part of this, MAPMAN program will be replaced by Density-fitness (https://github.com/PDB-REDO/density-fitness).

5.6 PDBe Tools for Ligand Analysis

5.6.1 Ligand Interactions

Approximately three-quarters of PDB entries contain complexes of biomacromolecules (proteins or nucleic acids) and small molecule ligands. These small molecules often have a biological role in the complex; however, they may also exist only as components of the experimental sample buffers. Biologically important small molecules in PDB entries include drugs, cofactors, metabolites, carbohydrates, and lipids. Pipelines developed at PDBe help to distinguish biologically important ligands and provide functional annotations to place them in their biological context (see Section 5.7 for details).

5.6.1.1 Classifying Ligand Interactions

It is important to identify the protonation state of a ligand in order to accurately define and classify its interactions with other molecules. However, the resolution of most PDB structures is not sufficient to support the modeling of hydrogen atoms. Therefore, a process must add hydrogen atoms before the identification of ligand interactions. For protonation of molecular structures, PDBe uses ChimeraX, [56] which supports the input of assembly mmCIF files, representing the whole molecular complex, rather than only the asymmetric unit for crystallographic entries.

After protonation, the PDBe process uses the Arpeggio software [57] to identify ligand interactions. There are four main categories of interactions determined by Arpeggio: (I) atom–atom interactions; (II) atom–plane interactions; (III)

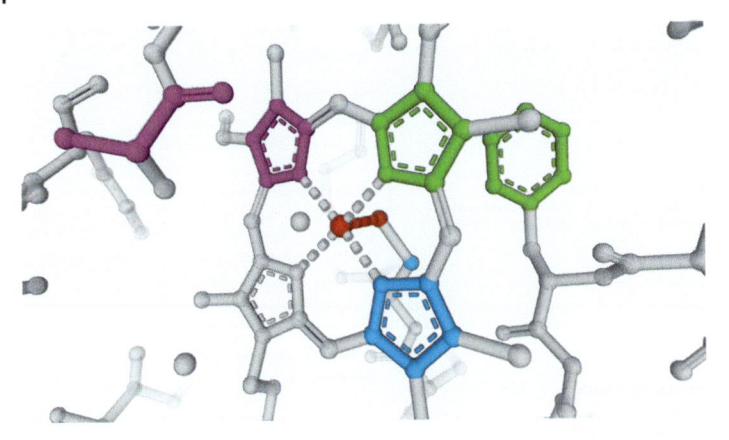

Figure 5.7 Image showing a heme ligand (HEM A 508) and its surroundings from PDB entry 1tqn (pdbe.org/1tqn). The structure is shown in ball and stick representation with atoms and bonds shown in grey by default. The colored atoms represent the following different examples of interactions between the ligand and neighboring amino acids: in red, atom–atom interaction of heme FE with SG atom of Cys 442; in blue, atom–plane interaction of heme atoms C1A, C2A, C3A, C4A, and NA with CB atom of Cys 442; in green, plane–plane interaction of heme atoms C1B, C2B, C3B, C4B, and NB with CD1, CD2, CE1, CE2, CG, and CZ atoms of Phe 435; in magenta, plane–group interaction of heme atoms C1C, C2C, C3C, C4C, and NC with C, CA, N, and O atoms of Ala 305.

plane–plane interactions, and (IV) plane–group interactions. Examples of each of these interactions are displayed in Figure 5.7. For a more comprehensive overview of the molecular interactions identified by Arpeggio, along with their description, please see the supplementary information of the Arpeggio manuscript.

5.6.1.2 Data Availability

Details on molecular interactions are available through the PDBe API (https://pdbe.org/aggregated-api). The API provides atomic-level information for individual ligand instances in a particular PDB entry and residue-level information aggregated for all PDB entries for a specific protein of interest. The protonated biological assemblies are also available through the PDBe ModelServer (https://www.ebi.ac.uk/pdbe/coordinates/index.html), a service, which allows dynamic access to atomic coordinates from PDB entries. Arpeggio uses these assemblies for computing interactions.

5.6.2 Ligand Environment Component

While a trained eye can often intuitively recognize significant partners of the molecular interactions within a binding site, it is helpful to visualize these interactions both in a 2D schematic way, and in a 3D viewer, particularly for less experienced users of PDB data. PDBe provides a schematic interactive visualization of ligand-binding sites in atom-level and residue-level detail that corresponds to the 3D conformation of the binding site. There are two levels of visualization,

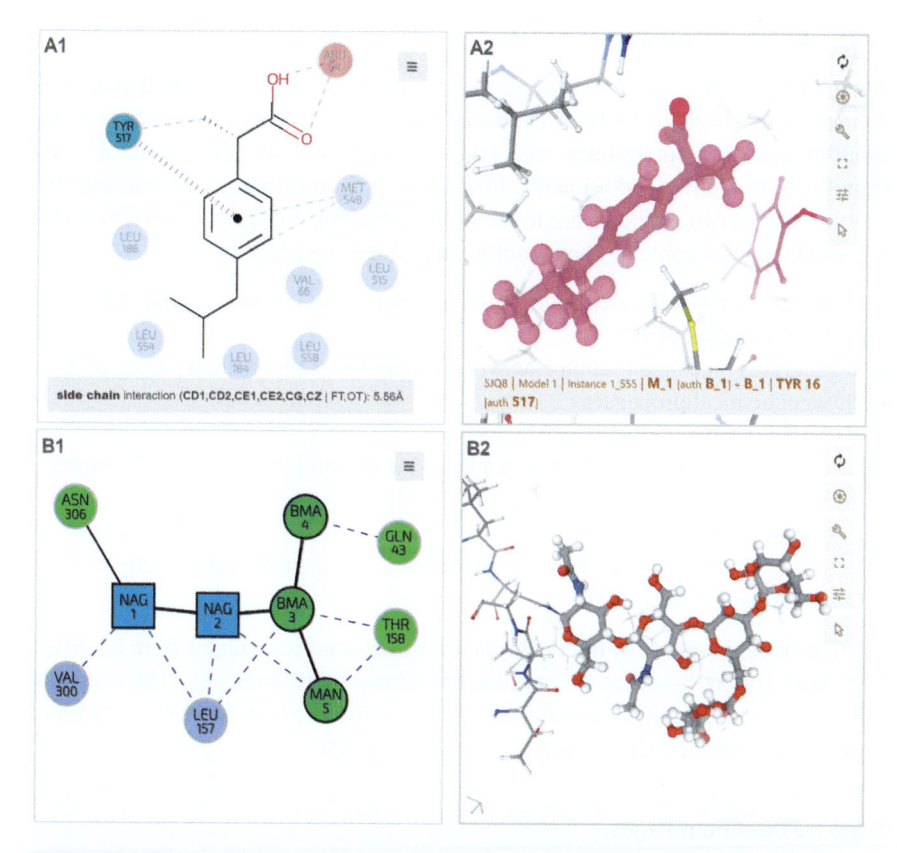

Figure 5.8 A1 and A2 display the binding site of ibuprofen (IBP) in the PDB entry 5jqb with the aromatic stacking interaction highlighted between tyrosine's side chain and phenyl ring in both ligand environment component (A1) and Mol* (A2). B1 and B2 display the binding site of a polysaccharide formed by 2 × NAG and 3 × BMA in the PDB entry 3d12 with SNFG annotations in the ligand environment component (B1) and Mol* (B2).

one for residue-level interactions of polysaccharides and another for atom-level interactions of ligands defined in the wwPDB CCD. This information is available for all PDB entries (Figure 5.8).

The ligand interactions component is interactive and seamlessly communicates with the 3D viewer Mol*[58] to better depict the spatial distribution of the residues forming a binding site. Users can export the underlying interactions from the 2D component in JavaScript Object Notation (JSON) format and the depiction in SVG format. All the ligands with atom-level information are displayed in the same conformation and orientation to support a straightforward comparison of the similar ligands across varying binding sites and PDB entries. Residues forming the binding site are color-coded. This color-coding is consistent with the PDBe-KB aggregated views of proteins pages and follows the Clustal X [59] scheme. Finally, the ligand interaction component depicts known glycans following the recommendations of the SNFG [34].

5.6.3 Chemistry Process and FTP

At the PDBe, there is a weekly process to generate 2D images of the small molecules defined in the wwPDB CCD. This process also produces representations of these small molecules in community-used data formats, which are not available directly from the PDB archive. Additionally, PDBe processes continuously update wwPDB CIF files with further annotations to better place these ligands in their broader chemical and biological context. These additional annotations include:

- Mapping of molecular identifiers to many other popular resources (e.g. ChEMBL [60] and PubChem [61])
- Regenerated "idealized" conformers (lowest energy conformation) using RDKit
- Physicochemical properties
- Murcko scaffolds
- Substructures (fragments) found in a ligand with pointers to three different fragment libraries
- Known synonyms
- Details of the ligand classification, properties, and possible known targets from the DrugBank database [11]

All the files generated by the PDBe chemistry process are available from the PDBe FTP area (http://ftp.ebi.ac.uk/pub/databases/msd/pdbechem_v2). The data are organized hierarchically in a tree-like directory structure (e.g. A/ATP/…). A list of example files for the CCD ID ATP is given in Table 5.3.

5.6.4 PDBeChem Pages

The long-established PDBeChem service (https://pdbe.org/chem) offers a generic browsing interface for all the ligands defined in the wwPDB CCD. A wide range of search options is available from the main page, including search by (I) CCD ID; (II) molecule name; (III) chemical formula; (IV) nonstereo SMILES, and (V) set of predefined fragments.

If the user provides a search input that is not specific to a single ligand ID, PDBeChem returns all results that match the search input as a list of ID codes, with the name, formula, and chemical image displayed. If the user searches for an exact CCD ID or molecule name, or clicks on a specific ligand ID in the search results, the page redirects to an entry page for that ligand.

5.7 Ligand-Related Annotations in the PDBe-KB

5.7.1 Introduction to PDBe-KB

The PDBe-KB (https://pdbe-kb.org) is a collaborative data resource established in 2018 [62]. It is developed and maintained by the PDBe team at EMBL-EBI. The mission of PDBe-KB is to place macromolecular structure data in their biological context, mapping biochemical-, biophysical-, and functional annotations to the

Table 5.3 Example files generated by the PDBe chemistry process for the CCD ID ATP.

Files in the pdbechem_v2 top directory

Filename	File format	Description
chem_comp.list	Text	List of processed wwPDB CCD ids
chem_comp_list.xml	XML	File containing all CCD entries, with additional metadata
components.cif	mmCIF	Aggregated file with all the CCD information
components_inchikeys.csv	CSV	Mapping between wwPDB CCD ids and InChIKey
pdbechem.tar.gz		The complete archive in the *.tar.gz format

Files in the specific chemical component directory (i.e. A/ATP/…)

Filename	File format	Description
ATP.cif	mmCIF	Standard wwPDB CCD file with the following enrichments: UniChem mapping, RDKit regenerated conformer, physicochemical properties, 2D coordinates, scaffolds, fragments, and other details
ATP_ideal.pdb	PDB	Ideal coordinates
ATP_ideal_alt.pdb	PDB	Ideal coordinates with atom alternate names
ATP_model.pdb	PDB	Model coordinates
ATP_model_alt.pdb	PDB	Model coordinates with atom alternate names
ATP_N.svg	SVG	2D depiction in $N \times N$ resolution. Where N is one of (100, 200, 300, 400, and 500)
ATP_N_names.svg	SVG	2D depiction in $N \times N$ resolution with atom names. Where N is one of (100, 200, 300, 400, and 500)
ATP_model.sdf	MOL	Model coordinates
ATP_ideal.sdf	MOL	Ideal coordinates
ATP.cml	CML	Component representation in the CML format
ATP_annotation.json	JSON	2D depiction in "natural format" (i.e. 50 px per 1 Å) with additional annotations. This file is consumed by the ligand environment comp interaction viewer

Table 5.4 Ligand-related annotations in PDBe-KB.

Name of the data provider	Types of annotations	Number of annotated PDB entries
Mechanism and Catalytic Site Atlas [63]	Catalytic sites	1,908
MetalPDB [64]	The biological relevance of bound metals	14,208
Arpeggio [57]	Calculated atomic-level interactions	130,553
canSAR [65]	Predicted druggable pockets	21,767
P2rank [18]	Predicted ligand binding sites	138,820
CATH-FunSites [66]	Predicted functional sites	20,673
3D LigandSite [17]	Predicted ligand binding sites	916
ChannelsDB [67]	Molecular channels	25,351
Covalentizer (in preparation)	Potential covalently binding small molecules	1,693

structural models that are archived in the PDB [1]. It is a collaborative effort between PDBe and an ecosystem of specialist data resources and scientific software that provides pieces of the biological context for proteins and nucleic acids. As of 2021, 31 data providers contribute over 800,000 annotations for over 170,000 PDB entries. These annotations are crucial to understanding the role and mechanism of small molecules that interact with proteins and nucleic acids (Table 5.4). Data providers deposit curated annotations, such as catalytic sites [63] and biologically relevant metal ions [64], and predicted annotations, such as druggable pockets [65] and predicted ligand binding sites [17, 18].

5.7.2 Data Access Mechanisms for Ligand-Related Annotations

Data contributors rely on the PDBe-KB deposition system, which consists of three main components (Figure 5.9): (I) a data exchange format; (II) an FTP area provided by EMBL-EBI; and (III) the data validation and conversion process responsible for the seamless integration of annotations with the core PDB data.

The data exchange format is a schema implemented as a JSON specification developed and maintained by the PDBe-KB consortium of data providers and software developers. It aims to capture the commonality of residue-level annotations by focusing on the minimally necessary amount of meta-information that users require to utilize the deposited annotations. The format captures the annotations of residues, their corresponding probabilities and confidence measures, the underlying evidence as defined by the Evidence Code Ontology [68], and links to where users may find more comprehensive datasets and meta-information that is specific to a given data provider. The schema is open access and is freely available at https://github.com/PDBe-KB/funpdbe-schema.

5.7 Ligand-Related Annotations in the PDBe-KB | 161

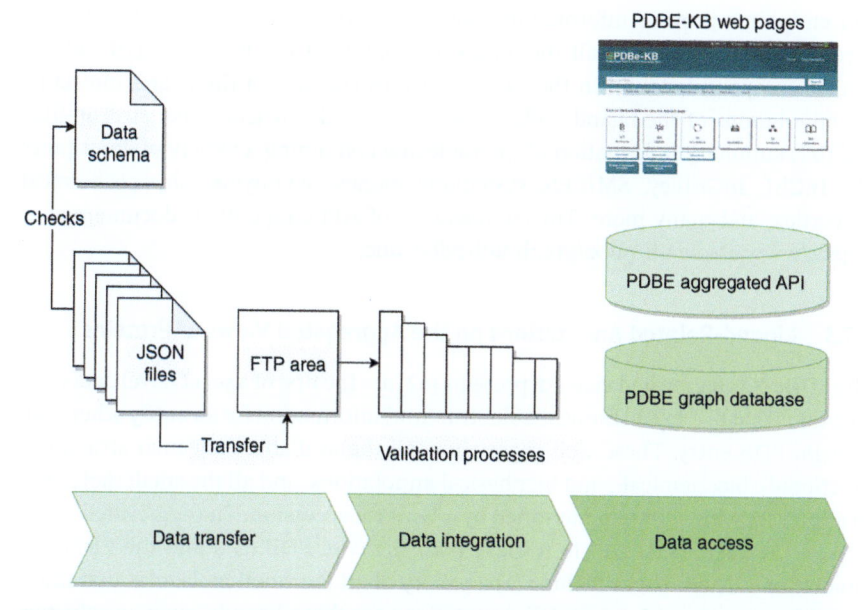

Figure 5.9 Mechanism of data transfer to PDBe-KB: the PDBe-KB consortium members prepare JSON files that record their annotations in a format that complies with the data exchange schema. Depositors transfer these files via File Transfer Protocol (FTP). A set of computational processes parse, validate, and convert the files in preparation for the integration with the core PDB data in the PDBe knowledge graph. The data are publicly accessible via the distributed graph database, the programmatic access points of the PDBe aggregated API, and the PDBe-KB web pages.

Data providers convert their annotations to comply with the data exchange format and transfer them via FTP. PDBe-KB then makes these raw JSON files containing the annotations available to the public at http://ftp.ebi.ac.uk/pub/databases/pdbe-kb/, together with standardized benchmarking datasets that the PDBe-KB consortium collates. The deposited data are used to regenerate the PDBe knowledge graph weekly, ensuring that PDB entries are up-to-date and integrated with the latest PDBe-KB annotations. This process validates the deposited JSON files, converts them into CSV format, and imports them into the PDBe knowledge graph.

The PDBe knowledge graph is a Neo4j (https://neo4j.com/) graph database that stores the core PDB data and PDBe-KB annotations. Users may download the database from https://www.ebi.ac.uk/pdbe/pdbe-kb/graph-download to install it locally and mine the PDBe knowledge graph for macromolecular structures and their ligand molecules, together with their functional annotations. The schema of the graph database is also openly accessible at https://www.ebi.ac.uk/pdbe/pdbe-kb/schema through an interactive schema explorer.

Users can access data from the graph database via a set of 80+ Application Programmatic Interface (API) endpoints. These API endpoints cover all the aspects of the information integrated into the knowledge graph. The endpoints are grouped into categories, such as those related to compounds, proteins (i.e. UniProt accessions), PDB entries or data validation. Specifically, the compound-related

API endpoints provide information about (I) all the PDB entries that contain a particular compound; (II) all the atoms and bonds of the molecule; (III) all the similar compounds found in the PDB; (IV) substructures of the ligand molecule; (V) annotations of the ligand molecule as cofactor-like, reactant-like or drug-like; and (VI) summary information of the molecule containing a variety of descriptors like InChI, InChIkey, SMILES, systematic names, synonyms, physicochemical properties, and many more. The complete set of API endpoints is documented at https://www.ebi.ac.uk/pdbe/graph-api/pdbe_doc.

5.7.3 Ligand-Related Annotations on the Aggregated Views of Proteins

The PDBe-KB aggregated views of proteins [62] are the first of a set of novel data visualizations that display all the available structural information for an entity other than a single PDB entry. These web pages show all the available molecular structures, functional-, biochemical-, and biophysical annotations, and all the small molecules that interact with a protein identified by a UniProt accession. The aggregated views rely on the aggregated API to retrieve both the core PDB data and the PDBe-KB annotations. These pages include (I) a gallery of all the small molecules that interact with a protein of interest; (II) annotations for these ligands, such as cofactors or reactants; (III) residue-level annotations of the binding sites (both experimentally observed/predicted), and (IV) an interactive 3D visualization of all the ligands superposed on all the available PDB structures for a protein of interest.

The "Ligands and Environments" section of these aggregated views contains ligand-related information (Figure 5.10). It has a gallery that displays all the small molecules found directly interacting with the protein of interest or observed in the PDB entry of the protein of interest but interacting with a different protein chain or nucleic acid (Figure 5.10a). The gallery displays a chemical structure of the compound, its 3-letter code ("HET" code in PDB nomenclature), its recommended name, and any available annotations, such as cofactor-like, reactant-like, or drug-like [62, 69]. The ligands are also clustered based on their scaffold, so that similar ligands are grouped together, making visual comparisons more convenient.

Users can download all the PDB entries containing a specific small molecule by clicking on the "download" button from the gallery. Clicking on any 2D representations will open an interactive 3D viewer, Mol* [58], to investigate the binding sites and the ligands in 3D. This section also includes a 2D sequence feature viewer (ProtVista [70]) that displays all the residues of the protein of interest that interact with a specific small molecule (Figure 5.10b). The more frequently and consistently interacting residues have a darker shade of blue, distinguishing them from other nonspecifically interacting residues (shown in light shade of blue). This view enables researchers to identify patterns in the binding events and elucidate common key binding residues at a glance. Finally, users can also download these annotations in CSV or JSON formats.

In addition to displaying individual binding sites using Mol* in the ligand gallery, the aggregated views also provide the option to display a superposed view of all the small molecules from all the PDB entries for a specific protein segment (Figure 5.11).

5.7 Ligand-Related Annotations in the PDBe-KB

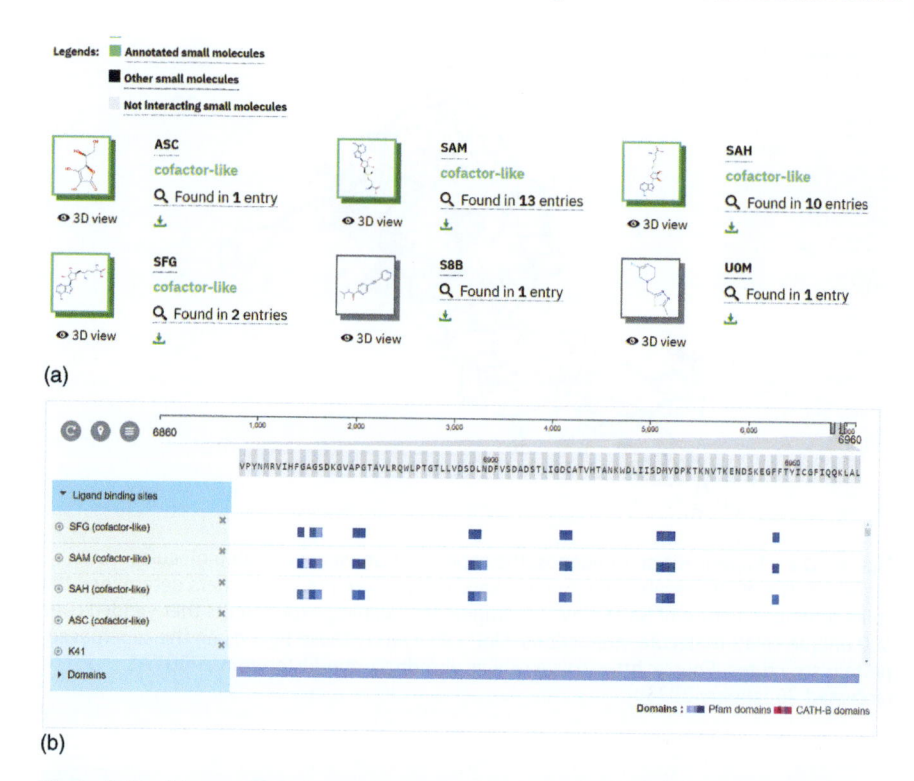

Figure 5.10 Ligand gallery and ligand binding site viewer: the ligand gallery (panel a) displays all the small molecules that interact with any of the processed proteins of the Replicase polyprotein 1ab of SARS-CoV-2 (https://www.ebi.ac.uk/pdbe/pdbe-kb/proteins/P0DTD1). It allows the users to download all the PDB entries that contain both the protein and a particular small molecule. Biologically relevant small molecules, such as cofactors, are displayed in green boxes. The gallery also displays a chemical structure of the ligand, and clicking on these images opens an interactive 3D molecular viewer, Mol*. The sequence feature viewer, ProtVista (panel b), displays all the protein residues, which directly interact with ligands.

This superposed view is available from the summary section of the web page by clicking on the "View all ligands" button. A representative PDB structure from each superposition cluster is displayed by default, together with all the small molecules found in any PDB entries for that segment (residue range). This view is most helpful for proteins where fragment screening experiments identified high numbers of interactions as superposition view can conveniently highlight all the binding pockets.

All the information on the PDBe-KB webpages is powered by the PDBe-KB graph API. Users can use these API endpoints to obtain various ligand-related data in a programmatic manner. For instance, users can get a list of all the ligands similar to the LOI using https://www.ebi.ac.uk/pdbe/graph-api/compound/similarity/:hetcode.

This API endpoint returns stereoisomers, ligands with the same scaffold, and ligands with similarity of over 60% defined by PARITY method [71]. Other API end-points can be explored from https://www.ebi.ac.uk/pdbe/graph-api/pdbe_doc.

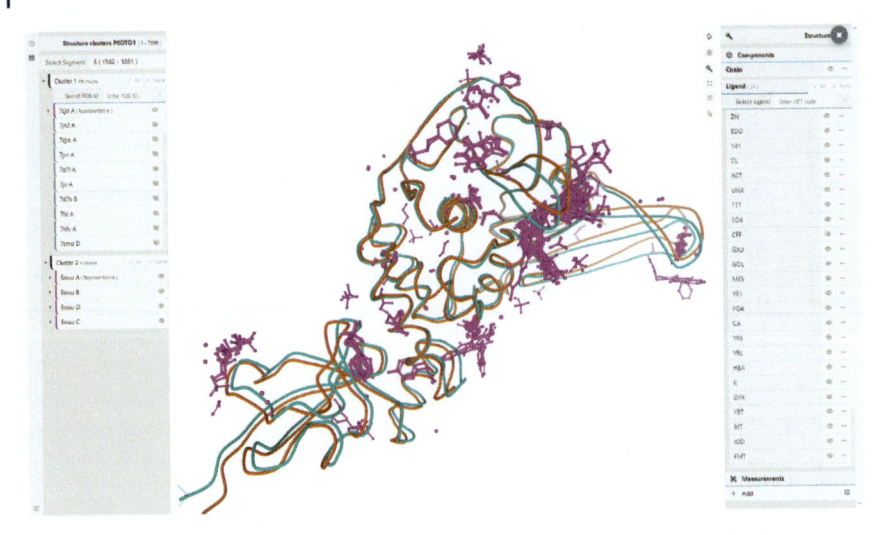

Figure 5.11 Superposition of ligands: the superposition view of small molecules highlights the most prevalent binding pockets. In this example, researchers determined the spike protein structure of SARS-CoV-2 in fragment screening experiments that yielded over 500 unique small molecule interactions. Mol* can overlay these ligands on the superposed protein structures. Source: https://www.ebi.ac.uk/pdbe/pdbe-kb/proteins/P0DTD1 (accessed 26 January 2023).

5.8 Case Study: Using PDB Data to Support Drug Discovery

There are many cases of PDB data being used to support drug discovery [12]. One of the most high-profile, recent cases is the COVID Moonshot consortium, an open-science collaboration aiming to use structure data for drug discovery of antiviral drugs to combat COVID-19 and potential future viral pandemics [72–77]. This worldwide consortium integrates several approaches to support the drug discovery process, based on data from structural biology, biochemistry, and molecular simulations, leading to identification of compounds that could be suitable for advancing into clinical trials.

The COVID Moonshot campaign focuses specifically on collecting data relating to the main protease protein (Mpro) from SARS-CoV-2, the virus that causes COVID-19 [74, 75]. This protein is required for processing of polyproteins and thus generation of all mature proteins in all coronaviruses. This is therefore a key target for disrupting viral activity and has the potential for generation of broad-spectrum antivirals acting across a number of different organisms.

Furthermore, the structure of Mpro was the first from SARS-CoV-2 to be made available in the PDB archive in early 2020, solved by Zihe Rao's group and colleagues in China [78]. This availability of experimental structural biology data, and the shared knowledge of how to effectively generate crystals of Mpro, allowed further structural biology, including fragment screening experiments, to proceed at pace

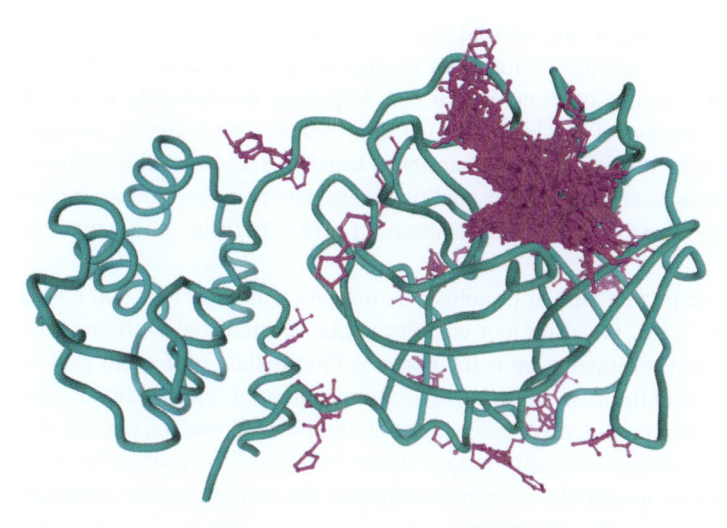

Figure 5.12 Aggregated structure data from PDBe-KB for a single protein chain of Mpro from SARS-CoV-2. Protein chain is displayed as ribbon and colored green, with a selection of bound ligands from fragment screening experiments displayed as ball and stick and colored pink. Data from pdbekb.org/proteins/P0DTD1.

[73]. This led to the identification of numerous chemical fragments that were further assayed to identify binding affinities (Figure 5.12).

After the identification of this host of chemical fragments that bound to Mpro, a number of other methods were used to enhance the compounds and support faster drug development. This included creation of an online crowdsourcing platform to allow worldwide participants to submit their own compound designs, based on these fragment screening hits [77]. The consortium also leveraged the use of machine learning techniques in order to design new compounds optimized for activity against SARS-CoV-2 Mpro [74]. In addition, another computational pipeline, covalentizer, was developed and used to identify modification to compounds that would allow covalent attachment to nearby cysteine residues to cause inhibition [75].

All these efforts have led to the rapid identification of a number of promising antiviral therapeutics, with the first of these now progressing to preclinical evaluation [77]. Despite this success, the consortium continues to pursue other potential compounds across different structural groups. Furthermore, they are making all data freely available, and all relevant compounds can be purchased from consortium partners. The hope is that this method of open data and collaboration in drug discovery will open up development of new drugs across more diseases, faster and more affordably than ever before [77].

5.9 Conclusions and Outlook

As the PDB archive continues to expand, both in quantity and diversity of structures, it becomes an increasingly valuable resource for drug design [12]. Furthermore, in addition to knowledge being derived directly from macromolecular structures in the PDB, this data are also being used to improve prediction of novel structures [79, 80]. Prediction of protein folds has improved dramatically in recent years, thanks to the use of machine learning approaches, which are increasingly successful thanks to the quality and quantity of training datasets available in the PDB [81, 82]. Thousands of these high-quality protein structure predictions are now publicly available from the AlphaFold Database at EMBL-EBI (https://alphafold.ebi.ac.uk) [83].

Despite these improvements in protein structure prediction, there is still a long way to go before large, novel protein complexes can be predicted with any confidence, though improvements are being made to the prediction of small protein complexes [84]. In addition, even the most accurate computational predictions are not precise enough to confidently model ligand binding sites, therefore, making this improvement of limited use for drug design. Therefore, it is still critical that the PDB provide high-quality, accessible structures to support the computational chemistry community and support drug discovery.

The data and tools provided by PDBe and PDBe-KB support researchers by providing a means to easily interpret binding sites in macromolecules, and validate this information based on experimental data. The standardization of small molecule information allows the easy comparison of binding sites across multiple structures and comparison of interactions between related small molecules. The visualization tools developed at PDBe and PDBe-KB allow users to easily interpret the data, guiding future research and developments in drug design.

5.9.1 Upcoming Features and Improvements

The team at PDBe-KB is currently working on the development of the PDBe-KB aggregated views of ligands. Following the same principles as the aggregated views of proteins, these pages will collate all the available data in the PDB for specific ligands of interest. This will allow users to easily find all the structures containing a specific ligand and view common interactions made by that ligand across multiple PDB entries. These pages will also highlight similar, related ligands in the PDB that share common scaffolds, while also providing a host of ligand properties and links to additional resources for even more in-depth analysis. The first iteration of the aggregated views of ligands is due to be released in late 2023.

Another project that is underway and aims to support the drug design community is the BioChemGraph project. This project is a collaboration between PDBe [4], ChEMBL [54], and Cambridge Crystallographic Data Center (CCDC) [45], and aims to improve the integration of data between these three vital chemistry resources. This collaboration will help to increase the coverage of ligand information beyond what is available in the PDB, while also adding even more functional annotations for small molecule ligands. Through the BioChemGraph project and the aggregated views of ligands, we aim to greatly improve access and interpretation of chemistry data in the PDB.

References

1 wwPDB Consortium (2019). Protein Data Bank: the single global archive for 3D macromolecular structure data. *Nucleic Acids Research* 47 (D1): D520–D528. https://doi.org/10.1093/nar/gky949.

2 Berman, H., Henrick, K., Nakamura, H., and Markley, J.L. (2007). The worldwide Protein Data Bank (wwPDB): ensuring a single, uniform archive of PDB data. *Nucleic Acids Research* 35 (SUPPL): 1. https://doi.org/10.1093/nar/gkl971.

3 Burley, S.K., Bhikadiya, C., Bi, C. et al. (2021). RCSB Protein Data Bank: powerful new tools for exploring 3D structures of biological macromolecules for basic and applied research and education in fundamental biology, biomedicine, biotechnology, bioengineering and energy sciences. *Nucleic Acids Research* 49 (D1): D437–D451. https://doi.org/10.1093/NAR/GKAA1038.

4 Armstrong, D.R., Berrisford, J.M., Conroy, M.J. et al. (2020). PDBe: improved findability of macromolecular structure data in the PDB. *Nucleic Acids Research* 48 (D1): D335–D343. https://doi.org/10.1093/NAR/GKZ990.

5 Kinjo, A.R., Bekker, G.J., Wako, H. et al. (2018). New tools and functions in data-out activities at Protein Data Bank Japan (PDBj). *Protein Science* 27 (1): 95–102. https://doi.org/10.1002/pro.3273.

6 Lawson, C.L., Patwardhan, A., Baker, M.L. et al. (2016). EMDataBank unified data resource for 3DEM. *Nucleic Acids Research* 44 (D1): D396–D403. https://doi.org/10.1093/nar/gkv1126.

7 Ulrich, E.L., Akutsu, H., Doreleijers, J.F. et al. (2008). BioMagResBank. *Nucleic Acids Research* 36 (SUPPL): 1. https://doi.org/10.1093/nar/gkm957.

8 Wilkinson, M.D., Dumontier, M., Jan Aalbersberg, I. et al. (2016). The FAIR guiding principles for scientific data management and stewardship. *Scientific Data* 3 (1): 1–9. https://doi.org/10.1038/sdata.2016.18.

9 Bourne, P.E., Berman, H.M., McMahon, B. et al. (1997). Macromolecular crystallographic information file. *Methods in Enzymology* 277: 571–590. https://doi.org/10.1016/S0076-6879(97)77032-0.

10 Adams, P.D., Afonine, P.V., Baskaran, K. et al. (2019). Announcing mandatory submission of PDBx/mmCIF format files for crystallographic depositions to the protein data bank (PDB). *Acta Crystallographica Section D: Structural Biology* 75. Wiley-Blackwell: 451–454. https://doi.org/10.1107/S2059798319004522.

11 Wishart, D.S., Knox, C., Guo, A.C. et al. (2006). DrugBank: a comprehensive resource for in silico drug discovery and exploration. *Nucleic Acids Research* 34 (Database Issue): D668-72. https://doi.org/10.1093/NAR/GKJ067.

12 Westbrook, J.D. and Burley, S.K. (2019). How structural biologists and the Protein Data Bank contributed to recent FDA new drug approvals. *Structure* 27 (2): 211–217. https://doi.org/10.1016/J.STR.2018.11.007.

13 Young, J.Y., Westbrook, J.D., Feng, Z. et al. (2017). OneDep: unified wwPDB system for deposition, biocuration, and validation of macromolecular structures in the PDB archive. *Structure* 25 (3): 536–545. https://doi.org/10.1016/j.str.2017.01.004.

14 Feng, Z., Westbrook, J.D., Sala, R. et al. (2021). Enhanced validation of small-molecule ligands and carbohydrates in the Protein Data Bank. *Structure* 29 (4): 393–400.e1. https://doi.org/10.1016/J.STR.2021.02.004.

15 Varadi, M., Anyango, S., Armstrong, D. et al. (2021). PDBe-KB: collaboratively defining the biological context of structural data. *Nucleic Acids Research* 50 (D1): D534–D542. https://doi.org/10.1093/NAR/GKAB988.

16 Mitsopoulos, C., di Micco, P., Fernandez, E.V. et al. (2021). CanSAR: update to the cancer translational research and drug discovery knowledgebase. *Nucleic Acids Research* 49 (D1): D1074–D1082. https://doi.org/10.1093/NAR/GKAA1059.

17 Wass, M.N., Kelley, L.A., and Sternberg, M.J.E. (2010). 3DLigandSite: predicting ligand-binding sites using similar structures. *Nucleic Acids Research* 38 (Web Server Issue): W469–W473. https://doi.org/10.1093/NAR/GKQ406.

18 Krivák, R. and Hoksza, D. (2018). P2Rank: machine learning based tool for rapid and accurate prediction of ligand binding sites from protein structure. *Journal of Cheminformatics* 10 (1): 1–12. https://doi.org/10.1186/S13321-018-0285-8/TABLES/4.

19 Velankar, S., Van Ginkel, G., Alhroub, Y. et al. (2016). PDBe: improved accessibility of macromolecular structure data from PDB and EMDB. *Nucleic Acids Research* 44 (D1): D385–D395. https://doi.org/10.1093/nar/gkv1047.

20 Nair, S., Váradi, M., Nadzirin, N. et al. (2021). PDBe Aggregated API: programmatic access to an integrative knowledge graph of molecular structure data. *Bioinformatics* 37 (21): 3950–3952. https://doi.org/10.1093/BIOINFORMATICS/BTAB424.

21 Kühlbrandt, W. (2014). The resolution revolution. *Science* 343 (6178): 1443–1444. https://doi.org/10.1126/SCIENCE.1251652/ASSET/71F1CC4C-5202-4323-A43C-1F8F1197BD97/ASSETS/GRAPHIC/343_1443_F1.JPEG.

22 Reif, B., Ashbrook, S.E., Emsley, L., and Hong, M. (2021). Solid-state NMR spectroscopy. *Nature Reviews Methods Primers* 1 (1): 1–23. https://doi.org/10.1038/s43586-020-00002-1.

23 Blakeley, M.P., Langan, P., Niimura, N., and Podjarny, A. (2008). Neutron crystallography: opportunities, challenges, and limitations. *Current Opinion in Structural Biology* 18 (5): 593. https://doi.org/10.1016/J.SBI.2008.06.009.

24 Badger, J. (2012). Crystallographic fragment screening. *Methods in Molecular Biology* 841: 161–177. https://doi.org/10.1007/978-1-61779-520-6_7.

25 Pearce, N.M., Krojer, T., Bradley, A.R. et al. (2017). A multi-crystal method for extracting obscured crystallographic states from conventionally uninterpretable electron density. *Nature Communications* 8 (1): 1–8. https://doi.org/10.1038/ncomms15123.

26 Westbrook, J.D., Shao, C., Feng, Z. et al. (2015). The chemical component dictionary: complete descriptions of constituent molecules in experimentally determined 3D macromolecules in the Protein Data Bank. *Bioinformatics* 31 (8): 1274–1278. https://doi.org/10.1093/bioinformatics/btu789.

27 Hoffmann-Ostenhof, O., Cohn, W.E., Braunstein, A.E. et al. (2002). A one-letter notation for amino acid sequences. Tentative rules. *Biochemistry* 7 (8): 2703–2705. https://doi.org/10.1021/BI00848A001.

28 Hawkins, P.C.D., Skillman, A.G., and Nicholls, A. (2007). Comparison of shape-matching and docking as virtual screening tools. *Journal of Medicinal Chemistry* 50 (1): 74–82. https://doi.org/10.1021/JM0603365/SUPPL_FILE/JM0603365SI20061004_124557.PDF.

29 Young, J.Y., Feng, Z., Dimitropoulos, D. et al. (2013). Chemical annotation of small and peptide-like molecules at the Protein Data Bank. *Database* 2013: https://doi.org/10.1093/DATABASE/BAT079.

30 Dutta, S., Dimitropoulos, D., Feng, Z. et al. (2014). Improving the representation of peptide-like inhibitor and antibiotic molecules in the Protein Data Bank. *Biopolymers* 101 (6): 659–668. https://doi.org/10.1002/BIP.22434.

31 Young, J.Y., Westbrook, J.D., Feng, Z. et al. (2018). Worldwide Protein Data Bank biocuration supporting open access to high-quality 3D structural biology data. *Database* 2018 (2018): https://doi.org/10.1093/database/bay002.

32 wwPDB, "PDBx/mmCIF Dictionary Resources," *wwPDB website*. https://mmcif.wwpdb.org/ (accessed 6 December 2021).

33 Shao, C., Feng, Z., Westbrook, J.D. et al. (2021). Modernized uniform representation of carbohydrate molecules in the Protein Data Bank. *Glycobiology* 31 (9): 1204–1218. https://doi.org/10.1093/GLYCOB/CWAB039.

34 Varki, A., Cummings, R.D., Aebi, M. et al. (2015). Symbol nomenclature for graphical representations of glycans. *Glycobiology* 25 (12): 1323–1324. https://doi.org/10.1093/GLYCOB/CWV091.

35 Neelamegham, S., Aoki-Kinoshita, K., Bolton, E. et al. (2019). Updates to the symbol nomenclature for glycans guidelines. *Glycobiology* 29 (9): 620–624. https://doi.org/10.1093/GLYCOB/CWZ045.

36 Thieker, D.F., Hadden, J.A., Schulten, K., and Woods, R.J. (2016). 3D implementation of the symbol nomenclature for graphical representation of glycans. *Glycobiology* 26 (8): 786–787. https://doi.org/10.1093/GLYCOB/CWW076.

37 Kleywegt, G.J. and Jones, T.A. (1998). Databases in protein crystallography. *Acta Crystallographica. Section D, Biological Crystallography* 54 (Pt 6 Pt 1): 1119–1131. https://doi.org/10.1107/S0907444998007100.

38 Kleywegt, G.J., Henrick, K., Dodson, E.J., and Van Aalten, D.M.F. (2003). Pound-wise but penny-foolish: how well do micromolecules fare in macromolecular refinement? *Structure* 11 (9): 1051–1059. https://doi.org/10.1016/S0969-2126(03)00186-2.

39 Kleywegt, G.J. (2007). Quality control and validation. *Methods in Molecular Biology (Clifton, N.J.)* 364: 255–272. https://doi.org/10.1385/1-59745-266-1:255.

40 Davis, A.M., St-Gallay, S.A., and Kleywegt, G.J. (2008). Limitations and lessons in the use of X-ray structural information in drug design. *Drug Discovery Today* 13 (19–20): 831–841. https://doi.org/10.1016/J.DRUDIS.2008.06.006.

41 Liebeschuetz, J., Hennemann, J., Olsson, T., and Groom, C.R. (2012). The good, the bad and the twisted: a survey of ligand geometry in protein crystal structures. *Journal of Computer-Aided Molecular Design* 26 (2): 169–183. https://doi.org/10.1007/S10822-011-9538-6.

42 Pozharski, E., Weichenberger, C.X., and Rupp, B. (2013). Techniques, tools and best practices for ligand electron-density analysis and results from their application to deposited crystal structures. *Acta Crystallographica. Section D, Biological Crystallography* 69 (2): 150–167. https://doi.org/10.1107/S0907444912044423.

43 Smart, O.S. and Bricogne, G. (2015). Achieving high quality ligand chemistry in protein-ligand crystal structures for drug design. *NATO Science for Peace and Security Series A: Chemistry and Biology* 38: 165–181. https://doi.org/10.1007/978-94-017-9719-1_13.

44 Deller, M.C. and Rupp, B. (2015). Models of protein-ligand crystal structures: trust, but verify. *Journal of Computer-Aided Molecular Design* 29 (9): 817–836. https://doi.org/10.1007/S10822-015-9833-8.

45 Read, R.J., Adams, P.D., Arendall, W.B. et al. (2011). A new generation of crystallographic validation tools for the Protein Data Bank. *Structure* 19 (10): 1395–1412. https://doi.org/10.1016/J.STR.2011.08.006/ATTACHMENT/E8FC7B5B-D2ED-4050-BABE-4974B4E60BE0/MMC1.PDF.

46 Montelione, G.T., Nilges, M., Bax, A. et al. (2013). Recommendations of the wwPDB NMR validation task force. *Structure* 21 (9): 1563–1570. https://doi.org/10.1016/J.STR.2013.07.021.

47 Henderson, R., Sali, A., Baker, M.L. et al. (2012). Outcome of the first electron microscopy validation task force meeting. *Structure(London, England:1993)* 20–330 (2): 205. https://doi.org/10.1016/J.STR.2011.12.014.

48 Adams, P.D., Aertgeerts, K., Bauer, C. et al. (2016). Outcome of the first wwPDB/CCDC/D3R ligand validation workshop. *Structure* 24 (4): 502–508. https://doi.org/10.1016/J.STR.2016.02.017.

49 Gore, S., Sanz García, E., Hendrickx, P.M.S. et al. (2017). Validation of structures in the Protein Data Bank. *Structure* 25 (12): 1916–1927. https://doi.org/10.1016/j.str.2017.10.009.

50 Feng, Z., Hsieh, S.-H., Gelbin, A., and Westbrook, J. (1998). MAXIT: macromolecular exchange and input tool. https://sw-tools.rcsb.org/apps/MAXIT/index.html

51 Bruno, I.J., Cole, J.C., Kessler, M. et al. (2004). Retrieval of crystallographically-derived molecular geometry information. *Journal of Chemical Information and Computer Sciences* 44 (6): 2133–2144. https://doi.org/10.1021/CI049780B.

52 Groom, C.R., Bruno, I.J., Lightfoot, M.P., and Ward, S.C. (2016). The Cambridge structural database. *Acta Crystallographica. Section B: Structural Science, Crystal Engineering and Materials* 72 (2): 171–179. https://doi.org/10.1107/S2052520616003954.

53 Global Phasing Ltd. (2011). BUSTER-Report,. https://www.globalphasing.com/BUSTER/wiki/index.cgi?BusterReport (accessed 8 December 2021).

54 Murshudov, G.N., Skubák, P., Lebedev, A.A. et al. (2011). REFMAC5 for the refinement of macromolecular crystal structures. *Acta Crystallographica Section D: Biological Crystallography* 67 (4): 355–367. https://doi.org/10.1107/S0907444911001314.

55 Kleywegt, G.J., Harris, M.R., Zou, J.Y. et al. (2004). The uppsala electron-density server. *Acta Crystallographica. Section D, Biological Crystallography* 60 (Pt 12 Pt 1): 2240–2249. https://doi.org/10.1107/S0907444904013253.

56 Pettersen, E.F., Goddard, T.D., Huang, C.C. et al. (2021). UCSF ChimeraX: structure visualization for researchers, educators, and developers. *Protein Science* 30 (1): 70–82. https://doi.org/10.1002/PRO.3943.

57 Jubb, H.C., Higueruelo, A.P., Ochoa-Montaño, B. et al. (2017). Arpeggio: a web server for calculating and visualising interatomic interactions in protein structures. *Journal of Molecular Biology* 429 (3): 365–371. https://doi.org/10.1016/J.JMB.2016.12.004.

58 Sehnal, D., Bittrich, S., Deshpande, M. et al. (2021). Mol* viewer: modern web app for 3D visualization and analysis of large biomolecular structures. *Nucleic Acids Research* 49 (W1): W431–W437. https://doi.org/10.1093/NAR/GKAB314.

59 Thompson, J.D., Gibson, T.J., Plewniak, F. et al. (1997). The CLUSTAL_X windows interface: flexible strategies for multiple sequence alignment aided by quality analysis tools. *Nucleic Acids Research* 25 (24): 4876–4882. https://doi.org/10.1093/NAR/25.24.4876.

60 Davies, M., Nowotka, M., Papadatos, G. et al. (2015). ChEMBL web services: streamlining access to drug discovery data and utilities. *Nucleic Acids Research* 43 (W1): W612–W620. https://doi.org/10.1093/NAR/GKV352.

61 Kim, S., Chen, J., Cheng, T. et al. (2021). PubChem in 2021: new data content and improved web interfaces. *Nucleic Acids Research* 49 (D1): D1388–D1395. https://doi.org/10.1093/NAR/GKAA971.

62 Varadi, M., Berrisford, J., Deshpande, M. et al. (2020). PDBe-KB: a community-driven resource for structural and functional annotations. *Nucleic Acids Research* 48 (D1): D344–D353. https://doi.org/10.1093/NAR/GKZ853.

63 Ribeiro, A.J.M., Holliday, G.L., Furnham, N. et al. (2018). Mechanism and Catalytic Site Atlas (M-CSA): a database of enzyme reaction mechanisms and active sites. *Nucleic Acids Research* 46 (D1): D618–D623. https://doi.org/10.1093/NAR/GKX1012.

64 Putignano, V., Rosato, A., Banci, L., and Andreini, C. (2018). MetalPDB in 2018: a database of metal sites in biological macromolecular structures. *Nucleic Acids Research* 46 (D1): D459–D464. https://doi.org/10.1093/NAR/GKX989.

65 Coker, E.A., Mitsopoulos, C., Tym, J.E. et al. (2019). canSAR: update to the cancer translational research and drug discovery knowledgebase. *Nucleic Acids Research* 47 (D1): D917–D922. https://doi.org/10.1093/NAR/GKY1129.

66 Ashford, P., Pang, C.S.M., Moya-García, A.A. et al. (2019). A CATH domain functional family based approach to identify putative cancer driver genes and driver mutations. *Scientific Reports* 9 (1): 263–263. https://doi.org/10.1038/S41598-018-36401-4.

67 Lukáš, L., Sehnal, D., Svobodová, R. et al. (2018). ChannelsDB: database of biomacromolecular tunnels and pores. *Nucleic Acids Research* 46 (D1): D399–D405. https://doi.org/10.1093/NAR/GKX868.

68 Chibucos, M.C., Mungall, C.J., Balakrishnan, R. et al. (2014). Standardized description of scientific evidence using the Evidence Ontology (ECO). *Database:*

The Journal of Biological Databases and Curation 2014: 1–11. https://doi.org/10.1093/DATABASE/BAU075.

69 Mukhopadhyay, A., Borkakoti, N., Pravda, L. et al. (2019). Finding enzyme cofactors in Protein Data Bank. *Bioinformatics* 35 (18): 3510–3511. https://doi.org/10.1093/bioinformatics/btz115.

70 Watkins, X., Garcia, L.J., Pundir, S., and Martin, M.J. (2017). ProtVista: visualization of protein sequence annotations. *Bioinformatics* 33 (13): 2040–2041. https://doi.org/10.1093/BIOINFORMATICS/BTX120.

71 Tyzack, J.D., Fernando, L., Ribeiro, A.J.M. et al. (2018). Ranking enzyme structures in the PDB by bound ligand similarity to biological substrates. *Structure* 26 (4): 565–571.e3. https://doi.org/10.1016/J.STR.2018.02.009.

72 Chodera, J., Lee, A.A., London, N., and von Delft, F. (2020). Crowdsourcing drug discovery for pandemics. *Nature Chemistry* 12 (7): 581–581. https://doi.org/10.1038/s41557-020-0496-2.

73 von Delft, F., Calmiano, M., Chodera, J. et al. (2021). A white-knuckle ride of open COVID drug discovery. *Nature* 594 (7863): 330–332. https://doi.org/10.1038/d41586-021-01571-1.

74 Morris, A., McCorkindale, W., Drayman, N. et al. (2021). Discovery of SARS-CoV-$_2$ main protease inhibitors using a synthesis-directed de novo design model. *Chem Commun (Camb)* 57 (48): 5909–5912. https://doi.org/10.1039/D1CC00050K.

75 Zaidman, D., Gehrtz, P., Filep, M. et al. (2021). An automatic pipeline for the design of irreversible derivatives identifies a potent SARS-CoV-$_2$ M^{pro} inhibitor. *Cell Chemical Biology* 28 (12): 1795–1806.e5. https://doi.org/10.1016/J.CHEMBIOL.2021.05.018/ATTACHMENT/20E5CE23-8FF0-4E1E-8F48-160104D17600/MMC4.XLSX.

76 Saar, K.L., Fearon, D., Consortium, T.C.M. et al. (2021). Turning high-throughput structural biology into predictive inhibitor design. *bioRxiv* e2214168120. https://doi.org/10.1101/2021.10.15.464568.

77 Consortium, T.C.M., Achdout, H., Aimon, A. et al. (2022). Open science discovery of oral non-covalent SARS-CoV-2 main protease inhibitor therapeutics. *bioRxiv* https://doi.org/10.1101/2020.10.29.339317.

78 Jin, Z., Du, X., Xu, Y. et al. (2020). Structure of M pro from SARS-CoV-$_2$ and discovery of its inhibitors. *Nature* 582 (7811): 289–293. https://doi.org/10.1038/S41586-020-2223-Y.

79 Jumper, J., Evans, R., Pritzel, A. et al. (2021). Highly accurate protein structure prediction with AlphaFold. *Nature* 596 (7873): 583–589. https://doi.org/10.1038/s41586-021-03819-2.

80 Baek, M., DiMaio, F., Anishchenko, I. et al. (2021). Accurate prediction of protein structures and interactions using a three-track neural network. *Science (1979)* 373 (6557): 871–876. https://doi.org/10.1126/SCIENCE.ABJ8754/SUPPL_FILE/ABJ8754_MDAR_REPRODUCIBILITY_CHECKLIST.PDF.

81 Simpkin, A.J., Sánchez Rodríguez, F., Mesdaghi, S. et al. (2021). Evaluation of model refinement in CASP14. *Proteins* 89 (12): https://doi.org/10.1002/PROT.26185.

82 Alexander, L.T., Lepore, R., Kryshtafovych, A. et al. (2021). Target highlights in CASP14: analysis of models by structure providers. *Proteins* 89 (12): https://doi.org/10.1002/PROT.26247.
83 Varadi, M., Anyango, S., Deshpande, M. et al. (2021, https://doi.org/10.1093/NAR/GKAB1061). AlphaFold protein structure database: massively expanding the structural coverage of protein-sequence space with high-accuracy models. *Nucleic Acids Research* 50 (D1): D439–D444.
84 Evans, R. O'Neill, M., Pritzel, A., et al. (2021). Protein complex prediction with AlphaFold-Multimer, *bioRxiv*, 2021-10.

6

The SWISS-MODEL Repository of 3D Protein Structures and Models

Xavier Robin[1,2], Andrew Mark Waterhouse[1,2], Stefan Bienert[1,2], Gabriel Studer[1,2], Leila T. Alexander[1,2], Gerardo Tauriello[1,2], Torsten Schwede[1,2], and Joana Pereira[1,2]

[1] *University of Basel, Biozentrum, Spitalstrasse 41, 4056, Basel, Switzerland*
[2] *SIB Swiss Institute of Bioinformatics, Computational Structural Biology, Spitalstrasse 41, 4056, Basel, Switzerland*

6.1 Introduction

Computer-Aided Structure-based Drug Design (SBDD) is the branch of Computer-Aided Drug Design, where the three-dimensional (3D) structure of a target protein is used to guide the computational design of drug-like molecules that strongly interact with it [1, 2]. Experimental structure determination has been the prime method for acquiring 3D structural information of targets for SBDD and the Protein Data Bank (PDB) [3] has been the major source of experimentally determined structures of proteins and their complexes. Since its origins in 1971, it archives and provides access to 3D macromolecular structures resulting from various biophysical methods such as X-ray crystallography, Nuclear Magnetic Resonance (NMR) spectroscopy, or Electron Microscopy (EM). The continuous development of such techniques, together with the availability of high-throughput methods for large-scale protein structure determination [4–6], promoted a rapid increase in the number of protein structures deposited in the PDB, with more than 192,000 available as of July 2022.

Despite this rapid increase, this number only represents a small fraction of all naturally occurring proteins. The rate by which protein sequence data becomes available is much higher than the rate by which proteins can be experimentally characterized, and computational structural modeling is the method of choice to cover this knowledge gap [7]. More recently, computational structure prediction methods became commonly applied in SBDD [8–10]. Over the last decades, two different computational structure prediction approaches emerged: (i) comparative methods based on homology [11] and (ii) *ab initio* techniques [12]. While homology-based modeling relies on the identification of a protein of known

Authors **Xavier Robin** and **Joana Pereira** contributed equally to this work

Open Access Databases and Datasets for Drug Discovery, First Edition.
Edited by Antoine Daina, Michael Przewosny, and Vincent Zoete.
© 2024 WILEY-VCH GmbH. Published 2024 by WILEY-VCH GmbH.

structure that is evolutionarily related to the desired target and using it as a template for modeling, *ab initio* methods exploit the sampling of structural fragments [13, 14], molecular dynamics [15], distance predictions from coevolution signals in deep multiple sequence alignments [16], or deep learning-based techniques [17, 18], to infer protein 3D models.

As the PDB is dedicated solely to archiving experimentally determined structures [19], published computational models generated by such approaches are usually stored in dedicated repositories, such as ModelArchive (https://www.modelarchive.org/) [20]. The increasing availability of high-performance computing facilities in both the academic and industrial sectors, as well as algorithmic improvements, considerably shortened computation time and allowed for the construction of high-throughput protein structure prediction pipelines whose results have extensive applications, including virtual screening. To make better use of computing time and provide easy access to high-quality, precomputed, and annotated models, the results of such large-scale efforts have typically been made available through dedicated databases, including the Genomic Threading Database (http://bioinf.cs.ucl.ac.uk/GTD/) [21, 22], ModBase (https://modbase.compbio.ucsf.edu/) [23], Genome 3D (http://www.genome3d.net/) [24], GPCRdb (https://gpcrdb.org/) [25], and the AlphaFold Protein Structure Database (AlphaFold DB; https://alphafold.ebi.ac.uk/) [26].

In this chapter, we review the SWISS-MODEL Repository (SMR: https://swissmodel.expasy.org/repository/) [27, 28], which provides access to annotated 3D protein models created by different modeling pipelines. Initially, SMR contained models generated by the SWISS-MODEL pipeline [29–31], and later included available experimental structures from the PDB. Recently, it evolved into a general database of annotated protein models for most sequences in the UniProt Knowledgebase (UniProtKB) [32] from multiple sources, including the AlphaFold DB and ModelArchive. UniProtKB is the major database of protein knowledge and gathers sequence and functional information for over 230 million entries, including those manually curated in Swiss-Prot and those automatically annotated in TrEMBL. The main goal of SMR is to provide life scientists with an up-to-date and annotated collection of high-quality protein structure models, both experimental and computational. Sequence-based and structural annotations, such as domains, variants, ligands, and transmembrane segments, help researchers to better analyze, and interpret those structures. SMR provides access to this information for every entry in UniProtKB. Proteins can be queried based on several criteria such as UniProtKB accession code (AC), protein name, or full-text search. Through a user-friendly web interface, SMR provides cross-referencing to the respective annotation databases, and the ability to transfer specific features from templates, such as protein–ligand interactions, allowing for the analysis and interpretation of structural models and inform approaches in SBDD.

6.2 SMR Database Content and Model Providers

This section describes sources of experimental and computational models in SMR, how they help complement the structural coverage of the database, their characteristics, respective strengths, and weaknesses, as well as aspects to watch out for before using them in SBDD projects. The list of data providers in SMR is continuously updated to reflect the latest method developments in structural biology. As of July 2022, SMR includes experimental structures from the PDB, homology models from SWISS-MODEL, predicted models from the AlphaFold Database, and a number of manually selected model sets from ModelArchive. The SMR team manually curates the list of model providers to have a set of well-established complementary methods and defines automatic filters to only include predictions of sufficiently high quality.

6.2.1 PDB

The PDB [3] contains experimentally derived models, including homo and heteromeric protein complexes and complexes of proteins with other types of biological macromolecules, including nucleic acids, polysaccharides, and ligands such as metal ions, small organic molecules, and peptides. The PDB is the gold standard that is used for the training of computational methods and is one of the major sources of structural information for SBDD [33]. Proteins in the PDB do not necessarily correspond directly or exactly to sequence entries in UniProtKB. Therefore, the "Structure Integration with Function, Taxonomy, and Sequence" (SIFTS) resource [34, 35] provides mappings between these structures and different databases, including UniProtKB. SMR uses this mapping to include and display experimental structures. In total, over 477,000 UniProtKB entries (including more than 47,000 Swiss-Prot entries) are currently covered, at least partially, by the experimental structures through the SIFTS mapping. This corresponds to more than 52,000 nonredundant sequences (including more than 30,000 in Swiss-Prot).

Although structures are generally of high quality and have undergone curation, they may still contain errors or inaccuracies driven by multiple factors, such as the quality or resolution of the experimental data. The PDB makes a significant effort in assessing the quality of the structures it publishes, as well as making this process transparent in the form of validation reports [36, 37]. Key quality metrics, the R values, assess the goodness-of-fit between the model and the underlying electron densities at the local and global levels, but these metrics can be challenging to interpret. The electron density score for individual atoms (EDIA) metric [38–40] is not included in SMR, and users must manually query this data from the ProteinsPlus server (https://proteins.plus), with a special focus on the desired binding sites. As SMR includes all PDB entries mapped via SIFTS and does not apply quality filtering, users are advised to assess the data quality independently, including the experimental data support of the protein and ligand atom coordinates, either through the ProteinsPlus server or the corresponding PDB validation report.

6.2.2 SWISS-MODEL

SWISS-MODEL is a fully automated protein structure modeling server, which implements a homology modeling pipeline [31]. The workflow encompasses six main steps: (i) homologous proteins with known structures to be used as templates are searched with BLAST [41] and HHblits, which is more sensitive and predicts better alignments for templates with low sequence identity [42], and the resulting alignment is retrieved; (ii) the oligomeric state is predicted from the target sequence(s) and the templates; (iii) one or more templates are selected, maximizing the length of the modeled region in the target sequence(s); (iv) a model is built for each selected template using the default homology modeling pipeline in the ProMod3 modeling engine [43], with additional models being progressively generated if new segments can be covered or if alternative models with different conformations (e.g. corresponding to different closed/open states) can be generated; (v) final models are then refined by energy minimization using the OpenMM molecular mechanics library [44]; and (vi) their quality evaluated with QMEANDisCo [45] so that only high-quality models are gathered in SMR. A local QMEANDisCo score is provided for each residue and ranges from 0 to 1 with a higher score indicating higher accuracy. The scores are trained to predict the all-atom lDDT score [46], which is described further below. SMR only includes models from SWISS-MODEL with a global QMEANDisCo (average of local scores) of at least 0.5.

In order to complement the PDB, SMR defines a set of species whose full proteomes are updated weekly with the SWISS-MODEL pipeline to consider new structures released in the PDB. The set of species is manually curated by the SMR team together with Swiss-Prot based on how often they get accessed in UniProt and on user requests. Currently, the set includes the following 13 species: *Homo sapiens, Mus musculus, Caenorhabditis elegans, Escherichia coli, Arabidopsis thaliana, Drosophila melanogaster, Saccharomyces cerevisiae, Schizosaccharomyces pombe, Caulobacter vibrioides, Mycobacterium tuberculosis, Pseudomonas aeruginosa, Staphylococcus aureus,* and *Plasmodium falciparum*. In addition, models for the remaining sequences of Swiss-Prot are regularly updated, and the results of automated modeling jobs requested by users for any protein from UniProtKB are also imported into SMR. This continuous update helps to ensure that (i) the target coverage is as complete as possible given the currently available templates, (ii) the models are built using the most recent sequence and template structure databases, and (iii) the continuous improvements of the underlying modeling pipeline are fully applied. Homology models allow increasing the structural coverage of UniProtKB significantly. SWISS-MODEL provides models for more than 3.4 million entries (1.2 million nonredundant sequences). Almost 90% of all Swiss-Prot entries (505,000), and 74% of the entries in the proteomes of the 13 "core" species (104,000) are, at least partially, covered. More than 385,000 high-quality models built by SWISS-MODEL contain ligands, and 483,000 are quaternary structure assemblies based on annotations from the PDB, both of which can be of relevance in SBDD.

Until recently, the highest prediction accuracy was reached for targets with homologous proteins of known structure, where template-based methods worked best [47, 48]. But with the latest developments in deep neural networks, high-accuracy models are now also available for targets without homologous template structures [48, 49]. Still, template-based methods remain widely used in SBDD and are very accurate for cases with high sequence identity to a known template. On average,

Reference structure	QMEANDisCo global: 0.85 local (BS): 0.84	QMEANDisCo global: 0.79 local (BS): 0.83	QMEANDisCo global: 0.74 local (BS): 0.68	QMEANDisCo global: 0.70 local (BS): 0.67	QMEANDisCo global: 0.54 local (BS): 0.44
(a)	(b)	(c)	(d)	(e)	(f)

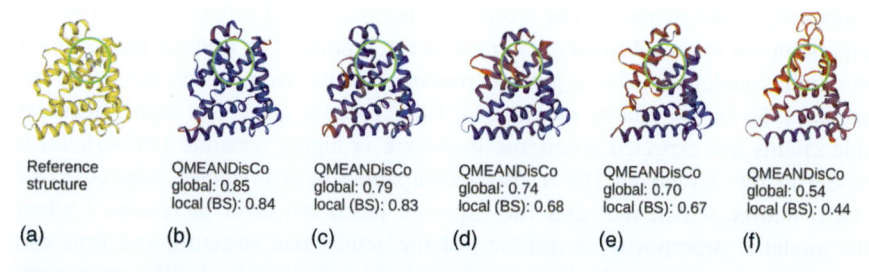

Figure 6.1 Models of the estrogen-related receptor gamma (P62508, ERR3_HUMAN) ligand-binding domain (Interpro: IPR000536) at decreasing levels of quality as indicated by QMEANDisCo coloring next to the reference structure (a) PDB entry 6I62 with the ligand (4,4'-(2,2,2-trichloroethane-1,1-diyl)diphenol). Models are based on PDB templates (b) 3D24; (c) 2A3I; (d) 3L0E; (e) 6CN5; and (f) 3P0U. The approximate position of the binding site is shown as a light green circle. Average QMEANDisCo local binding site (BS) scores were computed as the mean of the local scores of the 15 residues within 4Å of the ligand in 6I62.

side-chain placement is unreliable when the sequence identity to the template is lower than 70%, and overall model accuracy drops sharply when it is lower than 30% [50, 51]. However, sequence identity is a poor proxy for quality, and users should carefully check global and local quality scores before using these models.

Figure 6.1 shows a selection of models for the estrogen-related receptor gamma (P62508, ERR3_HUMAN) ligand-binding domain (Interpro: IPR000536), built from different templates and showing decreasing levels of predicted quality from left to right starting from the reference structure (PDB entry: 6I62, Figure 1.1a). The models built from PDB entry 3D24 (Figure 6.1b) and PDB entry 2A3I (Figure 6.1c), display very high QMEANDisCo global scores, and very high local quality scores (0.8 and above) in the binding site region (green circle). The remaining models (Figure 6.1d–f) show lower QMEANDisCo global scores, and in particular, the local qualities in the binding site start to deteriorate (around 0.6 or lower). These models should be used with caution for SBDD, like molecular docking, for instance.

6.2.3 AlphaFold Database

Recently, DeepMind and the EMBL's European Bioinformatics Institute (EBI) launched the AlphaFold DB [26]. It is an archive of protein models automatically generated by the AlphaFold modeling engine [18], a deep neural network, which was able to outperform all other participants at the CASP14 experiment, and in some cases even detected errors in the experimental structures [49].

So far, the AlphaFold DB provides models for proteins with 16 to 2700 residues. For human proteins with more than 2700 residues, models are made available for overlapping, 1400-residue-long fragments. AlphaFold DB does only provide one isoform per protein. For each Cα atom in each model, AlphaFold estimates the corresponding lDDT-Cα score, denoted predicted lDDT (pLDDT). The per-residue pLDDT scores are stored in the model file (B-factor column for PDB files or _ma_qa_metric categories for the ModelCIF files) and indicate the expected local confidence in the structure. The scores vary between 0 and 100, with higher values expressing an expected higher accuracy of the models. The average pLDDT over the entire model provides a general measure of the overall expected backbone accuracy. So far, no quality measure for side chains is given, but highly accurate side chains are expected when the backbone is highly accurate [18, 49]. Each model in the AlphaFold DB is also accompanied by a Predicted Aligned Error (PAE) matrix, which indicates the expected positional error at residue i when the model is superposed on residue j of the actual, real structure and thus can be used to assess the confidence in the relative orientation of different regions of the predicted model. The PAE matrix helps, for example, to assess the relative orientation, and corresponding modeled contacts, of different domains in the same chain, complementing the pLDDT scores.

As of August 2022, the AlphaFold DB contains models for over 200 million proteins, covering a large proportion of all catalogued protein sequences. This includes models for most entries in Swiss-Prot, most non-viral entries in UniProt, and the full proteomes of 48 species of particular scientific relevance, as model organisms or those related to global health. The AlphaFold DB allows for single-entry or bulk download of models, for example, those for specific proteomes. It also provides programmatic access through an API. SMR automatically retrieves the models with the 3D-Beacons API (https://3d-beacons.org) and displays them alongside the other computational models and experimental structures. All models in the AlphaFold DB meet the quality criteria for the inclusion in SMR.

AlphaFold models only include single proteins in their monomeric form, although research is actively ongoing to extend these possibilities, in particular, to model heteromers. Therefore, users that use these models should be aware that certain properties, like surface accessibility, might differ from those observed in a biological setting. In addition, disordered loops and regions are included in AlphaFold models, however the biological context, such as the presence of ligands or cofactors, is ignored. In the case of the Human B-raf kinase (P15056, BRAF_HUMAN), for instance, the protein contains a nucleotide binding site, and the corresponding binding pocket can be targeted by inhibitors, as shown in PDB entry 4E26 (Figure 6.2a). In the AlphaFold model of this protein (Figure 6.2b), careful inspection of local quality scores shows reduced accuracy of the nucleotide-binding site, with pLDDT values down to around 60. In addition, a disordered loop with pLDDT values at or below 30 is in close proximity and is modeled to pass through the binding site. Molecular recognition of inhibitors by the binding pocket becomes impossible if this loop is wrongly kept inside. The PAE matrix displayed in the AlphaFold DB (Figure 6.2c) also suggests that while the domains are modeled with high confidence, their relative orientation is uncertain and particularly so for the position of the disordered loop with respect to the rest of the protein. Reviewing these confidence metrics and careful visual inspection are critical before using AlphaFold models in SBDD projects.

6.2.4 ModelArchive

Finally, the SMR provides some manually selected, large-scale model sets from ModelArchive [20, 52, 53]. ModelArchive is an archive for theoretical models of

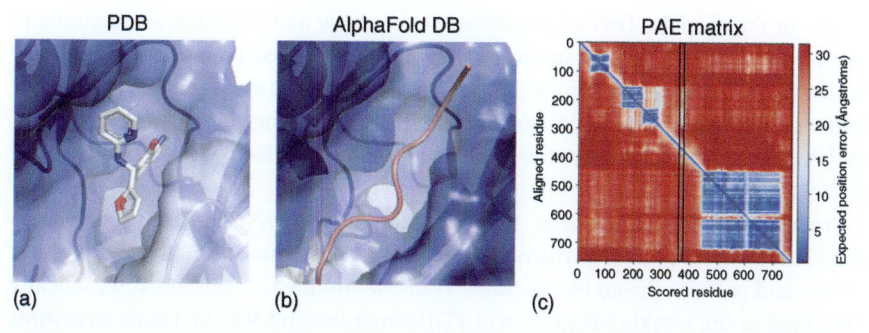

Figure 6.2 Binding pocket of the human B-raf protein kinase (P15056, BRAF_HUMAN). (a) Molecular surface of the binding site of inhibitor (5-chloro-7-[(R)-furan-2-yl(pyridin-2-ylamino)methyl]quinolin-8-ol) in PDB entry 4E26, and colored according to the B-factor. (b) The AlphaFold model of this protein with a disordered loop wrongly modeled to pass through the binding site, colored according to the per-residue pLDDT. (c) The Predicted Aligned Error (PAE) matrix for the AlphaFold model, where a black box marks the part covering the relative orientation of this disordered loop with the rest of the protein. In all panels, blue is used for regions of high confidence and red for low confidence, whatever the metrics.

macromolecular structures and complements the PDB for experimental structures and the PDB-Dev [54] for integrative structures, where experimental and computational methods are combined. Any researcher can deposit models in ModelArchive to make them available and supplement manuscripts for which the models were generated. As of July 2022, it contains more than 2800 models deposited on behalf of more than 110 researchers in computational structural biology worldwide. The models in the archive are automatically validated for their data format and manually checked by the ModelArchive team to ensure that they include a minimal level of method and quality annotations. However, their quality varies widely, and they represent a snapshot in time of the depositor's best effort to predict the protein structure.

Being generated by many different researchers using various methods, often these models do not fit the "high-quality" definition for model inclusion in SMR. However, some studies provide high-quality models with reliable quality metrics and are included on a case-by-case basis according to manual checks by the SMR team. For instance, the methods used to generate the set of models of protein–protein interactions across the *Saccharomyces cerevisiae* proteome deposited in ModelArchive by Humphreys et al. [55] have been thoroughly reviewed to ensure high quality and reliable quality estimates. They are therefore included in SMR.

6.3 Protein Feature Annotation and Cross-References to Computational Resources

6.3.1 Structural Features, Ligands, and Oligomers

To facilitate the interpretation of the structural models, SMR is cross-referenced with UniProtKB and InterPro [56], and users can manually add sequence features to any of the models. This allows different sequence and structure annotations to be mapped into the models and to provide a more detailed understanding of their molecular features. Annotations include protein domains and families, transmembrane segments and signal sequences, catalytic and binding sites, as well as natural variants. These are mapped at the sequence level and transferred into the structural model for visualization.

Properties of templates used to build models with SWISS-MODEL are also transferred where possible, which includes transmembrane annotations and orientation, and protein–ligand interactions. Transmembrane proteins are automatically identified in the weekly integration of PDB structures in SMR, and such structures are automatically displayed with dummy atoms that delimit a putative membrane region. This prediction is carried out based solely on structural information, by estimating the optimal membrane location for each biounit in the structure and classifying it based on energetic and geometric criteria as in Lomize et al. [57]. This membrane annotation is transferred to a model if at least 80% of all transmembrane residues in the template are aligned with the target sequence.

The relative coordinates of biologically relevant ligands, including not only small molecules but also metals and cofactors, are transferred from the template if the binding site is fully conserved and the resulting atomic interactions in the model are within the expected range for van der Waals interactions and water-mediated contacts. If this conservative homology transfer approach is too restrictive, the user can use an appropriate ligand docking tool such as SwissDock [58, 59] to predict the molecular interactions between the model and a ligand. When ligands are present in the model, seven types of noncovalent protein–ligand interactions are annotated with the Protein–Ligand Interaction Profiler (PLIP) [60] (i.e. hydrogen bonds, hydrophobic contacts, π–stacking, π–cation interactions, salt bridges, water bridges, and halogen bonds).

In biological settings, proteins do rarely operate in isolation. Many proteins will oligomerize by forming homo-oligomers, or assemble with other proteins into hetero-oligomeric complexes. SMR provides ways to visualize and navigate the partners when the information is available. Structures from the PDB often include such information. However, the automatic prediction of interaction partners still remains a challenge for automated methods, such as SWISS-MODEL or AlphaFold. Therefore, only a handful of experimentally supported or thoroughly validated heteromeric models are currently available in SMR, and cover pathogen–pathogen and human–pathogen interactions for SARS-CoV-2 proteins and multiple protein-interacting pairs from the *S. cerevisiae* interactome.

6.3.2 SWISS-MODEL associated tools

SMR is functionally linked with other parts of the interactive SWISS-MODEL workspace. The main link is to the SWISS-MODEL modeling engine, allowing users to submit modeling jobs for any UniProtKB entry, independently of whether there is a high-quality model already in SMR or not. Interactive remodeling can be useful to investigate the presence of ligands in the templates, to assess conformational changes of the protein (see Section 6.5 below), or to evaluate the presence of new templates for organisms, which are not part of the 13 regularly updated core species. The page of an entry provides a first-glance view of the model, showing the annotations described above, as well as global and local quality summaries, and target–template sequence alignment. Further insights can be gained by forwarding the model to the "Structure Assessment" and "Structure Comparison" tools.

The "Structure Assessment" page (Figure 6.3, https://swissmodel.expasy.org/assess) provides detailed structural information about the model. Together with the local and global quality estimates computed with QMEANDisCo, this page also displays the Ramachandran Plot (i.e. the distribution of Φ/Ψ dihedral angles, Figure 6.3a) for the model, as well as relevant scores provided by Molprobity [61], highlighting where residues of low quality are located in the model (Figure 6.3b). Additionally, amino acid residues from all protein polypeptide chains in the model are visualized in an interactive 3D view (Figure 6.3c) and a sequence display (Figure 6.3d), with each residue represented by its one-letter code below a bar chart displaying the QMEANDisCo local quality estimation value.

The "Structure Comparison" page (Figure 6.4a, https://swissmodel.expasy.org/comparison/), on the other hand, displays multiple models in a single view, automatically comparing them and highlighting structural variations. A model can be compared to other models for the same or similar proteins with a structural superposition based on the aligned sequences. The page shows the structure and sequence alignments and also performs the following analyses which allow for the detection of structural variations: (i) Ensemble Consistency, which measures the local deviation of a protein structure (or model) from the consensus established by all other structures being compared, similar to classical consensus approaches in protein model quality estimation [62] and (ii) Ensemble Variance, which assesses the variance of interatomic distances in the full ensemble [63].

6.3.3 Web and API Access

To enable a variety of usages in SBDD and other fields, SMR provides several ways to navigate, access, visualize and download its data: by (i) a web interface and dedicated per-entry pages, (ii) bulk downloads for any of the 13 SWISS-MODEL core proteomes, and (iii) programmatic access using a REST API.

The main entry point to the Repository is the web interface (https://swissmodel.expasy.org/repository/). A search bar at the top of every page (Figure 6.5a) allows direct access to an entry by entering its UniProtKB accession (for instance P9WJM9) or UniProtKB entry name (MSHC_MYCTU). In addition, the search bar enables free-text searches for protein names, descriptions, and keywords, as well as mnemonic protein identification codes and descriptions. The search results are sorted based on various criteria (e.g. the presence of the entry in Swiss-Prot or in one of the 13 core species), and show the ranges of the full-length protein that are structurally elucidated by experimental structures or computational models.

Each entry in UniProtKB has its own detailed page in SMR. A typical example page is shown in Figure 6.5b, corresponding to one entry identifier with links

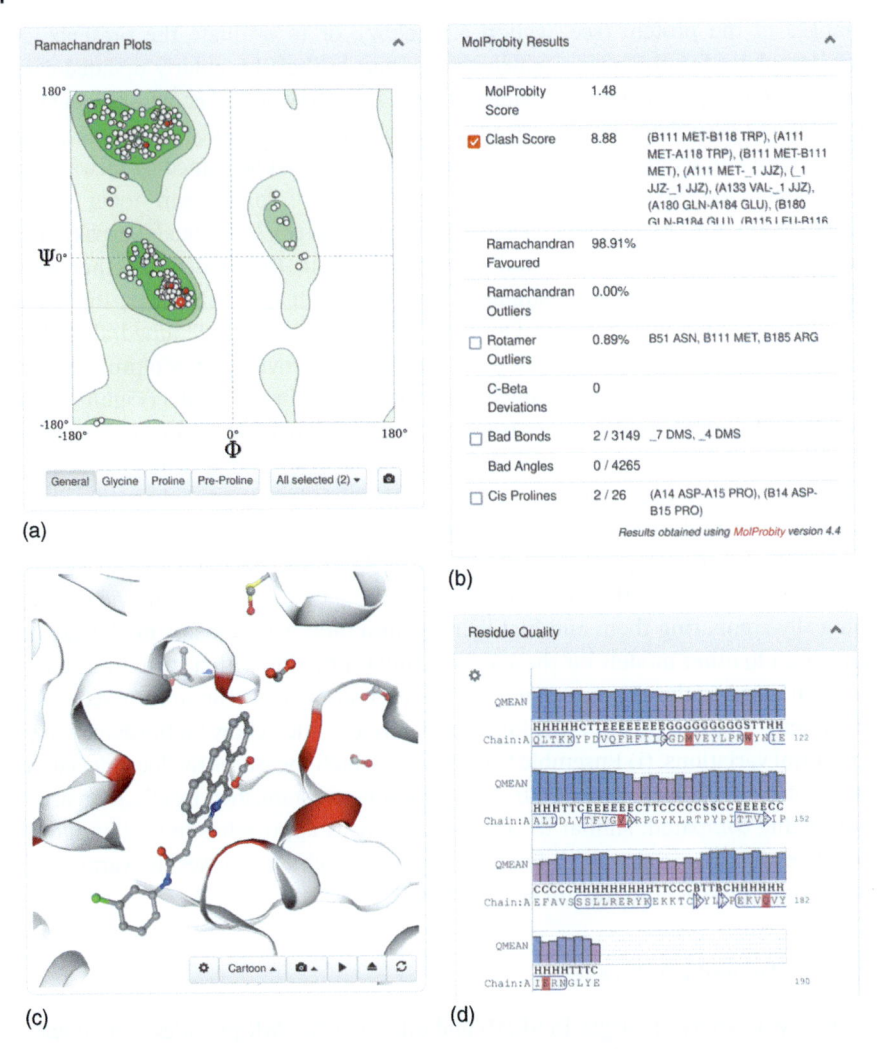

Figure 6.3 Structure Assessment tool results for PDB entry 3MLA. (a) A Ramachandran Plot shows the distribution of Φ/Ψ dihedral angles. (b) Molprobity results highlight residues of low quality. (c) Interactive view of the 3D model, highlighting selected residues of low quality found by MolProbity. (d) Bar chart displaying the QMEANDisCo local quality estimation above the sequence for every polypeptide chain. One-letter codes of the residues selected in Figure 6.3b are highlighted in red. The same analysis can be performed on a predicted model rather than a PDB structure.

that cross-reference to other databases (Figure 6.5b (1)). Figure 6.5b (2) displays the annotation tracks, which summarize which parts of the input sequence are covered by models or experimental structures, as well as the regions corresponding to multiple annotations (e.g. natural variants, protein domains, catalytic sites, or user-provided annotations). All regions are interactive and can be selected by clicking, and zoomed in or out by scrolling while pressing the control key. Figure 6.5b (3) provides detailed information about the template used for modeling (in the case of homology models), the version of the AlphaFold model, or the experimental

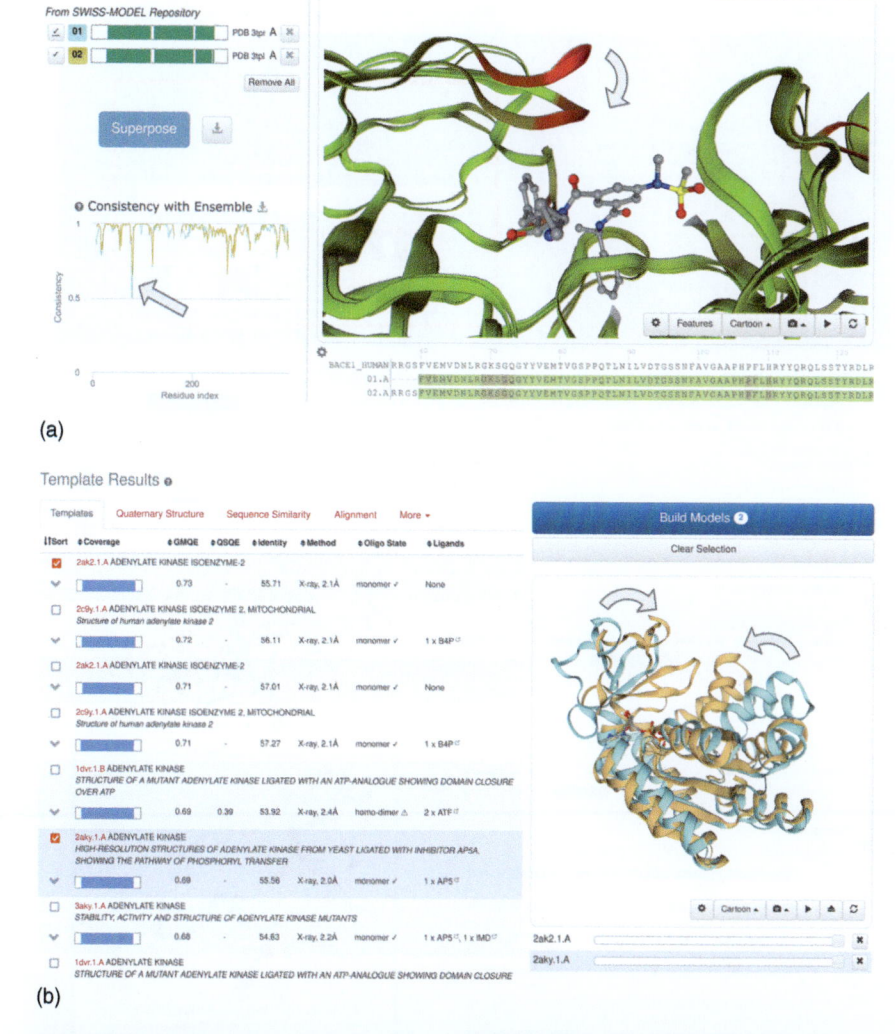

Figure 6.4 Assessment of conformational changes. (a) The Structure Comparison tool of SWISS-MODEL highlights conformational changes of apo (PDB entry 3TPL, model 02, yellow) and holo (PDB entry 3TPR, model 01, turquoise) states of Human Beta-secretase 1 (P56817, BACE1_HUMAN). This can be seen both in the 3D view (curved grey arrow) and in a local drop in the "Consistency with Ensemble" plot (straight grey arrow). (b) Template Search results for *D. discoideum* Adenylate kinase (Q54QJ9, KAD2_DICDI) show the presence of templates in both open (2AK2) and closed (2AKY) conformations depending on the ligands bound. The curved grey arrows show the main conformational change.

structure. It also includes information about global and local (per-residue) model confidence (for computational models) and on biologically relevant ligands as well as protein–ligand interactions (based on PLIP).

Figure 6.5b (4) provides the interactive 3D view of the structure where annotated regions are highlighted. If a ligand is present in the model, the protein–ligand interaction annotations can be displayed by clicking on the "Contains 2 ligands"

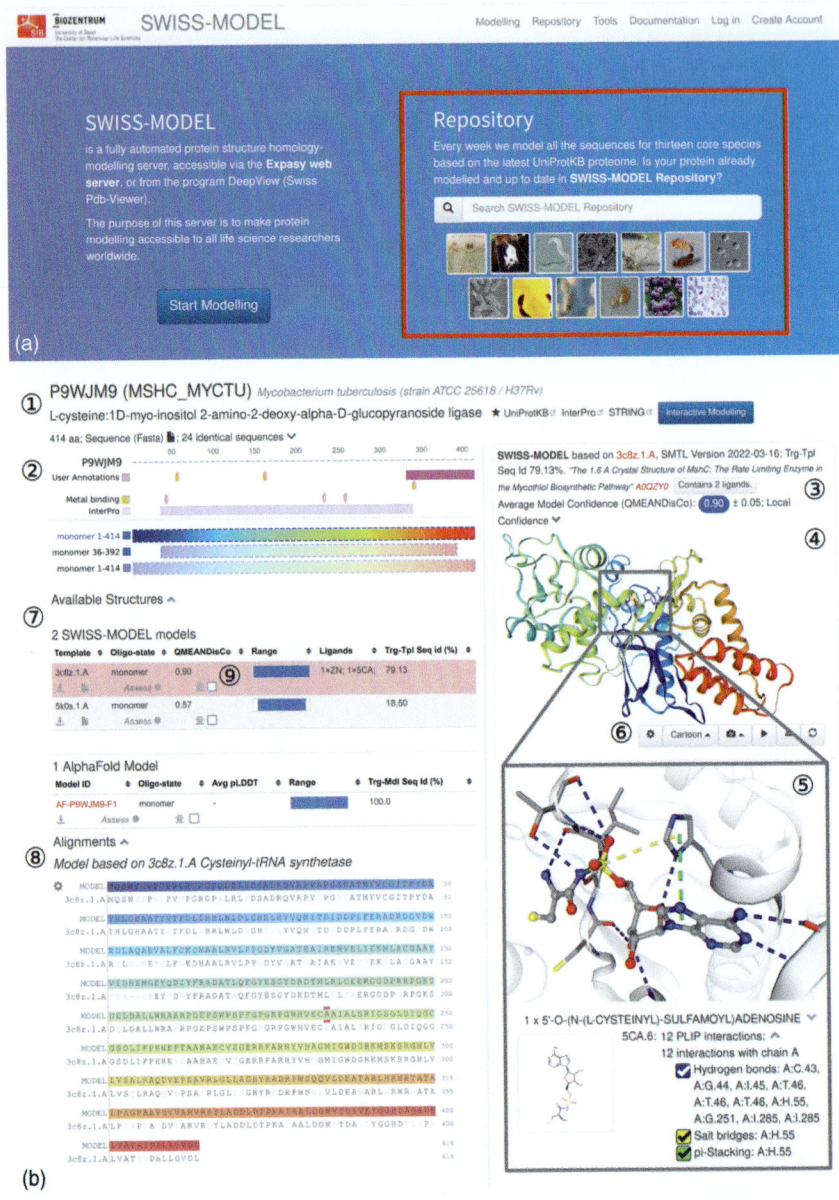

Figure 6.5 The SMR web interface (https://swissmodel.expasy.org/repository/). (a) A snapshot of the main landing page, highlighting its search field. (b) Example of a typical UniProtKB entry page is demonstrated here for the Mycothiol ligase from *Mycobacterium tuberculosis* (strain ATCC 25618/H37Rv) (UniProtKB AC: P9WJM9). Zoom into the ligand-binding site can be activated when a specific ligand is selected from the "Contains *n* ligands" button at the top of the protein view (here: *n* = 2). Circled numbers, from 1 to 7, indicate the different sections of the entry page: (1) the entry identifier and cross-reference to other databases, (2) the annotation tracks (including user-provided annotations), (3) information about the selected structure (here: template used and model confidence), (4) interactive view of the 3D model, (5) zoom in to an annotated ligand binding site, (6) tools to change figure representation and color options, (7) list of computational and experimental models, (8) sequence alignments as relevant for selected structure (here: target–template alignment), and (9) links to the Structure Assessment and Structure Comparison tools.

button (Figure 6.5b (3)), and selecting the ligand of interest with the down arrow. This will highlight the interacting residues in the model (Figure 6.5b (5)). The appearance of the protein model can be changed with the options in Figure 6.5b (6), which includes representation (e.g. cartoon or surface) and coloring mode (e.g. amino acid properties or local quality estimates, accessible with the cogwheel button).

Figure 6.5b (7) lists all models and experimental structures available for the target entry, and controls what is displayed in the viewer. The initial selection is based on several criteria: type of model (experimental or computational), oligomeric state, coverage range, experimental method, resolution, and model quality. Finally, Figure 6.5b (8) displays alignments between the target and the template (for homology models) or the alignment between the experimental structure and the UniProtKB sequence, or between the model and the UniProtKB sequence for other models. Here, the residues are colored according to the display in the 3D viewer (Figure 6.5b (4)) and their sequence numbering can be shown by hovering the alignment.

For users who require structural information for a large number of proteins, the repository provides two downloadable files for each of the 13 core species covered by SWISS-MODEL. They are available from the landing page of the repository (https://swissmodel.expasy.org/repository) and are updated shortly after every UniProtKB release. The first corresponds to the metadata, which contains an index of all the homology-based models and experimental structures available for that organism. It (i) lists information on the part of the protein that each model covers, (ii) provides a link for the download of the structure's atomic coordinates file, and (iii) provides template and model quality information for homology-based models. The same data are also available in tab-separated and JSON formats. The second file contains the atomic coordinates of all the homology-based models for the organism in PDB format. It does not contain experimental structures or models built by AlphaFold, but models that can be built with templates mapped via SIFTS are included. Those models can be useful even if the protein is covered in the PDB: (i) template selection aims to pick a high-quality structure if multiple exist; (ii) gaps will be filled; (iii) target sequence will be aligned with the UniProtKB sequence; and (iv) sidechains may be adjusted when sequence identity is below 100%. Users who require a large number of homology models for an organism that is not part of the 13 core species are free to contact the SWISS-MODEL help desk, who can generate a bulk download with recently updated homology models.

Programmatic access to the repository via the SMR REST API (https://swissmodel.expasy.org/docs/repository_help#smr_api) provides most flexibility, including detailed access to per-residue information on homology models and experimental structures. It follows the OpenAPI specifications (https://www.openapis.org/), and its full documentation is available on the Repository Help page. In addition, the 3D-Beacons (https://3d-beacons.org) API provides summary information per UniProtKB entry for several model providers, including those in SMR.

6.4 Quality Estimates and Benchmarking

SMR aims to only include high-quality models in its database. But what does high quality mean, especially in the context of SBDD? To answer such questions, the CAMEO benchmarking effort has been providing blind, weekly, automated benchmarking services for structure prediction methods since 2012 [63–66]. Based on the PDB pre-release data, which is part of the PDB release cycle, CAMEO participants are provided with a selection of sequences of proteins whose structures are going to be published in the following PDB release. The predictions are then compared to the newly released experimental structures, which are considered the *gold standard*.

To perform this comparison, several different metrics are used. Calculating the root-mean-square deviation (RMSD) of atomic positions between the reference structure and the model is a straightforward approach, but is strongly influenced by outliers in poorly predicted regions, is insensitive to missing parts of the model, and is strongly dependent on the superposition of the model with the reference structure [46]. Another approach that has been developed in the context of CASP is the Global Distance Test (GDT) score [67, 68], which quantifies the number of corresponding atoms in the model that can be superposed within a set of predefined tolerance thresholds to the reference structure. Although it is not sensitive to outliers and accounts for missing parts of the model, it is still dependent on superposition. In the case of flexible proteins composed of several domains, which can naturally change their relative orientation with respect to each other, a global rigid-body superposition is typically dominated by the largest domain, and as a consequence, the smaller domains may not correctly match, which can result in artificially unfavorable scores. In CASP, the effects of domain movement are mitigated by splitting the target into the so-called assessment units (AUs), which are evaluated separately. However, this process is based on visual inspection and remains mostly manual and often based on subjective criteria [46].

Superposition-free scores such as the local Distance Difference Test (lDDT) [46], which is a measure for the conservation of interatomic distances between the prediction and the reference structure, or the Contact Area Difference (CAD) score [69], based on differences in residue-residue contact area using Voronoi tessellation, have solved these problems. Both methods calculate a "local" (per-residue) score, which is often averaged into a "global" score representing the overall confidence in the model. The lDDT score and several field-specific variants have been developed. Of particular note in the context of SBDD is the lDDT-BS score, which assesses the accuracy of binding sites of biologically relevant ligands [64].

However, at the time of modeling, structure prediction methods do not know the correct answer, which prevents them from providing a direct metric of model quality. Thus, they typically report an estimation instead, which represents their expectation of the accuracy of the model. Of course, such estimations should be accurate, which is also assessed by CAMEO. Even for very good prediction methods, the quality of predictions can vary from one model to another, and even between regions within a single model. Therefore, CAMEO participants are tasked to provide reliable estimates of the quality of their predictions at a per-residue level, also known as "Model

Confidence" scores. The accuracy of the model confidence scores is evaluated by assessing the ability of those scores to distinguish between high-quality (lDDT ≥ 0.6) and low-quality (lDDT < 0.6) residues using an area under the receiver operating characteristic curve (ROC AUC) metric, which shows how sensitivity and specificity change as the decision threshold of local quality changes. Higher ROC AUC indicates more accurate predictions. Over the years, benchmarking of model quality estimation methods resulted in significant improvements in the performance of those methods [65], and has impacted internal model quality estimates too. Prediction of local lDDT scores has become a standard way to report internal model quality predictions, with both AlphaFold (pLDDT, which predicts lDDT-Cα, a variation of the lDDT score restricted to Cα atoms) and SWISS-MODEL (with QMEANDisCo which predicts the all-atom lDDT score) using comparable scores.

All computational models in SMR provide such a local confidence measure, with a method that has been critically benchmarked in CAMEO [65] and CASP [70]. Although all computational models are of high global quality (with criteria depending on the model provider), users should carefully review local quality information before attempting to use the model for SBDD. Docking a compound in a low-quality region is likely to produce wrong or misleading results. While there is no exact cut-off, users should be particularly cautious with any region where residues show local lDDT scores below 0.6.

6.5 Binding Site Conformational States

Most experimental structures and computational models are a snapshot in time and do not account for conformational changes and flexibility. However, proteins are dynamic in nature and their conformation can change, e.g. upon substrate binding. The aspartyl proteases [71], adenylate kinases [72], and cytochrome P450 [73] are three examples. In other cases, allosteric effects due to binding of a molecule outside the active site trigger structural changes in the binding site [74]. Thus, for computer-aided SBDD applications, it is essential to make sure that the predicted model or experimental structure represents the conformational state that is adequate for the specific downstream application.

With experimental structures from the PDB, such assessment is a relatively easy task and can be directly derived from the description and presence or absence of ligands in the structure. This can be illustrated in the example of the Human Beta-secretase 1 (P56817, BACE1_HUMAN). A wealth of experimental structures for this member of the aspartyl protease family is available for the bound (e.g. 3TPL) and unbound (e.g. 3TPR) states in both the PDB and SMR. The Structure Comparison tool (Figure 6.4a), available by clicking on the "compare" icon in the list of structures (Figure 6.5b 9), carries out a superposition, which highlights the structural differences to better inform the selection of a structure in the adequate conformation.

On the other hand, the homology models from SWISS-MODEL listed in SMR are built from automatically selected templates. They undergo minimal postprocessing and will adopt the binding site conformational state of the template regardless of the presence of a ligand in the final model. Because of its strict ligand transfer rules, SWISS-MODEL may produce a model of a bound state without the relevant ligand, even when the model is based on a template with relatively high sequence identity. Therefore, the absence of a ligand in a predicted structure is no guarantee that a conformation in the unbound state was built. Instead, users need to check whether ligands were present in the template used for modeling. They can do so by following the link to the template used for modeling (Figure 6.5b 3).

In cases where ligand binding causes significant structural changes, SWISS-MODEL can produce models for several of the conformations of the protein if corresponding template structures are available. The adenylate kinase from *P. aeruginosa* (Q9HXV4, KAD_PSEAE) is an illustrative example: since the conformational changes on ligand binding are rather large (more than 10Å after a superposition based on the target–template alignment), SWISS-MODEL built two models of the protein, one in each state (open and closed).

However, in other cases, the conformational changes may also be more subtle and not picked up automatically by the algorithm. Since there is no preferential conformation, models may represent either open (as in *Dictyostelium discoideum*, Q54QJ9, KAD2_DICDI) or closed (as in *S. cerevisiae*, P07170, KAD2_YEAST) states. Alternative conformational states of the target protein can be remodeled directly from within SMR by using the "Interactive Modeling" button above the 3D view (Figure 6.5b 3) and clicking on the "Search For Templates" button in the next window. In the resulting page (Figure 6.4b, which shows interactive template search results for *D. discoideum*, Q54QJ9, KAD2_DICDI), a selection of templates is presented which attempts to balance structural diversity with the predicted quality of the resulting model. Using the template descriptions (Figure 6.4b, left), bound ligands and 3D viewer (Figure 6.4b, right), users can explore the diversity of the template conformations and choose an appropriate selection of templates for modeling. Once that is done, clicking on the "Build Models" button (Figure 6.4b, top) will start the modeling process. If needed, models based on other templates can always be built at a later time point.

With AlphaFold models, the exact conformational state of a protein cannot be controlled. It has been shown that AlphaFold predicts the holo (bound) state of a protein in 70% of the cases [75] and users should exercise extra caution when using these models for docking studies.

6.6 SMR and Computer-Aided Structure-based Drug Design

Despite the recent astonishing results in protein structure prediction by the application of deep-learning-based methods [76, 77], homology-based modeling remains the most commonly used technique in SBDD due to its short response time, its direct relation to experimentally determined structures and well-established track record. One of the most recent applications of the SWISS-MODEL infrastructure was the generation of models for proteins from SARS-CoV-2, such as the spike protein for which a model was produced to accompany the publication of the sequenced genome of the virus [78]. To respond to the demand for such models, SMR introduced a dedicated page (https://swissmodel.expasy.org/repository/species/2697049) to make models for all single proteins and relevant protein complexes of SARS-CoV-2 publicly available. These models are generated and annotated following the same procedures and summary formats as regular SMR entries and are frequently updated. In addition, annotations for most "Variants of Interest" and "Variants of Concern" are available.

Since the outbreak of COVID-19, the SWISS-MODEL infrastructure and these models have been explored by multiple teams worldwide in the quest for a therapy, including the mapping of druggable cavities in diverse, therapeutically relevant SARS-CoV-2 proteins [79, 80], the search for possible drugs by virtual screening [81, 82] or drug repurposing [83–85], the design of vaccines by antibody [86, 87], and the analysis of variant effects [88–90]. In these studies, researchers used SMR as a source of protein structure models and their quality estimations and also utilized the SWISS-MODEL pipeline for the identification of ligand-binding sites or the modeling of specific targets or antibody scaffolds.

But the use of SMR and SWISS-MODEL predictions for SBDD goes beyond COVID-19. For example, in a study about the toxic effect of curcumin, a flavonoid derived from the traditional medicinal plant *Curcuma longa* L, on female reproduction and embryo development, high-quality structure predictions of several key curcuma-binding proteins of unknown structure were collected from SMR and used for molecular docking in order to analyze the curcuma-binding mode and estimate its affinity [91]. Watanabe et al. followed a similar approach in a recent study on the possible anticancer effect of rabdosianone I, a bitter diterpene extracted from the oriental herb *Isodon japonicus* Hara, but in this case, the authors opted to predict 3D structural models using their own selection of templates [92]. In another study, Kwarteng et al. used SWISS-MODEL and its quality estimation tools to obtain a single high-quality structural model of 5′-aminolevulinic acid synthase from the *Wolbachia* bacteria (wALAS) and used it for virtual screening over 3200 FDA-approved drugs in the quest of treatment of neglected tropical diseases caused by these endosymbionts and endemic in African and Latin American countries [93]. Finally, in a study about the unexpected secondary effects of two azole antifungals by the overseen, potential inhibition of human 11β-hydroxysteroid dehydrogenase 2 (11β-HSD2), Inderbinen et al. predicted structures for the human and mouse proteins with SWISS-MODEL using multiple user-selected templates and used different predicted models to inspect the effects of species-specific variations in the binding of the two ligands [94].

6.7 Conclusion and Outlook

SMR is a source of high-quality, experimental, and computational structural models of proteins from UniProtKB. These models come from various providers: the

PDB, ModelArchive, the AlphaFold DB, and the homology modeling pipeline implemented in SWISS-MODEL. The repository is updated frequently in order to assure a comprehensive, high-quality snapshot of the current experimental and computational structural knowledge is provided. The cross-references to protein sequence and structural feature annotation databases, the mapping of transmembrane segments, and the inclusion of ligand information transferred from templates of known structure allow for an integrative analysis of the models, which may aid and inform different approaches in SBDD.

Deep-learning-based methods, such as AlphaFold [18] and RoseTTAFold [17], are revolutionizing the field of protein structure prediction [48, 95], impacting various fields of research, and could have ripple effects on many others, including SBDD [96]. The high accuracy of such models for both proteins with and without homologs of known structure, accompanied by their increasing speed, allows researchers and companies to not only produce a model of their favorite protein in a timely manner but also the generation of large sets across entire proteomes. The availability of these models in online repositories such as ModelArchive or the AlphaFold DB makes it possible for a fast bridging of the protein sequence–structure gap, which was out of the reach of biophysical methods and homology modeling.

However, when it comes to SBDD, the impact of deep-learning-based methods is still unclear. While the accuracy of these methods is high, it is higher for the protein backbone than for the side chains [49], which may result in low-quality binding sites. Downstream methods that require a highly accurate binding site and do not account for conformational changes will fail [97]. It is thus imperative to inspect local quality estimates in binding sites and, especially for full-length protein models from the AlphaFold DB, watch out for predicted disordered regions and uncertain domain orientations. When homologs of known structure exist, homology modeling users can hand-pick their templates, which allows for some control over the orientation of side chains and overall conformational changes. Hence, our recommendation is to always check first if a template-based method can provide a high-quality model and possibly refine the model with a manually selected template, and then extend the structural coverage with models from AlphaFold if this is needed. For SBDD to make full use of the extended structural coverage provided by AlphaFold, docking tools able to better account for inaccurately modeled and flexible binding sites are needed.

Additionally, users must bear in mind that current structure prediction methods are not able to include and consider post-translational modifications (PTMs), such as phosphorylations and glycosylations, which may affect conformational states or surface accessibility. There are ongoing efforts to use deep neural networks for PTMs [98], as well as for reliably and accurately predicting and modeling protein–protein interaction pairs [55], and for the prediction and annotation of functional regions [99], ligand-binding sites [100] and variant effects [101]. We expect that the fast-paced development of structural and annotation methods will continue in the coming years, which will drive a rapid and continuous adaptation of model repositories and model quality estimators.

When using any model for downstream SBDD applications, such as docking, the most critical parameter is model accuracy [102], especially at the all-atom and side-chain conformation levels. SMR displays all PDB structures and AlphaFold DB models available for a given UniProtKB AC, and only high-quality homology models or manually curated models from ModelArchive. Quality is measured based on quality estimation metrics, such as QMEANDisCo, which predict the average conservation of interatomic distances in the neighborhood of a residue (lDDT) when compared to the "correct" structure. The integration of protein assemblies and the modeling of complexes with ligands and other macromolecules will likely require the development of quality estimation metrics beyond those currently employed to better account for protein interfaces. Future scores should also be able to distinguish regions with disorder and flexibility from modeling inaccuracies since currently both would be represented by low lDDT values. In addition, the development of clearer and comparable quality estimates is a must. We expect that the CASP experiment [48] and CAMEO [63] will act as major forces in that direction.

The field is developing rapidly, and significant developments will occur in the coming years. We expect that computational model repositories and automated method benchmarking will help researchers along this path and, by providing state-of-the-art annotated models to everyone, remain useful tools for those who are not directly involved in structure prediction method development.

References

1 Anderson, A.C. (2003). The process of structure-based drug design. *Chemistry & Biology* 10 (9): 787–797.
2 Sliwoski, G. et al. (2014). Computational methods in drug discovery. *Pharmacological Reviews* 66 (1): 334–395.
3 wwPDB consortium (2019). Protein Data Bank: the single global archive for 3D macromolecular structure data. *Nucleic Acids Research* 47 (D1): D520–D528.
4 Anderson, S. and Chiplin, J. (2002) 'Structural genomics: shaping the future of drug design?', *Drug Discovery Today*, 105–107. https://doi.org/10.1016/s1359-6446(01)02125-0.
5 Jones, M.M. et al. (2014). The structural genomics consortium: a knowledge platform for drug discovery: a summary. *Rand Health Quarterly* 4 (3): 19.
6 Schapira, M. (2010). Structural genomics, its application in chemistry, biology, and drug discovery. *Burger's Medicinal Chemistry and Drug Discovery* [Preprint]. https://doi.org/10.1002/0471266949.bmc135.
7 Schwede, T. (2013). Protein modeling: what happened to the "protein structure gap"? *Structure* 21 (9): 1531–1540.
8 Blundell, T.L. et al. (2006). Structural biology and bioinformatics in drug design: opportunities and challenges for target identification and lead discovery. *Philosophical transactions of the Royal Society of London Series B, Biological Sciences* 361 (1467): 413–423.

9 Grant, M.A. (2009). Protein structure prediction in structure-based ligand design and virtual screening. *Combinatorial Chemistry & High Throughput Screening* 12 (10): 940–960.

10 Mizuguchi, K. (2004). Fold recognition for drug discovery. *Drug Discovery Today: Targets* 3 (1): 18–23.

11 Hameduh, T. et al. (2020). Homology modeling in the time of collective and artificial intelligence. *Computational and Structural Biotechnology Journal* 18: 3494–3506.

12 Dhingra, S. et al. (2020). A glance into the evolution of template-free protein structure prediction methodologies. *Biochimie* 175: 85–92.

13 Ovchinnikov, S. et al. (2018). Protein structure prediction using Rosetta in CASP12. *Proteins* 86 (Suppl. 1): 113–121.

14 Wang, T. et al. (2019). Improved fragment sampling for *ab initio* protein structure prediction using deep neural networks. *Nature Machine Intelligence* 1 (8): 347–355.

15 Cheung, N.J. and Yu, W. (2018). De novo protein structure prediction using ultra-fast molecular dynamics simulation. *PLoS One* 13 (11): e0205819.

16 Hopf, T.A. et al. (2019). The EVcouplings python framework for coevolutionary sequence analysis. *Bioinformatics* 35 (9): 1582–1584.

17 Baek, M. et al. (2021). Accurate prediction of protein structures and interactions using a three-track neural network. *Science* [Preprint] https://doi.org/10.1126/science.abj8754.

18 Jumper, J. et al. (2021). Highly accurate protein structure prediction with AlphaFold. *Nature* 596 (7873): 583–589.

19 Berman, H.M. et al. (2006). Outcome of a workshop on archiving structural models of biological macromolecules. *Structure* 14 (8): 1211–1217.

20 Schwede, T. et al. (2009). Outcome of a workshop on applications of protein models in biomedical research. *Structure* 17 (2): 151–159.

21 McGuffin, L.J., Street, S. et al. (2004). The genomic threading database. *Bioinformatics* 20 (1): 131–132.

22 McGuffin, L.J., Street, S.A. et al. (2004). The genomic threading database: a comprehensive resource for structural annotations of the genomes from key organisms. *Nucleic Acids Research* 32 (Database issue): D196–D199.

23 Pieper, U. et al. (2014). ModBase, a database of annotated comparative protein structure models and associated resources. *Nucleic Acids Research* 42 (Database issue): D336–D346.

24 Lewis, T.E. et al. (2015). Genome3D: exploiting structure to help users understand their sequences. *Nucleic Acids Research* 43 (Database issue): D382–D386.

25 Kooistra, A.J. et al. (2020). GPCRdb in 2021: integrating GPCR sequence, structure and function. *Nucleic Acids Research* 49 (D1): D335–D343.

26 Varadi, M. et al. (2022). AlphaFold Protein Structure Database: massively expanding the structural coverage of protein-sequence space with high-accuracy models. *Nucleic Acids Research* 50 (D1): D439–D444.

27 Bienert, S. et al. (2017). The SWISS-MODEL repository—new features and functionality. *Nucleic Acids Research* 45 (D1): D313–D319.

28 Kopp, J. and Schwede, T. (2004). The SWISS-MODEL Repository of annotated three-dimensional protein structure homology models. *Nucleic Acids Research* 32 (Database issue): D230–D234.

29 Biasini, M. et al. (2014). SWISS-MODEL: modeling protein tertiary and quaternary structure using evolutionary information. *Nucleic Acids Research* 42 (Web Server issue): W252–W258.

30 Schwede, T. et al. (2003). SWISS-MODEL: an automated protein homology-modeling server. *Nucleic Acids Research* 31 (13): 3381–3385.

31 Waterhouse, A. et al. (2018). SWISS-MODEL: homology modelling of protein structures and complexes. *Nucleic Acids Research* 46 (W1): W296–W303.

32 UniProt Consortium (2021). UniProt: the universal protein knowledgebase in 2021. *Nucleic Acids Research* 49 (D1): D480–D489.

33 Burley, S.K. (2021). Impact of structural biologists and the Protein Data Bank on small-molecule drug discovery and development. *The Journal of Biological Chemistry* 296: 100559.

34 Dana, J.M. et al. (2019). SIFTS: updated structure integration with function, taxonomy and sequences resource allows 40-fold increase in coverage of structure-based annotations for proteins. *Nucleic Acids Research* 47 (D1): D482–D489.

35 Velankar, S. et al. (2013). SIFTS: structure integration with function, taxonomy and sequences resource. *Nucleic Acids Research* 41 (Database issue): D483–D489.

36 Feng, Z. et al. (2021). Enhanced validation of small-molecule ligands and carbohydrates in the Protein Data Bank. *Structure* 29 (4): 393–400.e1.

37 Gore, S. et al. (2017). Validation of structures in the Protein Data Bank. *Structure* 25 (12): 1916–1927.

38 Fährrolfes, R. et al. (2017). ProteinsPlus: a web portal for structure analysis of macromolecules. *Nucleic Acids Research* 45 (W1): W337–W343.

39 Meyder, A. et al. (2017). Estimating electron density support for individual atoms and molecular fragments in X-ray structures. *Journal of Chemical Information and Modeling* 57 (10): 2437–2447.

40 Schöning-Stierand, K. et al. (2020) 'ProteinsPlus: interactive analysis of protein–ligand binding interfaces', *Nucleic Acids Research*, W48–W53. https://doi.org/10.1093/nar/gkaa235.

41 Camacho, C. et al. (2009) 'BLAST+: architecture and applications', *BMC Bioinformatics*, 10. https://doi.org/10.1186/1471-2105-10-421.

42 Steinegger, M. et al. (2019) 'HH-suite3 for fast remote homology detection and deep protein annotation', *BMC Bioinformatics*, 20(1). https://doi.org/10.1186/s12859-019-3019-7.

43 Studer, G. et al. (2021). ProMod3-A versatile homology modelling toolbox. *PLoS Computational Biology* 17 (1): e1008667.

44 Eastman, P. and Pande, V.S. (2015). OpenMM: a hardware independent framework for molecular simulations. *Computing in Science & Engineering* 12 (4): 34–39.

45 Studer, G. et al. (2020). QMEANDisCo-distance constraints applied on model quality estimation. *Bioinformatics* 36 (8): 2647.

46 Mariani, V. et al. (2013). lDDT: a local superposition-free score for comparing protein structures and models using distance difference tests. *Bioinformatics* 29 (21): 2722–2728.

47 Baker, D. and Sali, A. (2001) 'Protein structure prediction and structural genomics', *Science*, 93–96. https://doi.org/10.1126/science.1065659.

48 Kryshtafovych, A. et al. (2021). Critical assessment of methods of protein structure prediction (CASP)-Round XIV. *Proteins* 89 (12): 1607–1617.

49 Pereira, J. et al. (2021). High-accuracy protein structure prediction in CASP14. *Proteins* [Preprint], (prot.26171). https://doi.org/10.1002/prot.26171.

50 Haddad, Y., Adam, V., and Heger, Z. (2020). Ten quick tips for homology modeling of high-resolution protein 3D structures. *PLoS Computational Biology* 16 (4): e1007449.

51 Pearce, R. and Zhang, Y. (2021). Toward the solution of the protein structure prediction problem. *The Journal of Biological Chemistry* 297 (1): 100870.

52 Behringer, D. et al. (2019) ModelArchive – a deposition system for persistent archiving of theoretical protein structure models. *F1000 Research Limited*. https://doi.org/10.7490/F1000RESEARCH.1117295.1.

53 Berman, H.M. et al. (2019). Federating structural models and data: outcomes from a workshop on archiving integrative structures. *Structure* 27 (12): 1745–1759.

54 Vallat, B. et al. (2021). New system for archiving integrative structures. *Acta Crystallographica Section D, Structural Biology* 77 (Pt 12): 1486–1496.

55 Humphreys, I.R. et al. (2021). Computed structures of core eukaryotic protein complexes. *Science* 374 (6573): eabm4805.

56 Blum, M. et al. (2021). The InterPro protein families and domains database: 20 years on. *Nucleic Acids Research* 49 (D1): D344–D354.

57 Lomize, A.L. et al. (2006). Positioning of proteins in membranes: a computational approach. *Protein Science: A Publication of the Protein Society* 15 (6): 1318–1333.

58 Grosdidier, A., Zoete, V. and Michielin, O. (2011a) 'Fast docking using the CHARMM force field with EADock DSS', *Journal of Computational Chemistry*, 2149–2159. https://doi.org/10.1002/jcc.21797.

59 Grosdidier, A., Zoete, V., and Michielin, O. (2011b). SwissDock, a protein-small molecule docking web service based on EADock DSS. *Nucleic Acids Research* 39 (Web Server issue): W270–W277.

60 Salentin, S. et al. (2015) 'PLIP: fully automated protein–ligand interaction profiler', *Nucleic Acids Research*, W443–W447. https://doi.org/10.1093/nar/gkv315.

61 Williams, C.J. et al. (2018). MolProbity: more and better reference data for improved all-atom structure validation. *Protein Science: A Publication of the Protein Society* 27 (1): 293–315.

62 Ginalski, K. et al. (2003). 3D-Jury: a simple approach to improve protein structure predictions. *Bioinformatics* 19 (8): 1015–1018.

63 Haas, J. et al. (2013). The protein model portal – a comprehensive resource for protein structure and model information. *Database: The Journal of Biological Databases and Curation* 2013: bat031.

64 Haas, J. et al. (2018). Continuous automated model evaluation (CAMEO) complementing the critical assessment of structure prediction in CASP12. *Proteins: Structure, Function, and Bioinformatics* 387–398. https://doi.org/10.1002/prot.25431.

65 Haas, J. et al. (2019). Introducing "best single template" models as reference baseline for the continuous automated model evaluation (CAMEO). *Proteins* 87 (12): 1378–1387.

66 Robin, X. et al. (2021). Continuous automated model evaluation (CAMEO)-perspectives on the future of fully automated evaluation of structure prediction methods. *Proteins* 89 (12): 1977–1986.

67 Zemla, A. et al. (2001). Processing and evaluation of predictions in CASP4. *Proteins* 5: 13–21.

68 Zemla, A. (2003). LGA: a method for finding 3D similarities in protein structures. *Nucleic Acids Research* 31 (13): 3370–3374.

69 Olechnovič, K., Kulberkytė, E., and Venclovas, C. (2013). CAD-score: a new contact area difference-based function for evaluation of protein structural models. *Proteins* 81 (1): 149–162.

70 Kwon, S. et al. (2021). Assessment of protein model structure accuracy estimation in CASP14: old and new challenges. *Proteins* 89 (12): 1940–1948.

71 Navia, M.A. et al. (1989). Three-dimensional structure of aspartyl protease from human immunodeficiency virus HIV-1. *Nature* 337 (6208): 615–620.

72 Schulz, G.E., Müller, C.W., and Diederichs, K. (1990). Induced-fit movements in adenylate kinases. *Journal of Molecular Biology* 213 (4): 627–630.

73 Raag, R. et al. (1993). Inhibitor-induced conformational change in cytochrome P-450CAM. *Biochemistry* 32 (17): 4571–4578.

74 Guo, J. and Zhou, H.-X. (2016). Protein allostery and conformational dynamics. *Chemical Reviews* 116 (11): 6503–6515.

75 Saldaño, T. et al. (2022) Impact of protein conformational diversity on AlphaFold predictions, *Bioinformatics*. 38 (10) 2742–2748.

76 Callaway, E. (2020). "It will change everything": DeepMind's AI makes gigantic leap in solving protein structures. *Nature* 588 (7837): 203–204.

77 Service, R.F. (2020). "The game has changed." AI triumphs at protein folding. *Science* 370 (6521): 1144–1145.

78 Wu, F. et al. (2020). A new coronavirus associated with human respiratory disease in China. *Nature* 579 (7798): 265–269.

79 Gervasoni, S. et al. (2020) 'A comprehensive mapping of the druggable cavities within the SARS-CoV-2 therapeutically relevant proteins by combining pocket and docking searches as implemented in pockets 2.0', *International Journal of Molecular Sciences*, 21(14). https://doi.org/10.3390/ijms21145152.

80 Sarkar, M. and Saha, S. (2020). Structural insight into the role of novel SARS-CoV-2 E protein: a potential target for vaccine development and other therapeutic strategies. *PLoS One* 15 (8): e0237300.

81 Idris, M.O. et al. (2021). Computer-aided screening for potential TMPRSS2 inhibitors: a combination of pharmacophore modeling, molecular docking and molecular dynamics simulation approaches. *Journal of Biomolecular Structure & Dynamics* 39 (15): 5638–5656.

82 Mirza, M.U. and Froeyen, M. (2020). Structural elucidation of SARS-CoV-2 vital proteins: computational methods reveal potential drug candidates against main protease, Nsp12 polymerase and Nsp13 helicase. *Journal of Pharmaceutical Analysis* 10 (4): 320–328.

83 Ginex, T. et al. (2021) 'Host-directed FDA-approved drugs with antiviral activity against SARS-CoV-2 identified by hierarchical in silico/in vitro screening methods', *Pharmaceuticals* , 14(4). https://doi.org/10.3390/ph14040332.

84 Santos-Beneit, F. et al. (2021). A metabolic modeling approach reveals promising therapeutic targets and antiviral drugs to combat COVID-19. *Scientific Reports* 11 (1): 11982.

85 Sugiyama, M.G. et al. (2021). Multiscale interactome analysis coupled with off-target drug predictions reveals drug repurposing candidates for human coronavirus disease. *Scientific Reports* 11 (1): 1–18.

86 Banerjee, A., Santra, D., and Maiti, S. (2020). Energetics and IC50 based epitope screening in SARS CoV-2 (COVID 19) spike protein by immunoinformatic analysis implicating for a suitable vaccine development. *Journal of Translational Medicine* 18 (1): 281.

87 Rahman, N. et al. (2020) 'Vaccine design from the ensemble of surface glycoprotein epitopes of SARS-CoV-2: an immunoinformatics approach', *Vaccine*, 8(3). https://doi.org/10.3390/vaccines8030423.

88 Garushyants, S.K., Rogozin, I.B., and Koonin, E.V. (2021). Template switching and duplications in SARS-CoV-2 genomes give rise to insertion variants that merit monitoring. *Communications Biology* 4 (1): 1343.

89 Jimenez Ruiz, J.A., Lopez Ramirez, C., and Lopez-Campos, J.L. (2021). A comparative study between Spanish and British SARS-CoV-2 variants. *Current Issues in Molecular Biology* 43 (3): 2036–2047.

90 Ortega, J.T., Jastrzebska, B. and Rangel, H.R. (2021) 'Omicron SARS-CoV-2 variant spike protein shows an increased affinity to the human ACE2 receptor: an in silico analysis', *Pathogens*, 45. https://doi.org/10.3390/pathogens11010045.

91 Lin, Z. et al. (2021). Curcumin mediates autophagy and apoptosis in granulosa cells: a study of integrated network pharmacology and molecular docking to elucidate toxicological mechanisms. *Drug and Chemical Toxicology* 1–13.

92 Watanabe, M. et al. (2021) 'Rabdosianone I, a bitter diterpene from an oriental herb, suppresses thymidylate synthase expression by directly binding to ANT2 and PHB2', *Cancers*, 982. https://doi.org/10.3390/cancers13050982.

93 Kwarteng, A. et al. (2021). In silico drug repurposing for filarial infection predicts nilotinib and paritaprevir as potential inhibitors of the Wolbachia 5′-aminolevulinic acid synthase. *Scientific Reports* 11 (1): 1–14.

94 Inderbinen, S.G. et al. (2021). Species-specific differences in the inhibition of 11β-hydroxysteroid dehydrogenase 2 by itraconazole and posaconazole. *Toxicology and Applied Pharmacology* 412: 115387.

95 Pereira, J. and Schwede, T. (2021). Interactomes in the era of deep learning. *Science* 1319–1320.
96 Tong, A.B. et al. (2021). Could AlphaFold revolutionize chemical therapeutics? *Nature Structural & Molecular Biology* 28 (10): 771–772.
97 Egbert, M. et al. (2021). Assessing the binding properties of CASP14 targets and models. *Proteins* 89 (12): 1922–1939.
98 Yang, H. et al. (2021). PhosIDN: an integrated deep neural network for improving protein phosphorylation site prediction by combining sequence and protein-protein interaction information. *Bioinformatics* [Preprint]. https://doi.org/10.1093/bioinformatics/btab551.
99 Littmann, M. et al. (2021). Clustering FunFams using sequence embeddings improves EC purity. *Bioinformatics* [Preprint]. https://doi.org/10.1093/bioinformatics/btab371.
100 Aggarwal, R. et al. (2021). DeepPocket: ligand binding site detection and segmentation using 3D convolutional neural networks. *Journal of Chemical Information and Modeling* [Preprint]. https://doi.org/10.1021/acs.jcim.1c00799.
101 Shin, J.-E. et al. (2021). Protein design and variant prediction using autoregressive generative models. *Nature Communications* 12 (1): 2403.
102 Batool, M., Ahmad, B. and Choi, S. (2019) 'A structure-based drug discovery paradigm', *International Journal of Molecular Sciences*, 20(11). https://doi.org/10.3390/ijms20112783.

7

PDB-REDO in Computational-Aided Drug Design (CADD)

Ida de Vries, Anastassis Perrakis, and Robbie P. Joosten

Oncode Institute and The Netherlands Cancer Institute, Department of Biochemistry, Plesmanlaan, 121 1066 CX Amsterdam, the Netherlands

PDB-REDO is both a pipeline that aims to optimize crystallographic macromolecular structure models and a databank offering optimized versions of Protein Data Bank (PDB) models. The automated decision-making system refines, rebuilds, and validates the models available in the PDB or provided by users, based on their original experimental diffraction data. It returns a new structure model with rich metadata on model quality and structural changes. Optimized PDB models are saved to the PDB-REDO databank, which contains "redone" structure models with their electron density maps and associated validation data. The PDB-REDO databank is a good resource for structure models in a computer-aided drug design (CADD) project.

7.1 History and Concepts

7.1.1 X-ray Structure Models

The most commonly used technique to obtain macromolecular structure models is X-ray crystallography (Figure 7.1). In the crystallographic process, the protein, DNA, RNA, or complex is crystallized and irradiated with X-rays. This results in a set of 2D diffraction images, which undergoes a series of complex operations to determine the intensity and the associated error of diffracted X-rays constrained by the symmetry of the crystal. This results into what we will refer to here as "experimental data," a list of intensities and their estimated errors. After the experimental data are available, crystallographers need to retrieve the missing phases of the diffracted X-rays by computational methods that involve prior knowledge about the nature of the macromolecular structure, often by collecting additional experimental data. The experimental data and the phase estimates allow the construction of a 3D electron density map, which is to construct an initial structure model [1]. Next, this atomic model is refined using refinement software [2–4] and validated against targets based on independent knowledge of the macromolecular structure [5]. Important steps in this process are defining the parameters for the refinement and judging the quality of

Open Access Databases and Datasets for Drug Discovery, First Edition.
Edited by Antoine Daina, Michael Przewosny, and Vincent Zoete.
© 2024 WILEY-VCH GmbH. Published 2024 by WILEY-VCH GmbH.

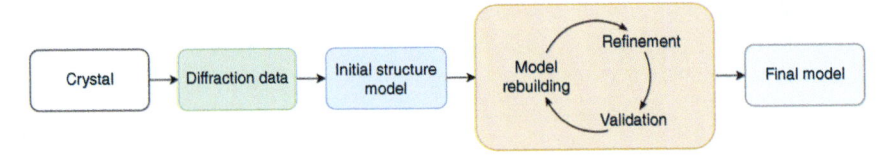

Figure 7.1 Workflow of an X-ray crystallographic experiment to obtain a macromolecular structure model.

the newly obtained model based on the validation. There are various software packages available for the refinement and validation [6–8], each with its own strengths and weaknesses. The rebuilding, refinement, and validation steps should be repeated because, due to the intricacies of the crystallographic process we briefly explained above, better estimates of the phases are computed and thus better electron density maps when the atomic model improves. After many iterations, the structure model cannot be improved any further and is then considered "optimal" [9]. This end-point remains highly subjective to date [10].

For several decades (50 years at the moment of writing [11, 12]), crystallographers have uploaded their structure models obtained from crystallography experiments to the PDB [13]. This databank contains over 180,000 structure models and has become a key resource for (computational) structural biology, biochemistry, and drug design with 1.3G downloads in 2020 alone. Experimental techniques and also the software used to analyze the diffraction data continue to develop and improve. This has resulted in overall more accurate models of macromolecular structures that were mostly deposited more recently [14]. Usually, crystallographers continue with other projects and do not update the deposited structure models after PDB deposition. As a result, especially older structure models are not as accurate as they could be with the current computational methods. Researchers interested in such a structure may choose to optimize the structure themselves when experimental data are available. The latter is not always the case, as only since 2008 the PDB has made it mandatory to upload the experimental data when depositing a new structure model to this database [5]. Nevertheless, 86% of all X-ray diffraction entries have their experimental data available. As crystallographic skills do not necessarily belong to the expertise of researchers in CADD, judging the quality of a structure model can become problematic. For such structural biology research purposes, but also to help active crystallographers determine better structures, the PDB-REDO procedure and the associated databank have been developed [15].

7.1.2 PDB-REDO Development

The PDB-REDO databank contains alternative versions of the X-ray crystallographic structure models deposited in the PDB that were updated with the PDB-REDO software pipeline using the original experimental data that is also deposited with most PDB entries. PDB-REDO entries (>155,000) are generally of better quality than their PDB counterparts in terms of fit to the experimental data and molecular geometry [15]. An additional and crucial benefit for CADD approaches is that the (methodological) uniformity of the structure models is substantially improved, as all models are generated using the same pipeline and validated against the same targets. Both overall model quality and model uniformity have made considerable steps forward over the course of PDB-REDO development.

7.1.2.1 First Uniformity

The first version of the PDB-REDO databank contained optimized coordinates of the structure models as well as the model parameters used in refinement for structures with a resolution of 2.70 Å or better [15]. R-free was used as a model quality indicator and the quality of the model coordinates was verified using WHAT_CHECK [8]. An important aspect of the process was that PDB-REDO optimized in a uniform way the relative weight of the experimental data and the so-called "geometric restraints." The latter consists of *a priori* expectations of the covalent geometry of amino acids and other chemical moieties that are found in macromolecular structures and in molecular simulations terminology can be thought of as a basic "force field." At least at that time, finding the optimal weight between these two factors, "experiment" and "geometry," has been often up to each user of each software package. Crucially, PDB-REDO was not only choosing the software package for optimization, but was also proposing an objective algorithm for determining this weighting factor. A key in the re-refinement process that was done for each entry was the uniform use of translation, liberation, and screw (TLS) displacement models [16] during the refinement [17]. The TLS models work on groups of atoms that behave as rigid bodies and provide a layer of information to the atomic displacement parameters. These parameters describe anisotropic movement by adding only 20 model parameters per group and without changing the characteristics of the input PDB entry in terms of e.g. ligands, rotamers, and amino acids. This was then followed by general model refinement that finetuned the atomic positions and B-factors. Although the structure models improved in terms of fit to the X-ray and to other model quality indicators, more gross modeling errors (e.g. side chains out of density) were not handled in this first version of the PDB-REDO databank. Manual inspection and adjustments were still required to resolve these errors [18].

7.1.2.2 Automatic Rebuilding of Protein Backbone and Side Chains

In further development of PDB-REDO, the programs *pepflip* and *SideAide* were adapted from the ARP/wARP package [19] and implemented in the pipeline [20]. These two were the first fully automated tools to systematically check, correct, and improve the protein with respect to the electron density maps if the electron density maps indicate that this is needed. As the name implies, *pepflip* systematically checks for all peptide planes (i.e. the planes consisting of the $C\alpha_i$, C_i, O_i, N_{i+1}, and $C\alpha_{i+1}$ backbone atoms) outside the cores of α-helices and β-strands whether alternative, flipped orientations improve the fit to the electron density as well as the position of the two involved residues on the Ramachandran plot. If so, the adjustment is kept, as it is considered to be an improvement of the model. *SideAide* was implemented to optimize amino acid side chain conformations. This tool searches for the rotamer conformation of a side chain that shows the best fit to the electron density map.

During this process, the correctly modeled parts of the structure model are kept rigid, so that no interference occurs. Furthermore, the Cα atoms are allowed to shift, increasing the sampled search space and thus the detection rate. The best rotamer is selected for each amino acid, after which refinement of the structure model against the electron density map is performed. Subsequent validation indicates whether the change in rotamer have indeed improved the structure [20]. Additionally, side chains of histidine, glutamine, and asparagine are flipped if this improves the local hydrogen bonding network.

It should be noted that PDB-REDO by default completes missing side chains in structure models even when the electron density is relatively poor. Although other methods of dealing with poor side chain density are also used by crystallographers (e.g. side chain truncation or manipulation of the occupancy of side chain atoms), the completion of side chains in the most plausible conformation has the advantage that interpretation is still possible even without having the complete structural model. The positional uncertainty of the added side chain atoms is, to a large extent, captured in the atomic B-factors.

7.1.2.3 Automated Model Completion Approaches

The addition of missing side-chains was a first step toward making structure models more complete. In further PDB-REDO development, *Loopwhole* was added to complete loops in protein models. When *Loopwhole* detects an unmodeled loop in the protein model (based on the deposited sequence), it looks for homologs of the protein that do contain a modeled loop at that position in the protein. If "homologous loops" are found, they are transferred to the structure model of interest by local structural alignment. After real-space optimization, the loop with the best fit to the electron density is retained when it is of sufficient quality in terms of geometry and fit to the density map [21]. Besides auto-completion of the protein part of structures, PDB-REDO also works on carbohydrates from N-glycosylation. Carbohydrates are often added to proteins as post-translational modifications and are important recognition parameters in several biological processes (e.g. protein folding). Modeling of the carbohydrates in protein structure models is often done relatively poorly [22, 23] because it has received little attention in the past, and interactive tools for handling carbohydrates were not well-developed (that is, handling polysaccharides required expertise far beyond normal use of the software available) and also because the task contains particular challenges. The experimental data are commonly less informative for carbohydrates than for protein and the tools for model building of carbohydrates are not as well established as those for proteins. Additionally, many carbohydrates present in structure models are often not the research interest of the depositor [24]. *Carbivore* was written and added to the PDB-REDO pipeline to overcome these challenges by automating the extension of existing carbohydrate trees [25] using, at that time, newly introduced functionality in the popular model-building software COOT [26, 27]. *Carbivore* is also able to build new trees at asparagine residues that are part of the so-called N-glycosylation sequon Asn-X-Ser/Thr [28]. Additionally, carbohydrates that do not fit any known glycosylation tree added *in vivo*, are deleted from the protein structure model and rebuilt.

7.1.2.4 Systematic Integration of Structural Knowledge

Besides the use of homologous proteins to complete loops in a protein, homolog structures are also used as an additional source of geometric restraints for the refinement of models with low-resolution experimental data [29]. This information is captured by comparing hydrogen bonds in the structure model to equivalent hydrogen bonds in close homologs (70% sequence identity or better). The mean hydrogen bond length in the homologs is used to set a distance restraint between the hydrogen bonding partners in the model. The standard deviation is used to set the relative weight of the restraints so that low standard deviations resulting from strong structural conservation and impose tight restrains, while large standard deviations cause loose restraints. The use of such restraints improves the geometric quality of the structure models [29]. Additionally, the use of such homology-based restraints increases the consistency of structural homologs, unless there is strong signal in the experimental data for structural differences. This makes it easier for users to assess the structural effect of moving a protein from one functional state to another, e.g. by binding different ligands.

The addition of new structural knowledge when refining structure models in PDB-REDO is not limited to proteins. Other specialized restraints are added for structural zinc binding sites [30] and for base pairs in nucleic acid structures [31].

7.1.2.5 Overview of PDB-REDO Pipeline

The input for the PDB-REDO pipeline (Figure 7.2) is an atomic coordinate file, the experimental data file, and the sequence. The pipeline checks if all required data are provided and determines various parameters that are used for the refinement with REFMAC [2]. Next, several parallel refinements of the structure model are executed with different combinations of parameters, and the best parameters for refinement are chosen. Then, the new model and electron density map are used for structure rebuilding with the tools we described above. The rebuilt model is refined once more, while fine-tuning the parameters from the previous round to obtain the final structure, i.e. the PDB-REDO model. This model is validated on overall structure parameters, e.g. R-free and Ramachandran Z-score. Nucleic acids are validated against their specific parameters and ligands are validated separately as well. The parameters, tools and software, the PDB-REDO model, maps, and validation data are all saved in the PDB-REDO databank for existing PDB entries. As a result of the

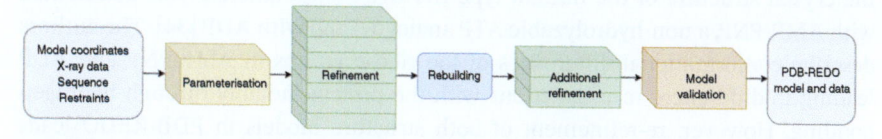

Figure 7.2 The fully automated decision-making PDB-REDO pipeline for optimization of macromolecular structure models that were obtained from X-ray crystallographic experiments. 3D boxes represent parallel computing.

PDB-REDO pipeline, more accurate descriptions of the structure models supported by the experimentally obtained electron density are obtained.

In order to optimize structure models in an effective and efficient manner, all the steps in PDB-REDO are fully automated. The tools in the PDB-REDO pipeline that enable the functionalities described above are tied together with many decision-making algorithms that together form a so-called "expert system," i.e. a framework that tries to mimic what a human expert would do [32]. Of course, the complexity of this system comes at a price in terms of speed and therefore many steps use parallel computing. As a result, a typical PDB-REDO calculation takes less than 30 minutes on a modern workstation whereas any manual approach might cost hours or even days.

7.2 Structure Improvements by PDB-REDO

To showcase the benefits of using PDB-REDO models, this section discusses specific examples that illustrate how updated macromolecular structure models can change the biological interpretation of a structure model. These cases are, therefore, interesting examples of the benefits that PDB-REDO can bring to CADD projects.

7.2.1 Parametrization and Rebuilding Effects on Small Molecule Ligands

Many macromolecular structures contain (small molecule) ligands, (metal) ions, or cofactors that are involved in protein function or structural integrity. Also, small molecules can be used to modulate the protein's function or to mediate protein–protein interactions. Such compounds are found in X-ray structure models and are treated distinctly during parameterization and refinement in the PDB-REDO pipeline [33]. Here, we illustrate how the specific and uniform treatment of such compounds, as well as the possible consequences of rebuilding in their proximity, can affect biochemical conclusions and thus CADD projects.

7.2.1.1 Re-refinement Improves Ligand Conformation

Type IIA DNA topoisomerases are ATP-dependent enzymes involved in cell growth and division by changing the coiling of DNA helices. These enzymes are the targets for antibiotics and antitumor agents. To obtain structural insights into the mechanism of ATP hydrolysis that is coupled to the topoisomerase function, the crystal structure of the human type IIA DNA topoisomerase was determined with AMP-PNP, a non-hydrolyzable ATP analogue, and with ADP [34]. The authors describe conformational differences of the ribose groups in AMP-PNP and ADP leading to differences in interactions with the protein, notably through hydrogen bonding. However, re-refinement of both structure models in PDB-REDO leads to conformational changes in the nucleotide, particularly in the ribose of ADP (Figure 7.3). The PDB-REDO procedure removed most of the differences in the ribose conformations and resulted to highly similar binding modes for ADP and

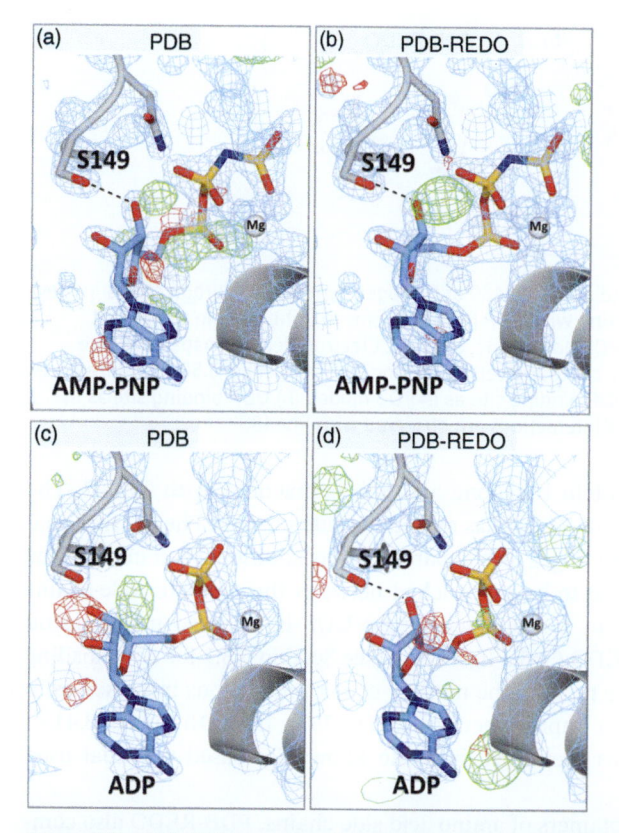

Figure 7.3 PDB-REDO results of the binding site of AMP-PNP and ADP (carbon atoms in light blue) in human type IIA DNA topoisomerase (grey, PDB entries 1zxm and 1zxn, chain A), side chains of SER149 and ASN150 are shown (carbon atoms in grey) and hydrogen bonds as black dotted lines. Electron density maps (blue) are oversampled at 0.5 for clarity, contour levels: 2.5σ for 2mF$_o$-DF$_c$ map 1zxm, 2.0σ for 2mF$_o$-DF$_c$ map 1zxn, 3.5σ for difference density (red and green). (a) Model as deposited in the PDB with AMP-PNP. (b) Model by PDB-REDO with the improved conformation of AMP-PNP. (c) Model as deposited in the PDB with negative difference density surrounding the O2′ and O3′ atoms of ADP. The ribose has a different conformation from that in AMP-PNP. (d) PDB-REDO model in which re-refinement has led to a change in ribose conformation removing the difference between ADP and AMP-PNP. The negative difference density surrounding the O2′ and O3′ atoms disappeared. Figure and all molecular graphics figures below were made with CCP4mg. Source: Adapted from McNicholas et al. [35].

AMP-PNP, contradicting the original interpretation of the authors. These models show the importance of proper refinement parameterization as used in PDB-REDO.

7.2.1.2 Side Chain Rebuilding Improves Ligand Binding Sites

Glycogen synthase-2 is involved in the biosynthesis of glycogen, which is one of the most important energy sources in eukaryotes. The basal state of this enzyme in complex with UDP was crystallized, which provided new structural insights into the activation of glycogen synthase-2 [36]. Inspection of the binding site in the PDB-deposited model shows that the uridine base is held in place by a

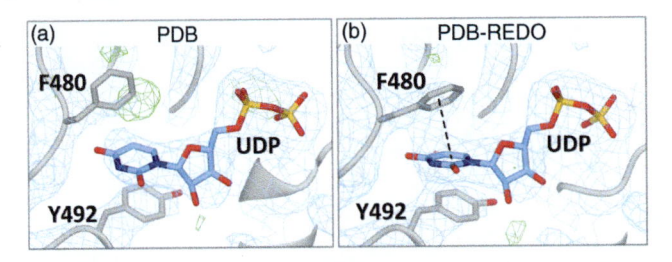

Figure 7.4 Side chain rebuilding of Phe480 of Glycogen synthase-2 (carbon atoms in grey) results in improved π–π stacking with UDP (carbon atoms in light blue) in the crystal structure of the basal state (PDB entry 3o3c, chain A). Electron density maps (blue) are oversampled at 0.5 for clarity, contour levels: 1.75σ for $2mF_o\text{-}DF_c$ map, 3.50σ for difference density (red and green). (a) UDP binding site as in PDB model. (b) UDP binding site as in PDB-REDO model, where π–π interactions are observed with Phe480.

hydrogen bond to the protein backbone and π–π interactions with Tyr492. The side-chain rebuilding in PDB-REDO has moved the side-chain of Phe480 such that its contribution to UDP binding is also apparent. It has additional π–π interactions with UDP causing the base to be sandwiched between the aromatic side-chains (Figure 7.4). The change in π–π interactions for UDP is recorded in the ligand validation data of PDB-REDO (3o3c_ligval.json (see Section 7.3.1 for downloading details)). In chain A of the protein, the number of π–π interactions increased from 3 to 6, with a π–π strength improvement of 0.69 (2.75 in the PDB model, 3.44 in the PDB-REDO model) as measured from the knowledge-based potential used in YASARA [37].

Besides changing the rotamers of amino acid side chains, PDB-REDO also completes residues in which the side-chains were left unmodeled. This is illustrated by the binding site of BRAF V600E mutant co-crystallized with vem-bisamide. This kinase is an oncoprotein in the mitogen-activated protein kinase (MAPK) signaling pathway that is found mutated in several forms of cancer. In melanoma for instance, the V600E pathogenic mutant is observed regularly and is often targeted in drug discovery. Vemurafenib is one of the compounds that resulted from such studies but can lead to so-called transactivation of wild-type BRAF. By chemical linkage of two vemurafenib molecules, vem-bisamide was developed to overcome this transactivation by forcing BRAF into an inactive dimeric conformation. One of the key residues in potency of inhibitors based on linked vemurafenib-moieties is Gln461 [38]. The interaction with this residue is nicely modeled in chain A of the crystal structure of BRAF-V600E in complex with vem-bisamide. However, in chain B the side-chain of Gln461 is not modeled, hiding a key protein–ligand interaction (Figure 7.5). In the PDB-REDO model, this residue Gln461 has been completed and the interaction with the ligand is made obvious (Figure 7.5).

7.2.1.3 Histidine Flip and Improved Ligand Parameterization

The crystal structure of the *E. coli* autoinducer-2 processing protein LsrF was obtained without and with the ligands ribose-5-phosphate (R5P) or

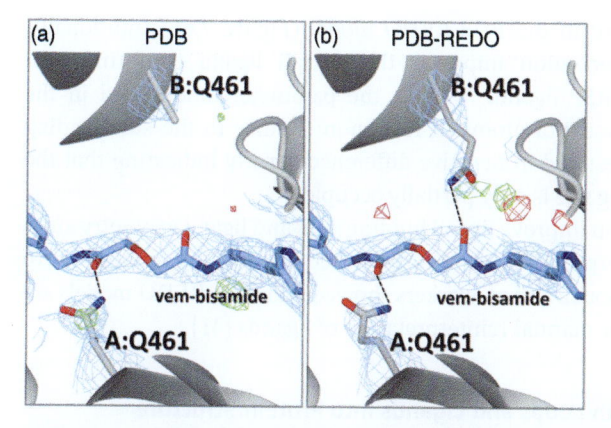

Figure 7.5 Vem-bisamide (carbon atoms in light blue, partially shown) is symmetrically bound by two copies of BRAF kinase (grey, PDB entry 5jt2). Electron density maps (blue) are oversampled at 0.5 for clarity, contour levels: 1.25σ for $2mF_o\text{-}DF_c$ map, 3.5σ for difference density (red and green). (a) In the PDB model, key interacting residue Gln461 (carbon atoms in grey) is only completely placed in one of the BRAF chains. (b) The missing side chain of the second Gln461 has been completed by PDB-REDO revealing the full interaction of VEM-BISAMIDE with BRAF.

ribulose-5-phosphate. These structures lead to the strong suggestion that LsrF belongs to class I aldolases, which are involved in maintaining bacterial expression of specific genes by catalyzing the formation or cleavage of C–C bonds [39]. The HSSP multiple sequence alignment [40] of LsrF shows that the binding pocket is highly conserved with His58 fully conserved among species. Therefore, it is most likely that this histidine is involved in binding of R5P. However, in the crystal structure of the autoinducer-2 as deposited in the PDB, His58 does not form any specific interaction with the ligand (Figure 7.6). As a result of the hydrogen bond optimization module in PDB-REDO, this histidine residue has been flipped to form

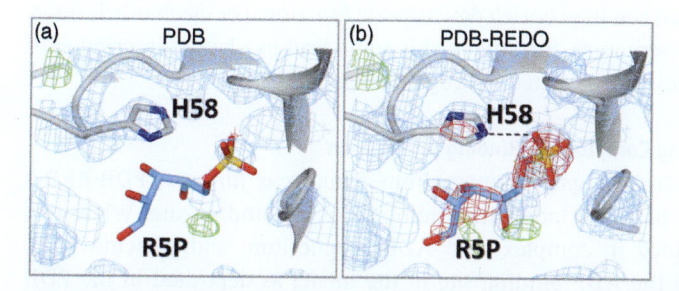

Figure 7.6 PDB-REDO improves the binding site of R5P (carbon atoms in light blue) in LsrF (grey, PDB entry 3glc, chain A) by flipping the His58 side chain (carbon atoms in grey). Additionally, the overall conformation of R5P is improved. Electron density maps (blue) are oversampled at 0.5 for clarity, contour levels: 1.5σ for $2mF_o\text{-}DF_c$ map, 3.5σ for difference density (red and green). (a) LsrF structure model as deposited in the PDB. (b) PDB-REDO model in which His58 has flipped and forms a hydrogen bond with the ligand (black dotted lines). The negative difference density indicates partial occupancy for ribose-5-phosphate.

a hydrogen bond with R5P in the PDB-REDO model (Figure 7.6). Additionally, the PDB-REDO parameterization improves the overall ligand conformational fit to the density of the R5P ligand. Notably, the parameterization used in the refinement made the B-factor of atoms in R5P more similar to the surrounding protein atoms. This has resulted in negative difference density indicating that the ribose-5-phosphate binding site is only partially occupied.

Although PDB-REDO can improve ligand binding sites and ligand geometry automatically, it cannot reinterpret the ligand to the level of providing an alternative compound. However, De Souza and co-workers showed that PDB-REDO models are a suitable starting point for manual reinterpretation of ligands [41].

7.2.2 Building of Protein Loops and Ligands into Protein Structure Models

Loops are the more flexible parts of a protein and tend to give weaker diffraction in crystallographic experiments. This results in poorer local quality of electron density maps and therefore loops are harder to model than other secondary structure elements such as α-helices and β-sheets. Incomplete protein structure models are deposited to the PDB, mostly for good reasons: when the experimental data do not support the modeling of explicit atoms, those should not be added to the model. However, the decision not to model a loop is invariably a personal one, and some unmodeled loops can be built with reasonable reliability into poor electron density if some prerequisites are met. PDB-REDO tries to solve this issue in two ways. First, the refinement steps in PDB-REDO typically lead to an improved atomic model, which in turn leads to better electron density maps than previously available. Second, the program *Loopwhole* reduces the vast number of possible loop conformations to the ones observed in experimental structures of the same or closely related proteins, which have a high probability of being correct. Combining both techniques allows PDB-REDO to add thousands of previously missing loops to PDB models. These more complete models can then enrich downstream functional or mechanistic interpretations of protein structure. Eventually, this could lead to a better description of potential binding sites to be targeted in drug discovery [21].

7.2.2.1 Loop Building Completes a Binding Site Region

In the crystal structure of galactokinase from *Pyrococcus furiosus*, PDB-REDO builds a substantial part of a loop surrounding the ADP binding site. While this structure was obtained in complex with ADP, magnesium, and galactose [42], the surroundings of the ADP binding site in the model as deposited in the PDB were left unmodeled. There is, however, density observed for this region of the protein (Figure 7.7). The automatic loop-building algorithm in the PDB-REDO pipeline improved this part of the protein structure by building the missing loop (residues 48–72) (Figure 7.7) with a good fit to the experimental data. Although new interactions between the built residues with ADP are not observed in the PDB-REDO model, the description of the protein is more complete, which is relevant for structure-based CADD.

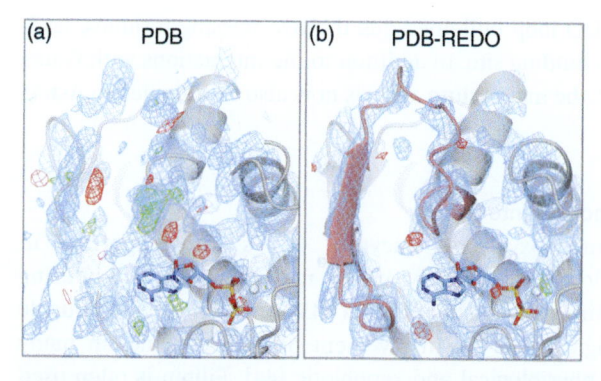

Figure 7.7 PDB-REDO builds loop surrounding the ADP (carbon atoms in light blue) binding site of the *Pyrococcus furiosus* galactokinase (grey, PDB entry 1s4e, chain B). Electron density maps (blue) are oversampled at 0.5 for clarity, contour levels: 1.0σ for $2mF_o\text{-}DF_c$ map, 3.5σ for difference density (red and green). (a) Model as deposited in the PDB with unmodeled density and difference density surrounding the ADP binding site. (b) PDB-REDO model with automatically built loop (residues 48–72, salmon pink ribbons) in the electron density to complete the chain.

7.2.2.2 Loop Building Results in Improved Binding Sites

Loop rebuilding in PDB-REDO can improve binding sites as showcased for the magnesium binding site of the geranyl diphosphate methyltransferase in complex with geranyl diphosphate (GPP) and sinefungin. This protein was used to provide insights in the methyl-group transfer mechanism, which is a common regulatory process in living organisms [43]. In the original model, magnesium interacts with the phosphate groups of GPP and with Glu89. However, the magnesium ion lacks an additional coordination ligand (Figure 7.8). This missing interaction could be explained by the unmodeled residues Val44 and Asn45, which are located in the magnesium

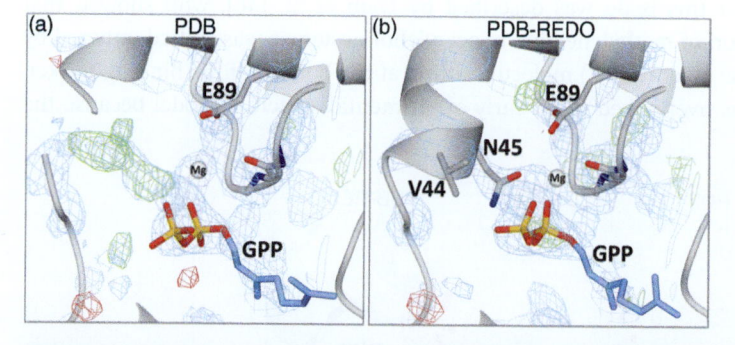

Figure 7.8 Addition of residues Val44 and Asn45 results in completing magnesium and GPP (carbon atoms in light blue) binding site in geranyl diphosphate methyltransferase (grey, PDB entry 4f86, chain H). Electron density maps (blue) are oversampled at 0.5 for clarity, contour levels: 1.75σ for $2mF_o\text{-}DF_c$ map, 3.5σ for difference density (red and green). (a) Model as deposited in the PDB with unmodeled residues 44 and 45. Magnesium is coordinated to GPP and Glu89 (carbon atoms in grey). (b) PDB-REDO model with added residues Val44 and Asn45 (carbon atoms in grey) resulting in more complete magnesium coordination.

binding site. The PDB-REDO loop building adds the two missing residues, leading to a proper magnesium binding site. In addition to the interactions with Glu89 and the phosphates of GPP, the magnesium atom is now also coordinated to Asn45 (Figure 7.8).

7.2.2.3 Building new Compounds into Density

The cytochrome P450 monooxygenase enzymes (CYPs) are important in post-polyketide modifications and thereby cause molecular diversity during metabolism. Insights into the mechanism of the CYP450 proteins provide valuable information for drug design, given the involvement of such enzymes in many metabolic processes, both physiological and xenobiotic [44]. Filipin is often used as probe for cholesterol binding sites in studies regarding this enzyme. One of such CYP450-filipin complex obtained by X-ray crystallography is the model of CYP105P1. Besides filipin, the structure also contains SO_4 ions and glycerol molecules that were used during the crystallization process [45]. When inspecting the model of this structure as deposited in the PDB, some well-defined density regions have no atoms modeled. Although this is not a feature that is employed by default, PDB-REDO can build missing compounds if provided a list of candidates. In the case of the CYP450-filipin complex, glycerol molecules and SO_4 were fitted (data not shown). Furthermore, one of the modeled water networks in the original structure (Figure 7.9) indicates that it might be replaced by a different compound present in the crystal and was indeed replaced by this compound in the PDB-REDO model (Figure 7.9).

These results show that, provided the input model has machine-readable metadata that describes other possible compounds, a model can be made more complete by automatically fitting compounds into the density. This becomes particularly important if a compound directly influences the binding pose of a ligand of interest. An example of this issue was described by Dym et al. [46], who showed that binding position of methylene blue in acetylcholinesterase was shifted outward by a poly-ethylene glycol (PEG) molecule sitting at the bottom of the binding pocket. This effect was overlooked in an early experimental structure model because the

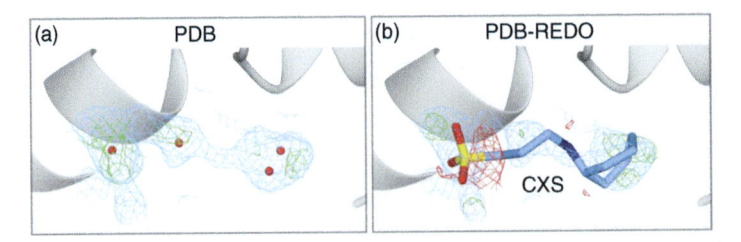

Figure 7.9 Original modeled water atoms (red spheres) are replaced by a buffer residue CSX (carbon atoms in light blue) in de PDB-REDO model of CYP105P1 (grey, PDB entry 3aba, chain A). Electron density maps (blue) are oversampled at 0.5 for clarity, contour levels: 1.0σ for $2mF_o$-DF_c map, 3.5σ for difference density (red and green). (a) Water network as present in the PDB model. (b) PDB-REDO model in which CXS has replaced the water network.

PEG was not fitted in the electron density, which caused conflicting results in downstream structural analyses.

Although crystallization additives and a buffer were used as examples, this approach can be used for ligands and fragments in experimental high-throughput (lead) drug discovery. This is available as a feature in the PDB-REDO software, which is currently being tested in real-life experimental settings.

7.2.3 Nucleic Acid Improvements by PDB-REDO

PDB-REDO also applies nucleic acid restraints and validation targets for nucleic acid-containing structure models. These parameters are limited to the most common structural features: Watson–Crick base pairs [31]. Overall nucleic acids are improved in both protein–nucleic acid complexes, as well as (mostly) nucleic acid structures such as ribosomal subunits. One of the first ribosomal structures that were deposited in the PDB is the 30S subunit that was used to study its interactions with antibiotics [47]. The antibiotic paromomycin is bound in such a way that it is surrounded by nucleotides, among which is G1494 (Figure 7.10). PDB-REDO restraints improve the orientation of this C–G base pair without changing the interactions of the nucleic acid structure with the ligand (Figure 7.10). The Z_{bpG}, a metric describing the relative orientation of the bases, is 3.63 in PDB and 2.04 in PDB-REDO, which is closer to an "ideal" C–G base pair with $Z_{bpG} = 0.0$. The strongest contribution to this improvement comes from reduced shearing between the bases. Additionally, the negative difference density on the ligand has disappeared.

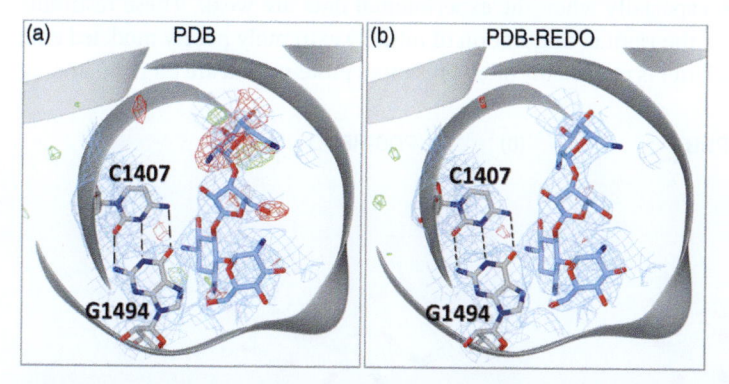

Figure 7.10 G1494-C1407 base pair (carbon atoms in grey) in the 30S ribosomal subunit (grey, PDB entry 1fjg) in complex with paromomycin (carbon atoms in light blue). Electron density maps (blue) are oversampled at 0.5 for clarity, contour level: 1.0 σ for 2mF$_o$-DF$_c$ map, 3.5 σ for difference density (red and green). Hydrogen bonds in the G–C base pair are indicated with black dotted lines. (a) Structure model as deposited in the PDB with suboptimal hydrogen bonds in the G–C base pair (2.7, 3.1, 3.3 Å, shear Z-score −8.85 Å). (b) Structure model as in PDB-REDO with improved base pair geometry (hydrogen bond distances 2.8, 2.9, 3.0 Å, shear Z-score -4.43) and the negative difference density on the ligand drastically reduced.

7.2.4 Glycoprotein Structure Model Rebuilding

Glycosylation is a common post-translational modification of proteins. The modifications are important in recognition of other proteins, stability, and formation of protein complexes [48]. In PDB models, the glycosylated parts of proteins are not always resolved properly, which indicates that there is sufficient room for model improvement. Initially, PDB-REDO worked on carbohydrates by improving model annotation and thereby helping model refinement to improve the atomic coordinates [49], but much more substantial improvements were achieved when automated (re)building of N-glycans was introduced [25]. The latter is illustrated through the crystal structure of the binding domain of SARS-CoV-2 spike, which contains a glycosylated Asn53 [50]. However, the electron density map suggests that the glycan tree can be extended (Figure 7.11). The PDB-REDO model indeed contains an additional NAG (Figure 7.11).

7.2.5 Metal Binding Sites

Description of metal binding sites is challenging in X-ray modeling software, especially at low resolution. The fact that metal binding sites have an enormous variety in geometries and possible interactors is one of the underlying causes. Many site geometries are too context-sensitive to reliably predict and restrain in model refinement, but there are common structural motifs around e.g. zinc, magnesium, and sodium, that are amenable to automated model improvement. The PDB-REDO pipeline includes a tool (*platonyzer*) that defines geometric restraints for structural zinc sites (i.e. ZnCys$_x$His$_y$ sites as found in zinc fingers and other motifs) and octahedral sodium and magnesium sites. The restraints impose regular geometry during refinement, especially when the experimental data are weak. These restraints can even recover the right configuration of initially extremely poorly modeled zinc atoms [30]. The latter is reasonably often present in proteins that are targeted in drug

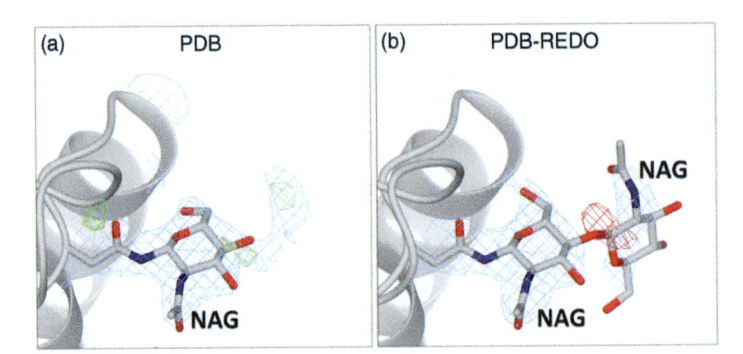

Figure 7.11 Extension of a glycan tree (carbon atoms in grey) by PDB-REDO in the SARS-CoV-2 spike receptor-binding domain bound with ACE2 (grey, PDB entry 6m0j, chain A). Electron density maps (blue) are oversampled at 0.5 for clarity, contour levels: 1.0σ for 2mF$_o$-DF$_c$ map, 3.5σ for difference density (red and green). (a) Model as deposited in the PDB that shows unmodeled density close to NAG. (b) PDB-REDO model which contains an extended glycan; no unmodeled density is observed.

discovery research. One such protein is the aspartate transcarbamoylase found in E. Coli [51], which in humans is an interesting drug target for malaria [52] and cancer [53]. The four cysteine side chains that are supposedly ligands for a zinc atom are apparently not, but instead, form an irrelevant "trisulfide" bond in the structure as deposited in the PDB (Figure 7.12). *Platonyzer* detects that this zinc binding site is not chemically correct, and generates restraints that will remodel the site during refinement. In this process, the model annotation describing incorrect disulfide bridges is removed. As a result, the zinc atom in the transcarbamoylase has the four cysteine side chains as ligands and thereby shows a correct coordination state (Figure 7.12). Additionally, the fit to the electron density maps has improved and both the positive and negative difference density disappeared.

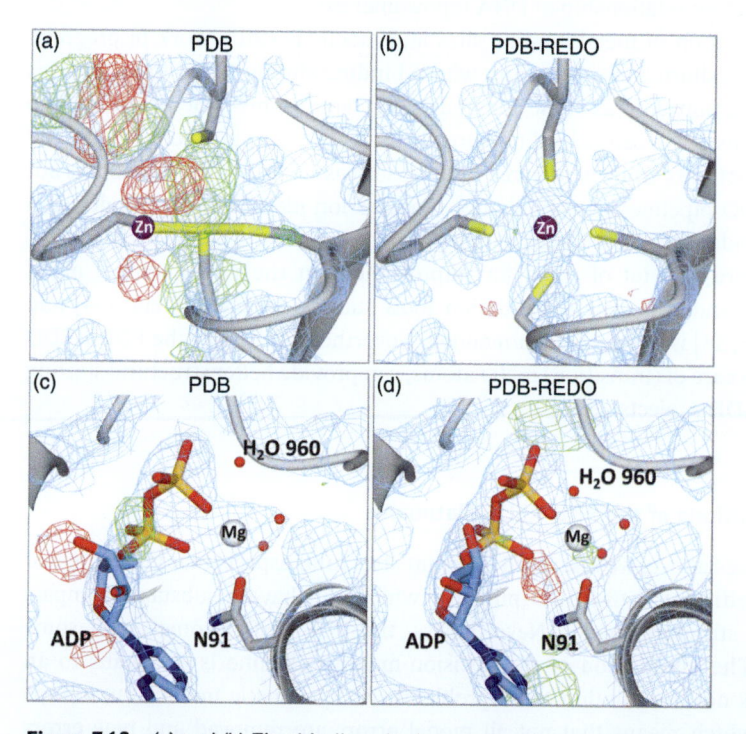

Figure 7.12 (a) and (b) Zinc binding site in aspartate transcarbamoylase (grey, PDB entry 1tug, chain D) is improved by the PDB-REDO pipeline. Electron density maps (blue) are oversampled at 0.5 for clarity, contour levels: 3.00σ for $2mF_o - DF_c$ map, 3.5σ for difference density (red and green). (a) Binding site as found in the original model wherein the cysteine side chains form a trisulfide bridge and the zinc atom does not have a valid number of ligands. (b) Improved zinc binding site in the PDB-REDO model where the cysteine side chains coordinate to the zinc atom that is now located in the middle of the binding site. (c) and (d) Magnesium binding site of the human type IIA DNA topoisomerase (grey, PDB entry 1zxn, chain A) is improved. Electron density maps (blue) are oversampled at 0.5 for clarity, contour levels: 2.00σ for $2mF_o-DF_c$ map, 3.5σ for difference density (red and green). (c) Magnesium site as in the original model in which water 960 is too far away to properly coordinate magnesium. (d) Magnesium binding site as in PDB-REDO model where water 960 has moved inward and describes a relevant magnesium site.

Besides structural zinc sites, *platonyzer* also evaluates magnesium and sodium binding sites with six-fold coordination. If these sites form (distorted) octahedrons, angle restraints are generated to clean up the site in refinement. Revisiting the DNA topoisomerase described in Section 2.1.1/Figure 7.3, but focusing on the magnesium site, which incorporates the ADP. The magnesium is coordinated to ADP phosphate groups (ADP O3B at 2.09 Å and ADP O2A at 2.01 Å), Asn91 OD1 at 2.01 Å, and two water molecules (H_2O 902 at 2.03 Å and H_2O 958 at 2.24 Å). The sixth ligand, H_2O 960, is improbably far away at 2.87 Å (Figure 7.12). In the PDB-REDO model, this water moves closer to the magnesium (1.99 Å), which makes the site more chemically realistic (Figure 7.12). This example illustrates the advantages of the PDB-REDO pipeline comprehensiveness: because both the ADP binding site and the magnesium coordination are improved, the user gets a clearer perspective on the structure–function relationship of DNA topoisomerase.

The identification of metal binding sites and metals is still a work in progress. Especially for sodium and magnesium whose binding sites are hard to distinguish in X-ray diffraction data as these ions have the same number of electrons. The coordination distances can help, if not directly used as restraints in refinement. The octahedral restraints from *platonyzer* help to unbias coordination distances, but the PDB-REDO pipeline does not change modeled ion identities yet. The decision about the ion identity thus still lies with the user.

Overall, there is a lot of room for improvement in the refinement of metal binding sites, and using metal validation tools such as CheckMyMetal [54] and MetalPDB [55, 56] is strongly recommended. Nevertheless, the way the PDB-REDO pipeline takes care of (transition) metal atoms, can provide better structural starting points for CADD projects.

7.2.6 Limitations of the PDB-REDO Databank

In the examples above, we discussed different structural aspects that are addressed by the very efficient PDB-REDO pipeline, which can have a substantial impact on the total structure model. Nevertheless, the PDB-REDO comes with some limitations. The automation of the decision-making pipeline is a "means to an end" but it is not the solution to all problems. No systematic manual curation is performed, which means that not all model errors are removed and new errors may be introduced by PDB-REDO. The software is designed to be conservative and to make only few mistakes, but with more than 150,000 structure models with tens of millions of residues in total, problems are unavoidable. The metadata of each PDB-REDO entry is designed to allow users to make an informed choice on which models are most suitable for their downstream studies. For detailed studies involving a few structure models, we recommend that users inspect the models carefully in the context of the provided electron density maps. For large-scale studies, filtering models by overall quality indicators such as R-factors and possibly local density fit metrics such as RSCC is important to construct the most suitable dataset [57].

Apart from the general problems linked to automation, there are few issues that need to be addressed separately. Firstly, some are regarding model annotation. PDB entries carry a lot of information that affects the way they are dealt with in PDB-REDO. Examples are descriptions of which (macromolecular) compounds were crystallized, which parts are modeled, residue and atom nomenclature, alternate conformers, R-factors, space groups, data quality indicators, *et cetera*. When these annotations are severely incorrect, the PDB-REDO process will either fail completely or will give very poor results. During PDB-REDO databank maintenance, errors like these are analyzed and if they can be solved by model reannotation, update requests are sent to wwPDB annotators. This process developed into a fruitful collaboration with the wwPDB by which many small and large issues in structure models have been solved at the source (i.e. the PDB) so that everyone, not just PDB-REDO users, can benefit.

A second issue is that not only new macromolecular structures but also new small molecule compounds are added to the PDB every week. Refinement of such compounds requires restraint targets that are not immediately available in the CCP4 monomer library [58], which is the key restraint source of the PDB-REDO pipeline. In such cases, restraints are generated "on the fly" based on the current atomic coordinates. This can lead to suboptimal restraints, which in turn lead to suboptimal molecular geometries. We collaborate with CCP4 developers to regularly update the CCP4 monomer library so that improved restraints become available to PDB-REDO users [59]. When users notice compounds with poor geometry in the PDB-REDO databank, brought on by poor restraints, they can request an update of the affected entry by clicking a link on the PDB-REDO entry page. Alternatively, they are welcome to contact the PDB-REDO developers directly.

A third issue that combines the problems of model annotation and geometric restraints is related to intermolecular linkages. Although the polymeric linkages between amino acids, nucleotides, and recently also saccharides [60] are well standardized by model annotation at the wwPDB and in the CCP4 monomer library [59], covalent bonds between ligands and the macromolecule are still a significant challenge. Generating the correct geometric restraints requires more information than is currently stored in structure model files. Currently, only *which* atoms are bound is stored, but not *how* they are bound. Changes in chemistry of the parent compounds, i.e. deleted atoms, changes in atom hybridization, and changes in bond orders, are not stored. This makes it challenging to generate correct restraints for covalent linkages without manual intervention [61]. Unfortunately, this phenomenon can be observed in some PDB-REDO entries and therefore users are advised to be vigilant when dealing with structure models that have such covalent linkages. Improvements to the standard data model used for macromolecules, the mmCIF format [62], are required to solve this issue permanently.

A final issue of note is technical. Due to the many practical limitations of the PDB file, this most commonly used data format for structure models, is being replaced by mmCIF. Most notably the size restrictions for models (99,999 atoms in one file, with 62 chains) and the limited extensibility to capture new metadata have led to this replacement. The mmCIF file format does not have these limitations and has been therefore chosen as the current standard for model handling in the PDB [63]. At the same time, the legacy of structural biology software, including software for CADD does not (fully) support the mmCIF format yet. This is also true for some of the software in the PDB-REDO pipeline. This means that even though PDB-REDO can use mmCIF formatted files as input and output, models are still described in PDB format within the pipeline. Because of this, 400 very large structure models could not be processed and are currently missing from the PDB-REDO databank. These will be added once all the software in the PDB-REDO pipeline becomes mmCIF compliant.

7.3 Access the PDB-REDO Databank and Metadata

7.3.1 Downloading and Inspecting Individual PDB-REDO Entries

All the models that are parsed through the PDB-REDO pipeline are stored in a databank that can be accessed at https://pdb-redo.eu/. The whole databank can be downloaded, but conveniently it is also possible to download a single entry. The latter can be done either through the website, or users can open the desired structure model directly in molecular graphics software YASARA [37], COOT [26], or CCP4mg [35]. These software packages have the utility to download and show the PDB-REDO model and corresponding density maps from their interface [64].

When using the PDB-REDO website, an entry page visualizing the metadata of the structure model is provided. An example for PDB entry 1lf2 [65] is shown in Figure 7.13. On top of the entry page, a table (Figure 7.13) provides crystallographic data such as space group, resolution, and R-factor of the structure model. Also, the links to download the PDB-REDO data for the structure are provided in this table. An additional table (Figure 7.13) containing metrics about the validation of the crystallographic refinement and model quality is provided. This table also indicates significant improvements or deteriorations of the PDB-REDO model compared to the model as deposited in the PDB, conveniently marked in green or red, respectively. Next, a Kleywegt-like plot is provided (Figure 7.13), showing changes in model geometry before and after PDB-REDO in terms of ϕ- and ψ-angles. The Ramachandran Z-scores are provided for both the PDB and PDB-REDO models, as well as details regarding residues in the preferred regions, allowed regions and outliers. In the subsequent panel (Figure 7.13) boxplots comparing the Z-score of the Ramachandran plot for both the PDB and PDB-REDO model with at least 1000 other structures that were obtained at similar resolutions are shown. This comparison is also provided for R-free and the rotamer quality as box plots. Additionally, a table (Figure 7.13) containing the significant model changes caused by PDB-REDO is provided. This table provides the counts of these changes, among which the number of rotamers changed, the number of side chains that were flipped, chiralities that were fixed, and also the improvement or deterioration of fit to the density. When a PDB-REDO entry is loaded into COOT, a button list is provided to users to quickly inspect all the changes in the structure model in 3D.

(a) PDB-REDO results

CRYSTAL STRUCTURE OF PLASMEPSIN II FROM P FALCIPARUM IN COMPLEX WITH INHIBITOR RS370

This entry was created with PDB-REDO version 7.36.

Crystallographic data

From PDB header

Spacegroup	I 2 2 2	a: 75.890 Å	b: 84.830 Å	c: 123.080 Å	α: 90.00°	β: 90.00°	γ: 90.00°
Resolution	1.80 Å	Reflections	32138	Test set	1675 (5.2%)		
R	0.1950	R-free	0.2580				

According to PDB-REDO

Resolution	1.80 Å	Reflections	32138	Test set	1675 (5.2%)	Twin	false

PDB-REDO files

Re-refined and rebuilt structure	Re-refined (only) structure	All files
PDB | mmCIF | MTZ	PDB | MTZ	(compressed)

Links

PDBe	RCSB PDB	3D bionotes	Proteopedia

(b) Validation metrics from PDB-REDO

	PDB	PDB-REDO
Crystallographic refinement		
R	0.2408	0.1737
R-free	0.2777	0.2112
Bond length RMS Z-score	0.738	0.436
Bond angle RMS Z-score	0.942	0.699
Model quality raw scores | percentiles		
Ramachandran plot normality	26	50
Rotamer normality	35	78
Coarse packing	73	76
Fine packing	29	46
Bump severity	41	44
Hydrogen bond satisfaction	25	38
WHAT_CHECK	Report	Report

(c) Kleywegt-like plot

Description	PDB	PDB-REDO
Ramachandran Z-score	-2.236	-1.122
Preferred regions	305	310
Allowed regions	15	13
Outliers	7	4

(d) Model quality compared to resolution neighbours

Boxplots: R-Free, Ramachandran Plot, Rotamer quality (PDB vs PDB-REDO, N=4061)

(e) Significant structural changes

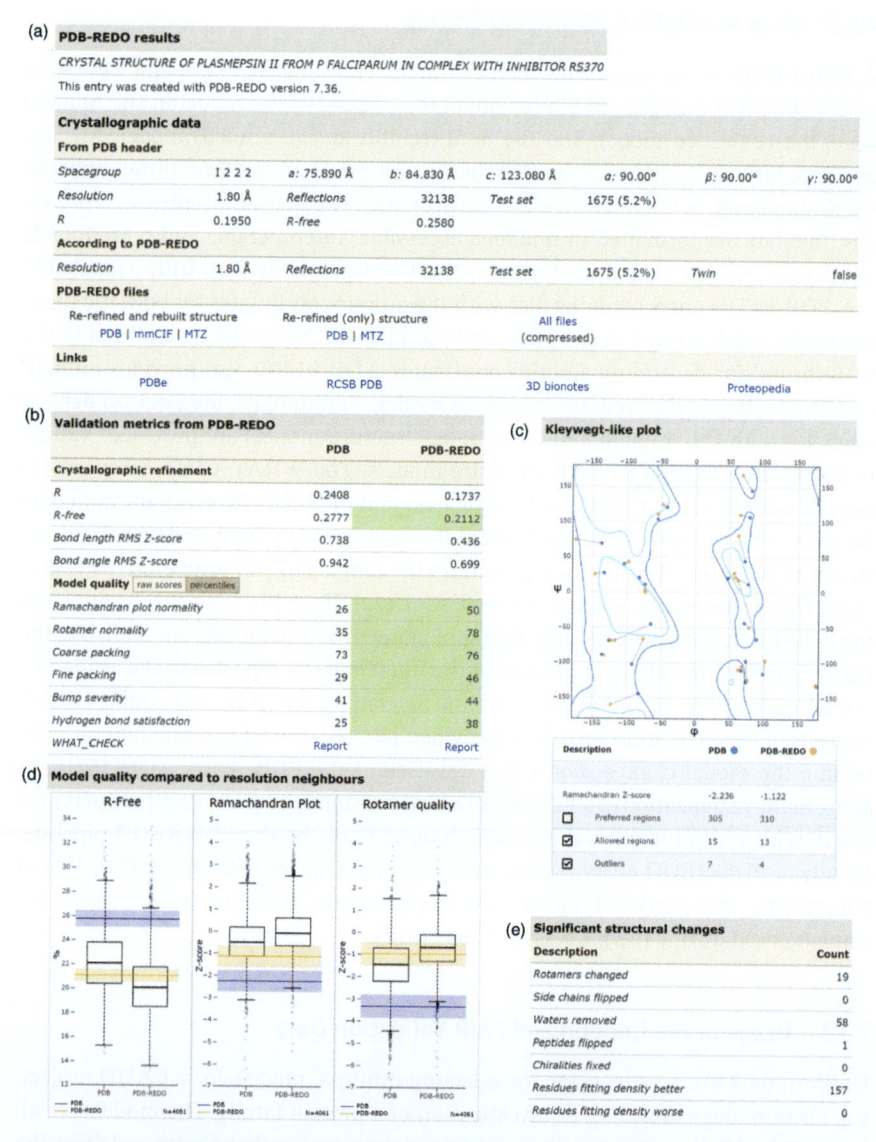

Description	Count
Rotamers changed	19
Side chains flipped	0
Waters removed	58
Peptides flipped	1
Chiralities fixed	0
Residues fitting density better	157
Residues fitting density worse	0

Figure 7.13 PDB-REDO entry interface for PDB entry 1lf2, which contains Plasmepsin 2, a potential antimalaria drug target bound to an inhibitor that can be found at https://pdb-redo.eu/db/1lf2. (a) Table containing crystallographic data. (b) Table containing the validation metrics used in PDB-REDO, while comparing to the model as deposited in the PDB. Green and red boxes indicate significant improvement or deterioration in the PDB-REDO model, respectively. (c) Kleywegt-like plot displaying changes of ϕ- and ψ-angles as a result of redoing the structure model. (d) Boxplots illustrating the model quality of the PDB and PDB-REDO models compared to models of similar resolution. (e) Table indicating the significant model changes obtained in the PDB-REDO model compared to the original model.

7.3.2 Data Available in PDB-REDO Entries

A PDB-REDO entry comes with the new model coordinates, maps, and validation details, but also contains all the metadata that describes the model in the original state, the re-refined model, and the final (rebuilt and re-refined) model. All files available for one entry are shown in Table 7.1. This data are uniform throughout the whole databank, as the same pipeline has been used to generate all entries. Additionally, the data are formatted in findable, accessible, interoperable and reproducible (FAIR) file formats. Both these features are advantages of the PDB-REDO databank.

A PDB-REDO entry contains files with the atomic coordinates for both the original model (as deposited in the PDB) and the PDB-REDO model. In addition to the PDB format for describing atomic coordinates, PDB-REDO also provides mmCIF coordinate files of the "redone" structure model. Additionally, the electron density maps for both the original and the redone structure models are provided. Validation data are available for both structure models. The WHAT_CHECK reports [8] provide comprehensive model validation data and the JSON files contain valid data for the macromolecular structure model that can be easily used in data mining for structure selection. If ligands are present in the entry, a ligand validation file is provided that contains the validation metrics for each ligand in both the original and the PDB-REDO structure models. If homologous structure models are available, the PDB identifiers and chain identifiers of the homologs are reported in the available_homologs.json file. Furthermore, a Define Secondary Structure of Proteins (DSSP) analysis of the PDB-REDO model is provided [40, 66] as well as a separate file containing the model change scores that are used at the PDBe entry pages [67]. For convenient visualization of a PDB-REDO structure model, a COOT [26] script is provided, which also indicates the model changes made by the PDB-REDO pipeline. Finally, a PDB-REDO entry comes with some descriptive data of the PDB-REDO parameters (data.json) and, for the sake of provenance tracking, versions of all the software used during the process (versions.json).

7.3.3 Usage of the Uniform and FAIR Validation Data

Uniform data are an advantage for selecting multiple models for a CADD project, e.g. for homology modeling or investigation of a protein family. The models are all generated with the same pipeline and parameters can easily be extracted from the (meta)data provided. The JSON format respects FAIR data requirements. For each JSON formatted file, the corresponding schema is provided on the PDB-REDO website, which includes detailed information about the descriptors. The files themselves are user-friendly regarding data analyses. Desired values are easily extracted, after which analyses such as calculating differences or sorting data can be performed using any computer scripting language. For example, one could extract the number of cation–π interactions for all ligands found in the PDB-REDO databank. In the ligval.json file, these counts are stored for each ligand in the model as deposited in the PDB and for the corresponding PDB-REDO model. Once the values for a PDB-ligand and PDB-REDO ligand are compared, the difference between the two values can

Table 7.1 All data files for a PDB-REDO entry.

PDB-REDO data files

Files regarding	Description	Typical URL
Atomic coordinates	Initial model	https://pdb-redo.eu/db/PDB identifier/PDB identifier_0cyc.pdb.gz
	Re-refined (only) model	https://pdb-redo.eu/db/PDB identifier/PDB identifier_besttls.pdb.gz
	Re-refined and rebuilt structure model	https://pdb-redo.eu/db/PDB identifier/PDB identifier_final.pdb
	Re-refined and rebuilt structure model with total B-factors (PDB)	https://pdb-redo.eu/db/PDB identifier/PDB identifier_final_tot.pdb
	Re-refined and rebuilt structure model with total B-factors (mmCIF)	https://pdb-redo.eu/db/PDB identifier/PDB identifier_final.cif
Electron density	Map coefficients for the original model	https://pdb-redo.eu/db/PDB identifier/PDB identifier_0cyc.mtz.gz
	Map coefficients for re-refined (only) model	https://pdb-redo.eu/db/PDB identifier/PDB identifier_besttls.mtz.gz
	Map coefficients for re-refined and rebuilt structure model	https://pdb-redo.eu/db/PDB identifier/PDB identifier_final.mtz
Validation data	WHAT_CHECK report for initial model	https://pdb-redo.eu/db/PDB identifier/wo/pdbout.txt
	WHAT_CHECK report for re-refined (only) model	https://pdb-redo.eu/db/PDB identifier/wc/pdbout.txt
	WHAT_CHECK report for re-refined and rebuilt model	https://pdb-redo.eu/db/PDB identifier/wf/pdbout.txt
	Ligand and ligand interaction data for the re-refined and rebuilt structure model	https://pdb-redo.eu/db/PDB identifier/PDB identifier_ligval.json (only for entries that contain ligands)
	Validation data for the initial and structure model	https://pdb-redo.eu/db/PDB identifier/PDB identifier_0cyc.json.gz
	Validation data for the re-refined and rebuilt structure model	https://pdb-redo.eu/db/PDB identifier/PDB identifier_final.json
	Fitting and geometry scores for reporting at PDBe	https://pdb-redo.eu/db/PDB identifier/pdbe.json
	COOT script to show model changes	https://pdb-redo.eu/db/PDB identifier/PDB identifier_final.py (Python) and https://pdb-redo.eu/db/PDB identifier/PDB identifier_final.scm (Scheme)
Descriptive data	PDB-REDO statistics for data mining (crystal parameters, R-factors, validation scores, etc.)	https://pdb-redo.eu/db/PDB identifier/data.json
	Homologous structures that are available for the structure model	https://pdb-redo.eu/db/PDB identifier/PDB identifier_available_homologs.json
	DSSP analysis of the re-refined and rebuilt structure model	https://pdb-redo.eu/db/PDB identifier/PDB identifier_final.dssp
	Software versions of all programs used	https://pdb-redo.eu/db/PDB identifier/versions.json

The files describe the structure model in the original, the re-refined, and the final re-built and refined state. Typical URLs of all the files are shown, using the fictitious PDB entry 9xyz as an example.

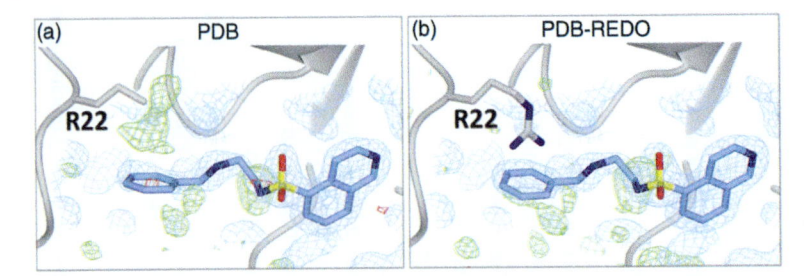

Figure 7.14 Completion of the Arg22 side chain (carbon atoms in grey) in the crystal structure of the catalytic subunit in protein kinase A (grey, PDB entry 5otg, chain A) results in cation–π interaction with ligand (carbon atoms in light blue). Electron density maps (blue) are oversampled at 0.5 for clarity, contour levels: 1.5σ for 2mF$_o$ − DF$_c$ map, 3.5σ for difference density (red and green). (a) Binding site of ligand with non-complete side chain modeled for Arg22 as found in the model as deposited in the PDB. (b) Binding site of ligand with rebuilt Arg22 side chain resulting in cation–π interaction with the ligand as seen in the PDB-REDO model.

be calculated and sorted in descending order to rank the ligands based on gained cation–π interactions. One of the ligands on top of this list is the AO8 ligand of the protein kinase A catalytic subunit from *Criteculus griseus* (PDB-ID 5otg). This ligand binds in the ATP binding site of the kinase, most likely to inhibit its function [68]. The AO8 ligand shows no cation–π interactions in the original model (Figure 7.14), whereas in the PDB-REDO model 7, such interactions are reported. This increase is due to the completed Arg22 side chain that is present in the binding pocket. The guanidinium cation is interacting with the π–electrons in the phenyl moiety of the ligand improving the binding mode with an interaction between protein and ligand (Figure 7.14) that was overlooked. For the sake of completeness, note that, the boronic acid of AO8 is not visible in the electron density. As boronic acids are known to be oxidatively unstable, most likely oxidation occurred during the experimental process [69].

7.3.4 Creating Datasets from the PDB-REDO Databank

Next to listing close homologs, PDB-REDO has a more in-depth way of creating datasets for CADD and method development for structural biology. At https://pdb-redo.eu/archive users can search the PDB-REDO databank based on all the model descriptors, validation scores, and crystallographic parameters stored in the databank, via program and property filters. The versions of all the programs used are also documented and stored to make a specific entry searchable. Complex queries can be built to perform successive filtering steps on the data. The final result can be downloaded as JSON file describing the dataset. To facilitate reproducible research, the description includes a persistent, version-specific identifier for each model so that even when a PDB-REDO model is updated (e.g. because of an algorithmic improvement) the exact model used in the study is referenced. Old versions of PDB-REDO databank entries are now archived to allow long-term access.

7.3.5 Submitting Structure Models to the PDB-REDO Pipeline

Besides the PDB-REDO databank, the PDB-REDO server is available, and also accessible through https://pdb-redo.eu/ [64]. The server provides the user with the ability to request an update for an existing PDB entry, or to upload their own structure model and diffraction data to the PDB-REDO pipeline. The server returns a new structure model with rebuilt parts, electron density maps, optimized refinement parameters, models-specific restraints, and a wealth of validation data.

7.4 Conclusions

The PDB-REDO databank contains optimized PDB entries that were obtained from X-ray crystallography. The underlying PDB-REDO pipeline refines, rebuilds, and validates the PDB models based on the original experimental data and returns the optimized structure models. PDB-REDO attempts to correct modeling errors, including the addition of missing side chain atoms, entire protein loops, or missing sugars in glycosylation sites. Besides model changes, a significant advantage of PDB-REDO entries is that they are uniformly treated. This is in sharp contrast to their counterpart entries in the PDB archive, which all reflect the idiosyncrasies of the software and the crystallographers that constructed them. Importantly, metadata and refinement, and validation parameters are provided for all entries, in FAIR data formats. Also, secondary structure information (DSSP analysis), ligand validation, and available homologous structures are provided. Either the entire databank or a single entry can be downloaded from https://pdb-redo.eu/. Single entries can also be directly opened in COOT, YASARA, or CCP4mg software packages.

Therefore, the PDB-REDO databank is a convenient starting point for structure selection in a CADD research project. For example, one of the key residues mutated in various subtypes of the SARS-CoV-2 spike protein, Asp501, is flipped in the PDB-REDO model compared to the model as deposited in the PDB. This residue is located in the receptor binding domain of the spike protein and the flip results in a hydrogen bond with Tyr41 in ACE2, spotting the importance of this residue in the protein complex [70]. Another study using structures available from the PDB-REDO databank involved docking in the ligand-binding pocket of β-lactoglobulin. The PDB-REDO models were selected for this study because of their improved fit to experimental X-ray data and overall model quality score compared to the models as deposited in the PDB [71]. Hydrogen bonding between a tryptophan and the ligand has been characterized in the hydrophobic binding pocket, which can be helpful in further investigation of this biopolymer involved in the transportation of hydrophobic nutrients. Similarly, in research describing the conformational flexibility of estrogen receptor α, the PDB-REDO structure of the monomer was selected as this model has been completed with several side-chains that were not present in the model as deposited in the PDB [72]. Besides using the models available from the PDB-REDO databank, the PDB-REDO pipeline can also be used during refinement and validation of an X-ray structure model as e.g. done by Min et al. and Musak et al.

in their works for designing inhibitors of programmed cell death-1/programmed death-ligand 1 [73] and the estrogen receptor [74], respectively.

Here, we have shown how PDB-REDO can contribute to CADD. At the moment this is limited to structures from X-ray crystallography, which represent the vast majority of experimental structure models, particularly those suited as drug targets. Cryo-electron microscopy (Cryo-EM) is an increasingly popular method for providing experimental structure models including those with bound ligands. This opens new possibilities for drug discovery including CADD. Developing new methods for Cryo-EM-based drug discovery is an active research field and will be for the foreseeable future. It is also part of the PDB-REDO research topics.

Acknowledgments and Funding

This work has been supported by iNEXT-Discovery, project number 871037, funded by the Horizon 2020 program of the European Commission and by EOSC-Life funding from the European Union's Horizon 2020 research and innovation program under grant agreement No. 824087.

List of Abbreviations and Symbols

2D	Two dimensional
$2mF_o$-DF_c map	The weighted electron density map
3D	Three dimensional
Å	Ångström
ADP	Adenosine diphosphate
AMP-PNP	Adenylyl-imidodiphosphate, a non-hydrolyzable ATP analogue
ATP	Adenosine triphosphate
Cα	C-alpha
CADD	Computer-Aided Drug Discovery
Cryo-EM	Cryo-Electron Microscopy
CYPs	Cytochrome P450 hydroxylase enzymes
CXS	CAPS buffer
DSSP	Define Secondary Structure of Proteins
GPP	Geranyl diphosphate
HSSP	Homology derived Secondary Structure of Proteins
MAPK	Mitogen-Activated Protein Kinase
NAG	*N*-acetylglucosamine
PDB	Protein Data Bank
PEG	Poly-ethylene glycol
R5P	Ribose-5-phosphate
RSCC	Real Space Correlation Coefficient
TLS	Translation, liberation, and screw
UDP	Uridine diphosphate
Z_{bgG}	Metric describing the relative orientation of nucleic acid bases

References

1 Taylor, G.L. (2010). Introduction to phasing. *Acta Crystallographica Section D* 66 (4): 325–338.
2 Murshudov, G.N., Skubák, P., Lebedev, A.A. et al. (2011). REFMAC5 for the refinement of macromolecular crystal structures. *Acta Crystallographica Section D* 67 (4): 355–367.
3 Blanc, E., Roversi, P., Vonrhein, C. et al. (2004). Refinement of severely incomplete structures with maximum likelihood in BUSTER-TNT. *Acta Crystallographica Section D* 60 (12): 2210–2221.
4 Liebschner, D., Afonine, P.V., Baker, M.L. et al. (2019). Macromolecular structure determination using X-rays, neutrons and electrons: recent developments in Phenix. *Acta Crystallographica Section D* 75 (10): 861–877.
5 Read, R.J., Adams, P.D., Arendall, W.B. et al. (2011). A new generation of crystallographic validation tools for the Protein Data Bank. *Structure* 19 (10): 1395–1412.
6 Chen, V.B., Arendall, W.B., Headd, J.J. et al. (2010). MolProbity: all-atom structure validation for macromolecular crystallography. *Acta Crystallographica. Section D, Biological Crystallography* 66 (Pt 1): 12–21.
7 Gore, S., García, E.S., Hendrickx, P.M.S. et al. (2017). Validation of structures in the Protein Data Bank. *Structure* 25 (12): 1916–1927.
8 Hooft, R.W.W., Vriend, G., Sander, C., and Abola, E.E. (1996). Errors in protein structures. *Nature* 381 (6580): 272–272.
9 Rupp, B. and Kantardjieff, K. (2010). *Biomolecular Crystallography: Principles, Practice, and Application to Structural Biology*. Garland Science 809 p.
10 Roversi, P. and Tronrud, D.E. (2021). Ten things I 'hate' about refinement. *Acta Crystallographica Section D: Structural Biology* 77 (12): 1497–1515.
11 (1971). Crystallography: Protein Data Bank. *Nature: New Biology* 233 (42): 223–223.
12 (2021). A celebration of structural biology. *Nature Methods* 18 (5): 427–427.
13 wwPDB consortium. (2019). Protein Data Bank: the single global archive for 3D macromolecular structure data. *Nucleic Acids Research* 47 (D1): D520–D528.
14 Joosten, R.P., Chinea, G., Kleywegt, G.J., and Vriend, G. (2013). Protein three-dimensional structure validation. In: *Reference Module in Chemistry, Molecular Sciences and Chemical Engineering [Internet]*. Elsevier [cited 2021 Dec 14]. Available from: https://www.sciencedirect.com/science/article/pii/B9780124095472025348.
15 Joosten, R.P., Salzemann, J., Bloch, V. et al. (2009). PDB_REDO: automated re-refinement of X-ray structure models in the PDB. *Journal of Applied Crystallography* 42 (3): 376–384.
16 Schomaker, V. and Trueblood, K.N. (1968). On the rigid-body motion of molecules in crystals. *Acta Crystallographica. Section B* 24 (1): 63–76.
17 Winn, M.D., Isupov, M.N., and Murshudov, G.N. (2001). Use of TLS parameters to model anisotropic displacements in macromolecular refinement. *Acta Crystallographica Section D* 57 (1): 122–133.

18 Joosten, R.P., Womack, T., Vriend, G., and Bricogne, G. (2009). Re-refinement from deposited X-ray data can deliver improved models for most PDB entries. *Acta Crystallographica Section D* 65 (2): 176–185.

19 Cohen, S.X., Morris, R.J., Fernandez, F.J. et al. (2004). Towards complete validated models in the next generation of ARP/wARP. *Acta Crystallographica Section D* 60 (12-1): 2222–2229.

20 Joosten, R.P., Joosten, K., Cohen, S.X. et al. (2011). Automatic rebuilding and optimization of crystallographic structures in the Protein Data Bank. *Bioinformatics* 27 (24): 3392–3398.

21 van Beusekom, B., Joosten, K., Hekkelman, M.L. et al. (2018). Homology-based loop modeling yields more complete crystallographic protein structures. *IUCrJ* 5 (5): 585–594.

22 Lütteke, T. (2009). Analysis and validation of carbohydrate three-dimensional structures. *Acta Crystallographica. Section D, Biological Crystallography* 65 (2): 156–168.

23 Agirre, J., Davies, G., Wilson, K., and Cowtan, K. (2015). Carbohydrate anomalies in the PDB. *Nature Chemical Biology* 11 (5): 303–303.

24 Joosten, R.P. and Lütteke, T. (2017). Carbohydrate 3D structure validation. *Current Opinion in Structural Biology* 44: 9–17.

25 van Beusekom, B., Wezel, N., Hekkelman, M.L. et al. (2019). Building and rebuilding N-glycans in protein structure models. *Acta Crystallographica Section D: Structural Biology* 75 (4): 416–425.

26 Emsley, P., Lohkamp, B., Scott, W.G., and Cowtan, K. (2010). Features and development of Coot. *Acta Crystallographica. Section D, Biological Crystallography* 66 (4): 486–501.

27 Emsley, P. and Crispin, M. (2018). Structural analysis of glycoproteins: building N-linked glycans with Coot. *Acta Crystallographica Section D* 74 (4): 256–263.

28 Stanley, P., Taniguchi, N., and Aebi, M. (2015). N-Glycans. In: *Essentials of Glycobiology* [Internet], 3rde (ed. A. Varki, R.D. Cummings, J.D. Esko, et al.). Cold Spring Harbor (NY): Cold Spring Harbor Laboratory Press [cited 2020 Apr 9]. Available from: http://www.ncbi.nlm.nih.gov/books/NBK453020/.

29 van Beusekom, B., Touw, W.G., Tatineni, M. et al. (2018). Homology-based hydrogen bond information improves crystallographic structures in the PDB. *Protein Science* 27 (3): 798–808.

30 Touw, W.G., van Beusekom, B., Evers, J.M.G. et al. (2016). Validation and correction of Zn-CysxHisy complexes. *Acta Crystallographica Section D: Structural Biology* 72 (Pt 10): 1110–1118.

31 de Vries, I., Kwakman, T., Lu, X.J. et al. (2021). New restraints and validation approaches for nucleic acid structures in PDB-REDO. *Acta Crystallographica Section D* 77 (9): 1127–1141.

32 Joosten, R.P., Joosten, K., Murshudov, G.N., and Perrakis, A. (2012). PDB_REDO: constructive validation, more than just looking for errors. *Acta Crystallographica. Section D, Biological Crystallography* 68 (4): 484–496.

33 Cereto-Massagué, A., Ojeda, M.J., Joosten, R.P. et al. (2013). The good, the bad and the dubious: VHELIBS, a validation helper for ligands and binding sites. *Journal of Cheminformatics* 5 (1): 36.

34 Wei, H., Ruthenburg, A.J., Bechis, S.K., and Verdine, G.L. (2005). Nucleotide-dependent domain movement in the ATPase domain of a human type IIA DNA topoisomerase. *Journal of Biological Chemistry* 280 (44): 37041–37047.

35 McNicholas, S., Potterton, E., Wilson, K.S., and Noble, M.E.M. (2011). Presenting your structures: the CCP4mg molecular-graphics software. *Acta Crystallographica Section D* 67 (4): 386–394.

36 Baskaran, S., Roach, P.J., DePaoli-Roach, A.A., and Hurley, T.D. (2010). Structural basis for glucose-6-phosphate activation of glycogen synthase. *Proceedings of the National Academy of Sciences of the United States of America* 107 (41): 17563–17568.

37 Krieger, E. and Vriend, G. (2014). YASARA View—molecular graphics for all devices—from smartphones to workstations. *Bioinformatics* 30 (20): 2981–2982.

38 Grasso, M., Estrada, M.A., Ventocilla, C. et al. (2016). Chemically linked vemurafenib inhibitors promote an inactive BRAFV600E conformation. *ACS Chemical Biology* 11 (10): 2876–2888.

39 Diaz, Z., Xavier, K.B., and Miller, S.T. (2009). The crystal structure of the *Escherichia coli* autoinducer-2 processing protein LsrF. Valdivia RH. *PLoS ONE* 4 (8): e6820.

40 Touw, W.G., Baakman, C., Black, J. et al. (2015). A series of PDB-related databanks for everyday needs. *Nucleic Acids Research* 43 (D1): D364–D368.

41 Oliveira de Souza, J., Dawson, A., and Hunter, W.N. (2017). An improved model of the *Trypanosoma brucei* CTP synthetase glutaminase domain-acivicin complex. *ChemMedChem* 12 (8): 577–579.

42 Hartley, A., Glynn, S.E., Barynin, V. et al. (2004). Substrate specificity and mechanism from the structure of *Pyrococcus furiosus* galactokinase. *Journal of Molecular Biology* 337 (2): 387–398.

43 Ariyawutthiphan, O., Ose, T., Minami, A. et al. (2012). Structure analysis of geranyl pyrophosphate methyltransferase and the proposed reaction mechanism of SAM-dependent C-methylation. *Acta Crystallographica Section D* 68 (11): 1558–1569.

44 Zhao, M., Ma, J., Li, M. et al. (2021). Cytochrome P450 enzymes and drug metabolism in humans. *International Journal of Molecular Sciences* 22 (23): 12808.

45 Xu, L.H., Fushinobu, S., Takamatsu, S. et al. (2010). Regio- and stereospecificity of filipin hydroxylation sites revealed by crystal structures of cytochrome P450 105P1 and 105D6 from *Streptomyces avermitilis**. *Journal of Biological Chemistry* 285 (22): 16844–16853.

46 Dym, O., Song, W., Felder, C. et al. (2016). The impact of crystallization conditions on structure-based drug design: a case study on the methylene blue/acetylcholinesterase complex. *Protein Science* 25 (6): 1096–1114.

47 Carter, A.P., Clemons, W.M., Brodersen, D.E. et al. (2000). Functional insights from the structure of the 30S ribosomal subunit and its interactions with antibiotics. *Nature* 407 (6802): 340–348.

48 Arnaud, J., Audfray, A., and Imberty, A. (2013). Binding sugars: from natural lectins to synthetic receptors and engineered neolectins. *Chemical Society Reviews* 42 (11): 4798–4813.

49 van Beusekom, B., Lütteke, T., and Joosten, R.P. (2018). Making glycoproteins a little bit sweeter with PDB-REDO. *Acta Crystallographica. Section F* 74 (8): 463–472.

50 Lan, J., Ge, J., Yu, J. et al. (2020). Structure of the SARS-CoV-2 spike receptor-binding domain bound to the ACE2 receptor. *Nature* 581 (7807): 215–220.

51 Stieglitz, K., Stec, B., Baker, D.P., and Kantrowitz, E.R. (2004). Monitoring the transition from the T to the R state in *E.coli* aspartate transcarbamoylase by X-ray crystallography: crystal structures of the E50A mutant enzyme in four distinct allosteric states. *Journal of Molecular Biology* 341 (3): 853–868.

52 Wang, C., Krüger, A., Du, X. et al. (2022). Novel highlight in malarial drug discovery: aspartate transcarbamoylase. *Frontiers in Cellular and Infection Microbiology* [Internet] [cited 2022 Jul 5];12. Available from: https://www.frontiersin.org/articles/10.3389/fcimb.2022.841833.

53 Lei, Z., Wang, B., Lu, Z. et al. (2020). New regulatory mechanism-based inhibitors of aspartate transcarbamoylase for potential anticancer drug development. *The FEBS Journal.* 287 (16): 3579–3599.

54 Zheng, H., Cooper, D.R., Porebski, P.J. et al. (2017). CheckMyMetal: a macromolecular metal-binding validation tool. *Acta Crystallographica Section D* 73 (3): 223–233.

55 Putignano, V., Rosato, A., Banci, L., and Andreini, C. (2018). MetalPDB in 2018: a database of metal sites in biological macromolecular structures. *Nucleic Acids Research* 46 (D1): D459–D464.

56 van Beusekom, B., Damaskos, G., Hekkelman, M.L. et al. (2021). LAHMA: structure analysis through local annotation of homology-matched amino acids. *Acta Crystallographica Section D: Structural Biology* 77 (1): 28–40.

57 van Beusekom B, Perrakis A, Joosten RP. Data mining of macromolecular structures. In: Carugo O, Eisenhaber F, *Data Mining Techniques for the Life Sciences* [Internet]. New York, NY: Springer; 2016 [cited 2021 Apr 10]. p. 107–38. (Methods in Molecular Biology). Available from: https://doi.org/10.1007/978-1-4939-3572-7_6

58 Vagin, A.A., Steiner, R.A., Lebedev, A.A. et al. (2004). REFMAC5 dictionary: organization of prior chemical knowledge and guidelines for its use. *Acta Crystallographica Section D* 60 (Pt 12 Pt 1): 2184–2195.

59 Nicholls, R.A., Wojdyr, M., Joosten, R.P. et al. (2021). The missing link: covalent linkages in structural models. *Acta Cryst* D77.

60 Shao, C., Feng, Z., Westbrook, J.D. et al. (2021). Modernized uniform representation of carbohydrate molecules in the Protein Data Bank. *Glycobiology* 31 (9): 1204–1218.

61 Nicholls, R.A., Joosten, R.P., Long, F. et al. (2021). Modelling covalent linkages in CCP4. *Acta Crystallographica Section D* 77 (6): 712–726.

62 Westbrook, J.D., Young, J.Y., Shao, C. et al. (2022). PDBx/mmCIF ecosystem: foundational semantic tools for structural biology. *Journal of Molecular Biology* 434 (11): 167599.

63 Adams, P.D., Afonine, P.V., Baskaran, K. et al. (2019). Announcing mandatory submission of PDBx/mmCIF format files for crystallographic depositions to the Protein Data Bank (PDB). *Acta Crystallographica Section D* 75 (4): 451–454.

64 Joosten, R.P., Long, F., Murshudov, G.N., and Perrakis, A. (2014). The PDB_REDO server for macromolecular structure model optimization. *IUCrJ* 1 (4): 213–220.

65 Asojo, O.A., Afonina, E., Gulnik, S.V. et al. (2002). Structures of Ser205 mutant plasmepsin II from Plasmodium falciparum at 1.8 Å in complex with the inhibitors rs367 and rs370. *Acta Crystallographica Section D* 58 (12): 2001–2008.

66 Kabsch, W. and Sander, C. (1983). Dictionary of protein secondary structure: Pattern recognition of hydrogen-bonded and geometrical features. *Biopolymers* 22 (12): 2577–2637.

67 Velankar, S., Alhroub, Y., Alili, A. et al. (2011). PDBe: Protein Data Bank in Europe. *Nucleic Acids Research* 39 (Database issue): D402–D410.

68 Müller, J., Kirschner, R.A., Geyer, A., and Klebe, G. (2019). Conceptional design of self-assembling bisubstrate-like inhibitors of protein kinase A resulting in a boronic acid glutamate linkage. *ACS Omega* 4 (1): 775–784.

69 Graham, B.J., Windsor, I.W., Gold, B., and Raines, R.T. (2021). Boronic acid with high oxidative stability and utility in biological contexts. *Proceedings of the National Academy of Sciences of the United States of America* 118 (10): e2013691118.

70 Laffeber, C., de Koning, K., Kanaar, R., and Lebbink, J.H.G. (2021). Experimental evidence for enhanced receptor binding by rapidly spreading SARS-CoV-2 variants. *Journal of Molecular Biology* 433 (15): 167058.

71 Chakraborty, B., Sengupta, C., Pal, U., and Basu, S. (2020). Probing the hydrogen bond involving acridone trapped in a hydrophobic biological nanocavity: integrated spectroscopic and docking analyses. *Langmuir* 36 (5): 1241–1251.

72 Schneider, M., Pons, J.L., and Labesse, G. (2021). Exploring the conformational space of a receptor for drug design: an ERα case study. *Journal of Molecular Graphics & Modelling* 108: 107974.

73 Muszak, D., Surmiak, E., Plewka, J. et al. (2021). Terphenyl-based small-molecule inhibitors of programmed cell death-1/programmed death-ligand 1 protein–protein interaction. *Journal of Medicinal Chemistry* 64 (15): 11614–11636.

74 Min, J., Nwachukwu, J.C., Min, C.K. et al. (2021). Dual-mechanism estrogen receptor inhibitors. *Proceedings of the National Academy of Sciences* 118 (35): e2101657118.

8

Pharos and TCRD: Informatics Tools for Illuminating Dark Targets

Keith J. Kelleher[1], Timothy K. Sheils[1], Stephen L. Mathias[2], Dac-Trung Nguyen[1], Vishal Siramshetty[1], Ajay Pillai[1], Jeremy J. Yang[2], Cristian G. Bologa[2], Jeremy S. Edwards[2], Tudor I. Oprea[2,3], and Ewy Mathé[1]

[1] National Center for Advancing Translational Science, 9800 Medical Center Drive, Rockville, MD 20850, USA
[2] University of New Mexico Health Sciences Center, Department of Internal Medicine, Translational Informatics Division, MSC09-5025, 1 University of New Mexico, Albuquerque, NM 87131, USA
[3] Expert Systems Inc., 12760 High Bluff Dr Ste 370, San Diego, CA 92130, USA

8.1 Introduction

The current focus of translational and biomedical research tends to be dominated by a relatively small number of well-studied proteins. According to one estimate, around 10% of human proteins receive 75% of the focus of research [1]. Another study reported that at least one-third of the human proteome is understudied, based on mined information from PubMed or the granted patent corpus, antibody count, NIH-funded R01 grants, and other criteria [2].

A recent analysis found that much of the reason for this bias can be attributed to the publication history of a target and the availability of chemical probes for targets [3]. As such, there is a need to incentivize more diversity in the range of targets under investigation, such that more novel targets are featured in publications, and to develop molecular probes (e.g. chemicals or antibodies) and genetic constructs for them. This process of illumination can have a ripple effect – as more targets are studied and data are generated, similar understudied targets may receive additional focus. To address this bias and expand our knowledge of understudied proteins, the National Institutes of Health (NIH) initiated the Illuminating the Druggable Genome (IDG) Consortium [4] in 2013 to shed light on these understudied targets, oftentimes referred to as the "dark genome."

In this chapter, we use the term target to generically refer to both the characteristics of the gene and the protein in a drug discovery context: drug targets are macromolecules to which the drug (or its bioactive derivative) binds to exert the intended therapeutic effect [5].

As a primary step in guiding research toward understudied targets, the IDG Consortium defined a categorical metric called the Target Development Level (TDL) [6]. Each target protein is classified into one of four categories, which describe the degree of progress and available knowledge for these targets in terms of their chemistry, biology, and clinical activity. The four categories and their requirements are:

- **Tdark** proteins satisfy two or more of the following requirements:
    - A PubMed score [7] less than five
    - Three or fewer documented GeneRIFs (Reference Into Functions)
    - No more than 50 commercially available antibodies[2]
- **Tbio** proteins satisfy one of the following requirements:
    - Fail to satisfy two or more of the criteria for **Tdark**
    - Have a documented Gene Ontology Molecular Function or Biological Process with an experimental evidence code
- **Tchem** proteins must have:
    - At least one active small molecule documented by ChEMBL [8] or DrugCentral [9] that must be one of the following measures: IC_{50}, K_i, K_b, K_d, EC_{50}, AC_{50}, XC_{50}, and K_m. Depending on the target type, the activities must also satisfy the following potency cutoffs:
        - GPCRs and nuclear hormone receptors: 100nM
        - Kinases: 30nM
        - Ion Channels: 10µM
        - All others: 1µM
- **Tclin** proteins must have:
    - A documented activity for an approved drug, with a known mechanism of action (MoA).

Figure 8.1 shows the yearly distribution of the number of targets at each TDL, and how the generation of new knowledge has changed the distribution of the TDLs over time. Specifically, the number of Tdark proteins dramatically decreased from 9199 (December 2013) to 5932 (July 2022), indicating an increased awareness of the dark genome and the need to further study associated proteins (see also Figure 8.1).

As part of the IDG program, the Target Central Resource Database (TCRD) and Pharos were created to provide free, public access to information on targets and associated annotations [6, 10]. TCRD, accessible at http://juniper.health.unm.edu/tcrd/download/, is an aggregating database of 79 data sources and Pharos (https://pharos.nih.gov/) is the interactive web-based frontend that allows users to browse, search, filter, and analyze the rich information contained within TCRD. Users can log in via pre-established social media credentials, such as Google, Twitter, and GitHub, to save lists of targets, diseases, or ligands that are available upon return. Other than the ability to save custom lists, all functionalities are available without registration. Since its first publication, TCRD has had 27 new releases, and Pharos has a bimonthly release cycle. TCRD has had approximately 22,000 database downloads as of 31 March 2022. Pharos receives more than 2500 new visitors every month.

TCRD and Pharos are tailored to a broad range of user types, from those that need full access to the data available to others that may only be interested in a specific dataset for a select group of targets. Other types of users may generate tools or other web components that query Pharos' GraphQL API.

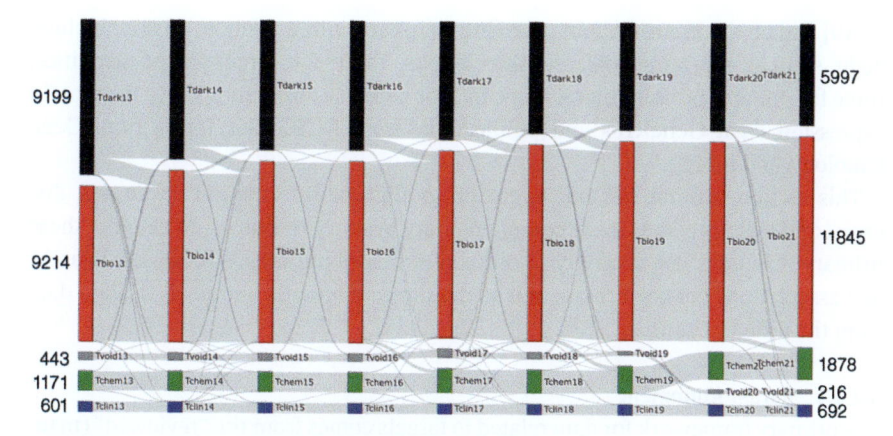

Figure 8.1 Changes in the TDL distribution over time.

- This Sankey plot represents TDL transition for proteins, as assigned in different versions of TCRD between December 2013 and December 2021.
- The counts of targets in each group at the endpoints are shown on the left and right sides of the plot.
- The last two-digit number indicates the year. An additional category, "Tvoid," was introduced for this plot to trace target transition for protein identifiers that have been obsoleted (e.g. pseudogenes) or more recently introduced in UniProt.

While many primary resources within TCRD already have a web portal where the data can be accessed, there is a clear benefit in database aggregators such as Open-Targets [11], GeneCards [12], or Pharos. These tools display detailed information about a target on a single page, allowing a user to learn about different aspects of target biology at once, a role that is also filled by Pharos' details pages (Section 8.2.3.2). In addition, the visualizations and analysis functionality offered by Pharos' list pages (Section 8.2.3.1) opens up a range of new possibilities for research questions that capitalize on the wide breadth of knowledge in the database. The use cases (Section 8.3) illustrate how generating lists in different ways, performing calculations, and constructing visualizations can help address different scientific questions, and reveal patterns in the data.

This chapter provides details on the methods (data organization, analysis, and programmatic access), gives an overview of the content and navigation, and exemplifies the utility and usage of Pharos through use cases. Our goal is to highlight and demonstrate how Pharos empowers users to gain chemical, biological, and clinical insight on targets, with the ability to analyze and visualize lists of targets, diseases, or ligands, and the ability to generate those lists in interesting and relevant ways.

8.2 Methods

8.2.1 Data Organization

TCRD is a relational database compiled from 79 datasets from various knowledge domains. Further details about each resource can be found in previous publications

[6, 10] and on the Pharos About page (https://pharos.nih.gov/about). Those include eight sources for target–disease associations, three for target–ligand activities, three for protein–protein interactions, five for pathway annotations, five for protein expression data, GeneRIFs and publications from NCBI, GO Terms from Gene Ontology, and more.

This section summarizes our approach to aligning information on targets, diseases, and ligands across these complementary primary resources. In general, these primary resources use a variety of ontologies describing targets, diseases, ligands, and associations between them, and so require a systematic approach to align data from the different sources.

8.2.1.1 Target Alignment

The primary framework for data related to targets comes from the "reviewed" (manually curated) human proteins described by UniProt [13]. TCRD maps protein and gene-related data to this dataset given the target identifiers used by each dataset, i.e. gene symbols, ENSG IDs, and UniProt IDs, and mapped to the synonyms that UniProt provides for each target.

8.2.1.2 Disease Alignment

Eight data sources [7, 9, 14–19] provide target–disease associations for TCRD and use seven different ontologies, including DO, UMLS, MESH, OMIM, Orphanet, AmyCo, and NCBIGene [20–25]. Pharos relies on the MONDO Disease Ontology (DO) [18] to align disparate input source types into a common disease annotation. For example, when one source reports an association between APP and "Cerebral amyloid angiopathy, APP-related (OMIM:605714)," and another source reports an association between APP and "APP-related cerebral amyloid angiopathy (DOID:0070028)," Pharos correctly reports those two associations as the same disease.

Overall, the eight data sources provide data for 26,418 unique disease IDs and 17,989 unique disease names among the set of documented target–disease associations. By aligning equivalent terms through the MONDO mappings, Pharos has been able to consolidate data down to 13,704 unique disease entities.

8.2.1.3 Ligand Alignment

Three data sources for activity data on ligands are used, including ChEMBL [8], DrugCentral [9], and Guide to Pharmacology [26]. Each source could represent a given ligand using a different SMILES string. To standardize molecules, Pharos uses Layered Chemical Identifier (LyChI – https://github.com/ncats/lychi), a hierarchical hash key representation for chemical structures. LyChI is a lexicographically meaningful four-layered hash key that is generated after standardization of the chemical structure, which involves valency check, kekulization, tautomerization, salt/solvent removal, protonation (or deprotonation), followed by perception of mobile charges and stereochemistry. Briefly, the hash keys are generated from SMILES, and all activities associated with each ligand across different targets are grouped based on that unique hash key.

8.2.1.4 Data and UI Updates

TCRD and the Pharos web portal are living resources that are constantly being updated. TCRD releases occur approximately twice a year. The list of data sources is constantly changing to meet the research community's needs and to track new trends and advances in methods and technologies. New data sources are chosen based on the quality and utility of the data source, with the focus on data sources that will help in the project's main focus, which is to illuminate less well-studied areas of the proteome. Pharos follows a bimonthly release cycle that incorporates new changes from TCRD and adds new functionality and analysis methods.

8.2.2 Programmatic Access and Data Download

Pharos queries TCRD using a Node.js server (https://nodejs.org/) running a GraphQL API (https://graphql.org/). GraphQL is a powerful tool for generating easily extensible queries that are ideal for hierarchical data. For example, top-level information about a ligand can be fetched alongside a list of targets for which the ligand has an activity. The query can easily retrieve further information about targets, such as affected pathways, protein classes, or associated diseases for those targets. External developers can use GraphQL to fetch only data they are interested in, making lighter payloads instead of a traditional REST API where the Pharos developers would dictate what data are returned from a request.

Users can query our GraphQL API directly through the website (https://pharos.nih.gov/api) or programmatically (https://pharos-api.ncats.io/graphql). Pharos' API page has several Example Queries to help get started querying the API.

Beyond querying the API, users can also download data through the UI, or download complete dumps of the SQL database TCRD from http://juniper.health.unm.edu/tcrd/download/.

The Pharos web application constructs GraphQL queries based on user input. The web server component is currently written in Angular 13 (https://angular.io/), using Server Side Rendering and pre-rendering for slow-loading pages. Each details page and list page provides a link to download data for offline analysis. Users can build a download query that includes any related data fields, such as Pathways for a target list or GWAS data for a disease list. The download builder can also help SQL users of TCRD to understand the table structure of the underlying database, as it presents the SQL query that will be used to execute the download query. The downloaded zip file will also contain a metadata file that reviews the version information at the time of the download, a summary of the downloaded fields, and the SQL query used to generate the download. Downloads are limited to 250,000 rows for this functionality. Users, who need more data, should download a full version of TCRD as described above.

8.2.3 UI Organization

This section provides a broad overview of the information layout in Pharos without going into detail about the data and functionality of each component. Many of the components and features will be introduced during the course of the use cases that will follow in Section 8.3. Regardless, each component has a help panel that provides those details to users as they need them (Figure 8.2 panel L and Figure 8.3 panel D).

There are two main types of pages that contain the bulk of biological data from TCRD, those being list pages (Section 8.2.3.1), which provide pageable lists of entities for browsing and population analysis, and details pages (Section 8.2.3.2), which present detailed data and source information for a single entity. List pages and details pages are available for all targets, diseases, and ligands in the database.

All Pharos pages contain a top menu with links to the homepage, the main list pages for targets, diseases, and ligands, as well as the About page, FAQ page, and Use Case page (Figure 8.2 panel A). Also from the toolbar, users can search the database, which will be discussed in more detail in Section 8.2.3.3. Rounding out the top menu are buttons to submit feedback to the Pharos development team and to Sign In via a number of social authentication providers (e.g. Google and GitHub). Signing into Pharos is optional, but is useful for users who will be saving their own custom lists (see section 8.3.2 "Uploading a Custom Ligand List") since they will be able to return to Pharos and access those lists later.

8.2.3.1 List Pages

List pages are browsable listings of targets, diseases, or ligands, that can be filtered by a number of data fields. The example in Figure 8.2 shows a list filtered to include only the 683 targets that have a TDL of Tclin. List pages can be toggled between Table View, where results are shown in a table, and List Analysis View, which offers functionality to show visualizations and perform calculations at the population level. More details on the functionality provided in the List Analysis tab are shown in context in Section 8.3.

The filter panel (Figure 8.2 panel E), shows the counts of entries in the list that have each filter value. Each list page provides the ability to upload a custom list and download data for all entries currently on the list.

The lower right quadrant, labeled Figure 8.2 panel K, is where the entries of the list are shown. Target list pages show each entry in a card view, which highlights some summary data for each target in the list. Disease list pages show a more simplified table of data, while ligand list pages show a card view including the chemical structure of each compound. The lists are pageable, and each entry will link to a details page for the entry. A popup information panel will explain the data behind each data point on the cards.

8.2.3.2 Details Pages

As mentioned above, each entry on the list pages will link to a corresponding details page. Figure 8.3 shows an example of a target details page. This example page, as well as all disease and ligand details pages, will have a header that includes the name of the entry, and a link to download data for the given entry. The left panel is a clickable table of contents that highlights, which sections have data and which do not, while the right panel shows the primary data in distinct components. All headers and data labels will show a tooltip on hover that helps the user understand the data and its context. A popup information panel can also be accessed for this information. There

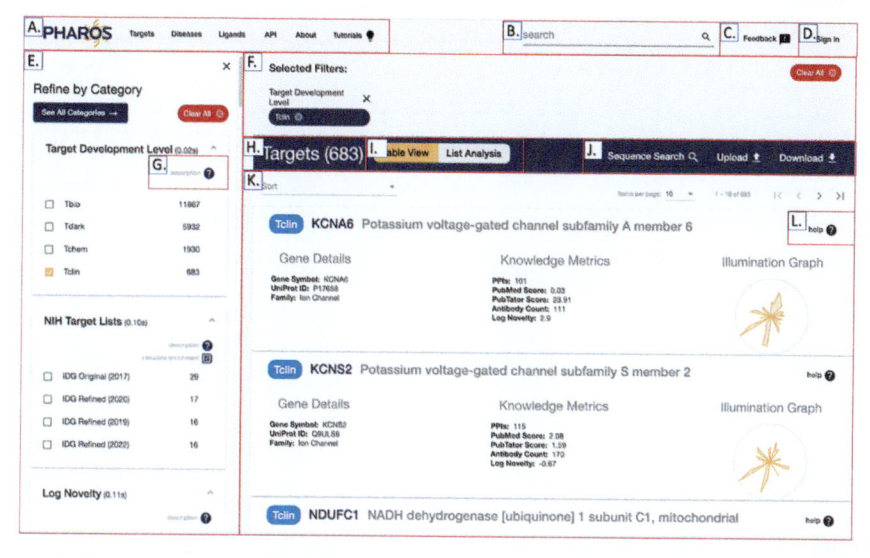

Figure 8.2 Overview of a list page.

A. Top Menu Bar. All pages contain links to the list pages for targets, diseases, and ligands, as well as a link to the API page, the About pages, and Tutorials.
B. Search bar. Search the database from the top menu bar of all pages. Suggestions will appear as users type based on common searches.
C. Feedback button. Provide feedback or report bugs to the Pharos team.
D. Sign In button. Signing in via social media credentials is available, but is optional. Users who create their own custom lists will likely want to sign in so that they can access their lists on subsequent visits.
E. Filter Panel. This panel is available on all list pages and displays the counts of entries in the list that have each filter value. In this example, the Target Development Level filter shows counts of targets at each TDL. This list is currently filtered to targets with a TDL of Tclin.
F. Selected Filters Panel. A complete listing of all filters applied to the list.
G. Filter Description. An expandable section that shows a description of the filter and where the data came from.
H. Table Header. Shows the type of list, and count of entries in the list.
I. View Toggle Button. Toggles the panel to show the Table View (the current view) or List Analysis View, which displays visualizations and functionality for analyzing a population
J. Other Buttons. All list pages contain buttons in this section to allow the user to Upload their own list of targets, diseases, or ligands, as well as to Download data for entries in the list. Target lists (shown here) will have a button to initiate targets in the database based on an amino acid sequence. Ligand lists (not pictured) will have a button for initiating a search for compounds in the database based on a chemical structure.
K. Data Table. A pageable listing of data for each entry in the list. Note: Disease lists have a more simplified Table View of the list, and ligand lists have a card view with the rendered chemical structure.
L. Info Panel Button. A button that triggers a panel of information describing each piece of data on the card.

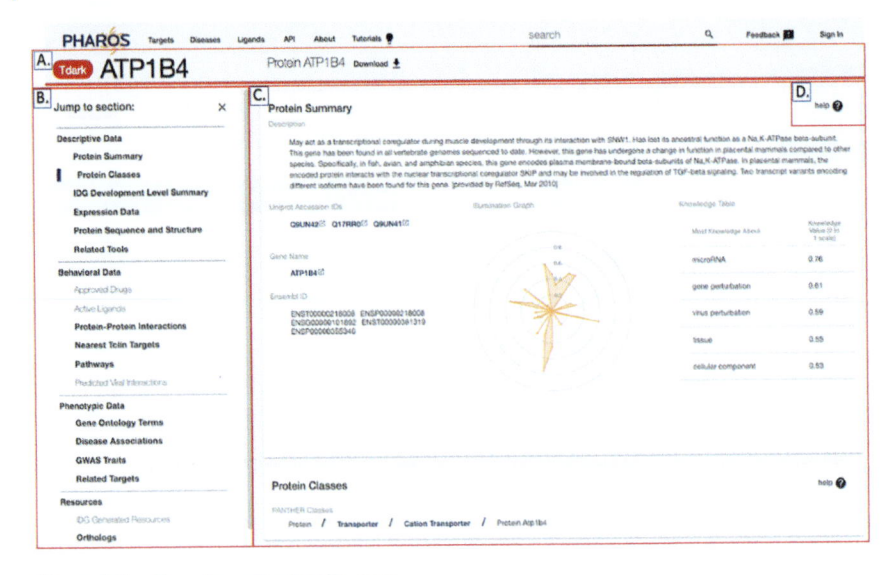

Figure 8.3 Overview of a details page.

A. Details Page Header. Details pages show the name of the main entity of the details page, as well as a download button, where users can download any piece of information shown on the page.
B. Table of Contents. Target details pages (shown here) and disease details pages (not pictured) will show this navigable menu for the different components on the details page. Bolded entries are components that have data. Ligand details pages do not have a table of contents due to the small number of components on the pages.
C. Main Panel is the scrollable region that holds the page's main content.
   - The Protein Summary component shows descriptions and aliases. The radar graph (Illumination Graph) from Harmonizome, quantifies the amount of data available for a target on a large number of dimensions.
   - Protein Classes as annotated by PANTHER and Drug Target Ontology appear in this section when they are available.
D. Info Panel Button. A button that triggers a panel of information describing each piece of data on the component, and some details about the data source. Some components may also display a button to launch a tutorial for understanding data in the component.

are many types of data on the details pages, especially the target details components, and many of them will be explained in more detail in the context of the use cases in Section 8.3.

8.2.3.3 Search

The search bar from either the top menu or the home page (Figure 8.4), will auto-complete partial queries with common searches. Users can navigate directly to matching details pages when the autocompletion match is to that of a name or common symbol for a target, disease, or ligand. When the autocompletion match is to that of a common filter value, such as a GO Term or a pathway, an option will be presented to navigate directly to a listing page filtered to entries that match that filter value. The bottom of Figure 8.4 shows the result of a general text search, which occurs when the user does not select an autocompletion match, or selects

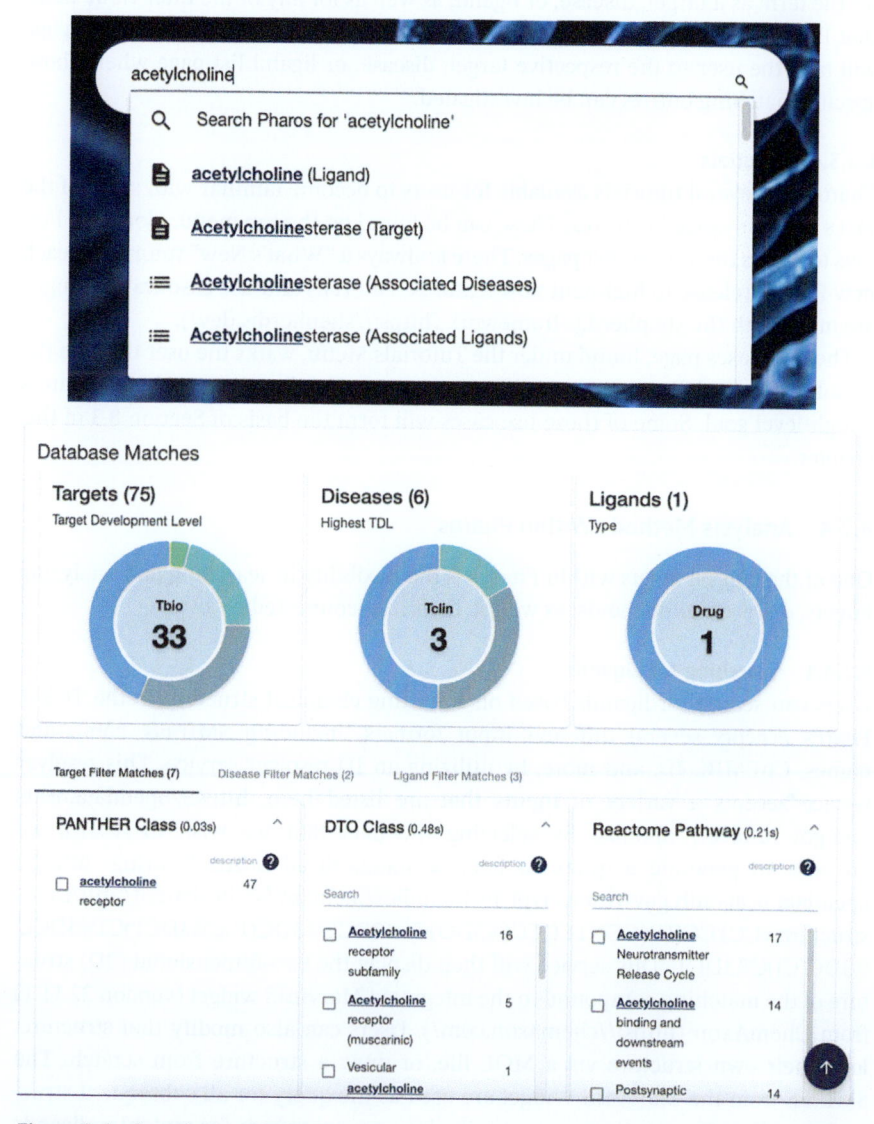

Figure 8.4 Search functionality.

- Top: Autocomplete suggestions based on the user's input will take the user directly to a details page, or a relevant list page. The user input, in this case, is "acetylcholine" and the suggestions include the ligand "acetylcholine" and the target "Acetylcholinesterase."
- Bottom: By selecting the "Search Pharos…" option, the search will be done for the term in many locations of the database. Matching targets, diseases, and ligands are profiled, as well as matching text within a variety of filters, such as the PANTHER Class for "acetylcholine receptor."

the "Search Pharos for..." option. That search page provides the results for a search for the term as a target, disease, or ligand, as well as for any of the filter value fields that Pharos searches. Selecting one of the Donut Charts on the search result page will take the user to the respective target, disease, or ligand list page where those specific matching entries can be investigated.

8.2.3.4 Tutorials

Pharos has several tutorials available for users to become familiar with some of the tool's more advanced features. These can be found on the top menu, alongside buttons to access the various list pages. There is always a "What's New" tutorial for each new Pharos release to highlight new features. Tutorials and use case walkthroughs are made with the shepherd.js framework (https://shepherdjs.dev/).

The Use Cases page, found under the Tutorials Menu, walks the user through the use of Pharos and illustrates how different functions can be used together to address a high-level goal. Some of those use cases will form the basis of Section 8.3 of this chapter.

8.2.4 Analysis Methods Within Pharos

One of the biggest assets within Pharos is the flexibility in searching and analyzing targets, diseases, and ligands, as well as their interconnectedness.

8.2.4.1 Searching for Ligands

Users can search for ligands based on a starting chemical structure in the TCRD. Pharos accepts several different input formats, including SMILES, compound names, ChEMBL ID, and more, by utilizing an ID resolver service. This resolver service accepts a variety of inputs that are listed here: https://opendata.ncats.nih.gov/resolver/_options. By selecting the data that we wish to return, we are able to generate a query to fetch a standardized SMILES string: https://opendata.ncats.nih.gov/resolver/pt/lychi/smiles/inchikey/smilesParent/unii/cas?structure=CC1CC(O)(CCN1CCCC(%3DO)C1%3DCC%3DC(F)C%3DC1)C1%3DCC%3DC(Cl)C%3DC1. This service will then display the two-dimensional (2D) structure of the matching compound in the integrated MarvinJS widget (version 22.11.1) from ChemAxon (https://chemaxon.com/). Users can also modify that structure, load their own structure via a MOL file, or draw a structure from scratch. The SMILES from the MarvinJS Widget are used as the query for all subsequent structure searches. Once the query is specified, users can search for matching ligands in TCRD based on an Apache Lucene-based structure index of all TCRD ligands. The structure index is based on an internally developed inverted index of chemical graphs that enables rapid structure searching. The source code for a self-contained implementation of this structure indexer is available at: https://github.com/ncats/structure-indexer.

Similarity Search finds ligands that are similar to the query, whereas substructure search finds all ligands that contain the query as a substructure. In both cases, the search results are sorted according to Tanimoto coefficient [27] between ChemAxon's Chemical Hashed Fingerprints.

8.2.4.2 Finding Targets by Amino Acid Sequence

Targets can be searched based on protein sequence alignment with a query sequence using the BLAST (blastp) algorithm [28]. Specifically, NCBI's dockerized BLAST image (https://github.com/ncbi/docker/tree/master/blast version 2.12) is used to query the UniProt human protein database [13] using default parameters. Search results are displayed within Pharos as a target list. A density plot of matching amino acid residues is constructed for matching targets in the list against the query sequence. Users can navigate to each matching target to view primary documentation, utilize the list analysis capabilities of the list pages highlighted in Section 8.3.1.2 and Section 8.3.2.2, or download data for the target list, including details of the alignments from blastp [28].

8.2.4.3 Finding Targets with Similar Annotations

The "Find Similar Targets" links generate target list pages consisting of other targets in TCRD that have overlapping annotations with the target of interest. For example, for a target with ten associated diseases, the list of similar targets will consist of all targets that are associated with any of those ten diseases. The sorting of the resulting list is based on the *Tanimoto coefficient* calculated between the two sets of associated diseases. Specifically $J(A,B) = |A \cap B| / |A \cup B|$ [29].

As such, identical sets of diseases correspond to a Tanimoto coefficient of 1. Decreasing the overlap between the two sets or increasing the size of either set will result in a lower Tanimoto coefficient. Compared to itself, the target of interest will have a Tanimoto coefficient of 1 and be sorted to the top of the list, followed by other targets with a high degree of overlap in the selected data field.

8.2.4.4 Finding Targets with Predicted Activity

Starting with a ligand structure, as described in Section 8.2.4.1, users can search for targets predicted to have an activity similar to that of the query structure. These results are based on a set of Quantitative structure-activity relationship (QSAR) models provided by NCATS Predictor [30]. See https://predictor.ncats.io/predictor/ for details or to download datasets and models.

8.2.4.5 Enrichment Scores for Filter Values

When a listing page is showing a filtered list, i.e. not the full list of all targets, diseases, or ligands, it makes sense to calculate enrichment scores for values returned after filtering. This functionality is featured in the use case in section "Filter Value Enrichment".

Enrichment scores are calculated using Fisher's Exact Test [31]. Significance is determined according to the adjusted p-value, using the Benjamini–Hochberg procedure to limit the False Discovery Rate to $\alpha = 0.05$ [32], For example, the degree of overrepresentation for an associated disease in a target list can be calculated to help users understand whether the count of targets associated with a particular disease is due to random chance [32].

8.3 Use Cases

We present these use cases to introduce the reader to some of the many data sources underlying Pharos, as well as the powerful visualizations and population analysis tools. These walkthroughs are intended to illustrate how a new Pharos user could navigate through the tool and accomplish common scientific tasks. The three use cases center around the three main Pharos entities: targets, ligands, and diseases.

8.3.1 Hypothesizing the Role of a Dark Target

The first step in learning about a dark target would be browsing the details page for primary documentation (https://pharos.nih.gov/targets/ATP1B4). For dark targets, information tends to be sparse, and finding ways to expand the search for relevant documentation is one way to generate hypotheses for what the target may be involved in. When data are sparse, the user can change the line of inquiry from "what does this target do?" to "what do similar, or related, targets tend to do?"

To exemplify this functionality, we focus on the ATP1B4 target, a dark target that has very little direct documentation, as will be discussed in Section 8.3.1.1. Unless mentioned otherwise, screenshots for this use case using data for ATP1B4.

8.3.1.1 Primary Documentation

Components of the target details pages are divided into sections that group components into similar types of data. The Descriptive Data section provides basic information about a given protein and where it is expressed. The section "Behavioral Data" provides information related to low-level questions about what the protein binds to, and to what pathways it belongs. The Phenotypic Data section includes the data from TCRD that addresses the higher-level questions of what cellular functions it is involved in, and what traits or diseases it has been associated with.

Descriptive Data

The *Protein Summary* component (Figure 8.3 panel C) presents general information and descriptions of the target. These descriptions are retrieved from UniProt and NCBI, as are the many other terms by which a target is known. The Illumination Graph is a high-level visual representation of the information available for a target across multiple knowledge domains, as categorized by and quantified by the Harmonizome Project [33]. For ATP1B4, the user learns from the description that the target has some ancestral relation to Na,K-ATPase beta-subunits but may no longer function in that capacity. There are a number of links to external sites for follow-up.

When annotations are available, the *Protein Classes* (Figure 8.3 panel C bottom) component includes classifications of a target from PANTHER [34] or Drug Target Ontology (DTO) [5]. The documented classes in this section are all links that bring the user to a target list page, consisting of all targets that share that annotation. In this example, PANTHER has annotated this target as a *cation transporter*, and following that link will show all targets that have been deemed to be cation transporters.

IDG Development Level Summary

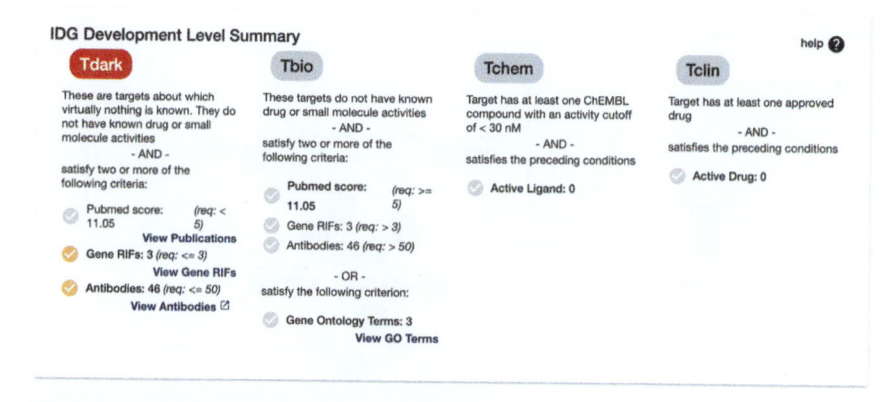

Tdark
These are targets about which virtually nothing is known. They do not have known drug or small molecule activities
- AND -
satisfy two or more of the following criteria:
- ✓ Pubmed score: (req: < 5) 11.05
  View Publications
- ✓ Gene RIFs: 3 (req: <= 3)
  View Gene RIFs
- ✓ Antibodies: 46 (req: <= 50)
  View Antibodies

Tbio
These targets do not have known drug or small molecule activities
- AND -
satisfy two or more of the following criteria:
- ✓ Pubmed score: (req: >= 5) 11.05
- ✓ Gene RIFs: 3 (req: > 3)
- ✓ Antibodies: 46 (req: > 50)
- OR -
satisfy the following criterion:
- ✓ Gene Ontology Terms: 3
  View GO Terms

Tchem
Target has at least one ChEMBL compound with an activity cutoff of < 30 nM
- AND -
satisfies the preceding conditions
- ✓ Active Ligand: 0

Tclin
Target has at least one approved drug
- AND -
satisfies the preceding conditions
- ✓ Active Drug: 0

Figure 8.5 IDG development level summary.

- This component summarizes criteria that led to a given target's TDL classification.
- The colored TDL is the assigned classification for this target, and the highlighted criteria are the ones that led to this classification.

Next, users will find the *IDG Development Level Summary* component (Figure 8.5), which briefly outlines the target's TDL. This explicitly shows which criteria pass and fail for the TDL assignment. Interpreting this component, we can see that ATP1B4 satisfies the Tdark criteria by having only three GeneRIFs, and less than 50 antibodies available. It fails the third criterion, having a PubMed score of less than 5, so this target is actually on the cusp of Tbio.

The *Expression Data* component is included as Descriptive Data and is aggregated from four primary data sources and one aggregating data source (Figure 8.6). Two of the primary datasets provide RNA expression data: GTeX [35] and HPA-RNA [36] datasets, which provide high throughput measurements of RNA expression in a wide variety of tissues. The other two primary datasets provide Protein expression data: HPA Protein [36], which measures protein expression through antibody labeling, and HPM Protein [37], which measures protein expression through mass spectrometry. Lastly, the JensenLab TISSUES resource [38] provides an aggregated view of data from many sources, including text mining, to provide a third avenue for understanding the expression patterns of targets. Tissues are aggregated based on the UBERON ontology [39], and details of each tissue and data source can be fetched by interacting with the heat map, circle plot, or anatomogram.

Continuing the review of primary documentation, the *Protein Sequence and Structure* component displays a density plot of amino acid counts in the protein sequence, as well as an interactive view of sequence and structure information. This component is built using EBI's Nightingale Web Components (https://ebi-webcomponents.github.io/nightingale/#/) [40]. The widget loads and displays all available structures from PDB [41] and AlphaFold [42, 43], and selecting different annotated domains in the sequence viewer will highlight the corresponding residues on the structure viewer. For our example protein, the user learns that there are no experimentally determined structures. There is an AlphaFold structure prediction

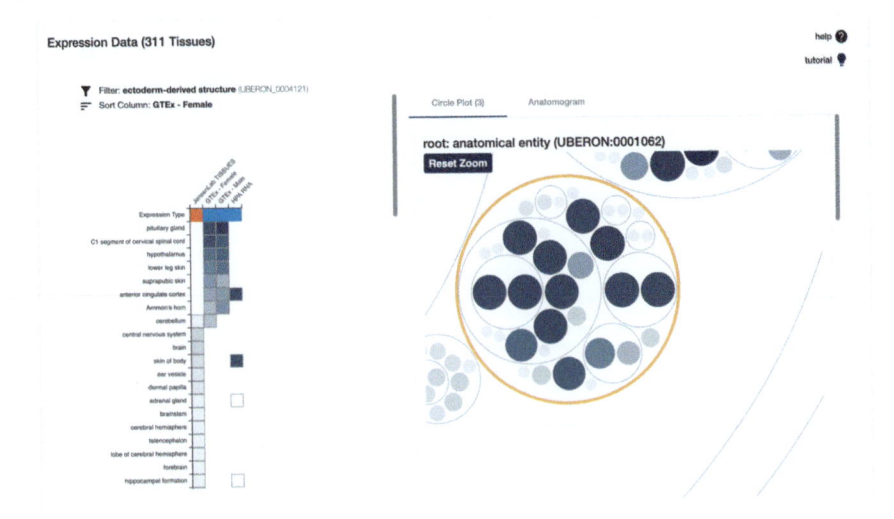

Figure 8.6 Expression data.

- Compiled expression data view that displays each source that has reported data for each tissue type. The Expression Type row delineates sources that report an aggregated score (red), RNA expression (blue), and protein expression (yellow, not pictured).
- Tissues can be found and filtered based on the name, or based on the UBERON ontology. The example shows a filtered heat map for tissues derived from the ectoderm, which includes the brain and spinal cord.
- The right panel has tabs for a circle-pack plot that groups tissues based on the UBERON hierarchy, and an anatomogram, where expression levels are projected onto a human form. The circle-pack plot is useful for identifying expression patterns where multiple tissues in the same category have high expression levels.

that claims high confidence for a large portion of the protein, and moderate/low confidence for another region.

Behavioral Data

Pharos displays an *Approved Drugs* component for targets that have appropriate drugs and an *Active Ligands* component where ligands are known (Figure 8.7 – Example CACNA2D1). These sections differ only in the approval status of the active compounds. Each component contains a pageable card list of the active compounds, a summary of the activity, and an image of the chemical structure. Buttons in these sections allow the user to switch from the target details page to a ligand list page, which allows the user to browse and analyze the list of compounds in a filterable list page. For our example dark target, we find no approved drugs or active ligands, as it has no compound activities above the potency threshold described in Section 8.1.

Protein–Protein Interactions are aggregated from STRING [44], Reactome [45], and BioPlex [46] and are shown in a pageable card list (Figure 8.8), showing some relevant features of the interaction. This component also includes a button to show the list of interacting proteins in a target list page, which opens the door to the same analysis and visualization options available for all list pages. For our example target, there

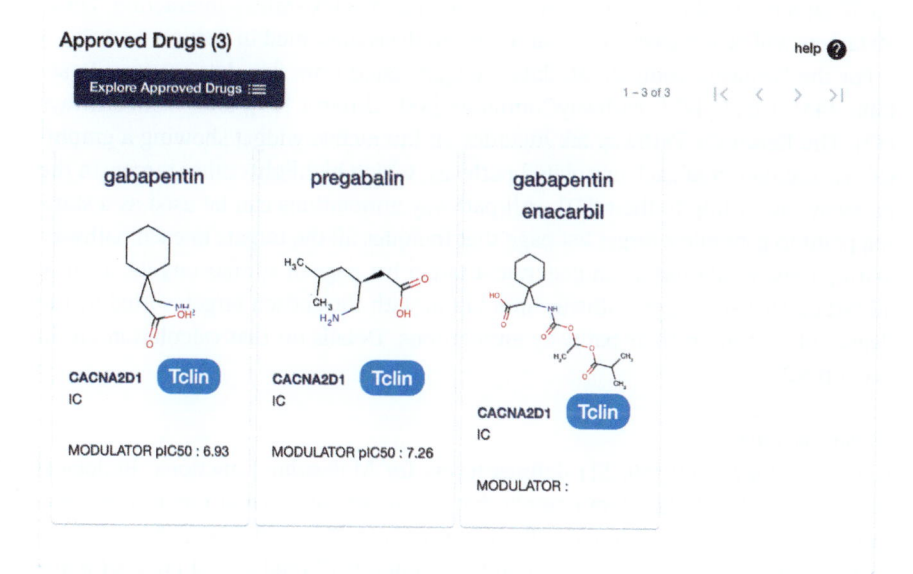

Figure 8.7 Drugs and ligands components.

- A pageable table of approved drugs for the current target. The 2D structure of each compound is rendered, as well as the measured activity against the target. A corresponding listing of other Active Ligands is shown on Pharos as well.
- The Explore Approved Drugs button will take the user to a ligand list page for this set of compounds, for further analysis.

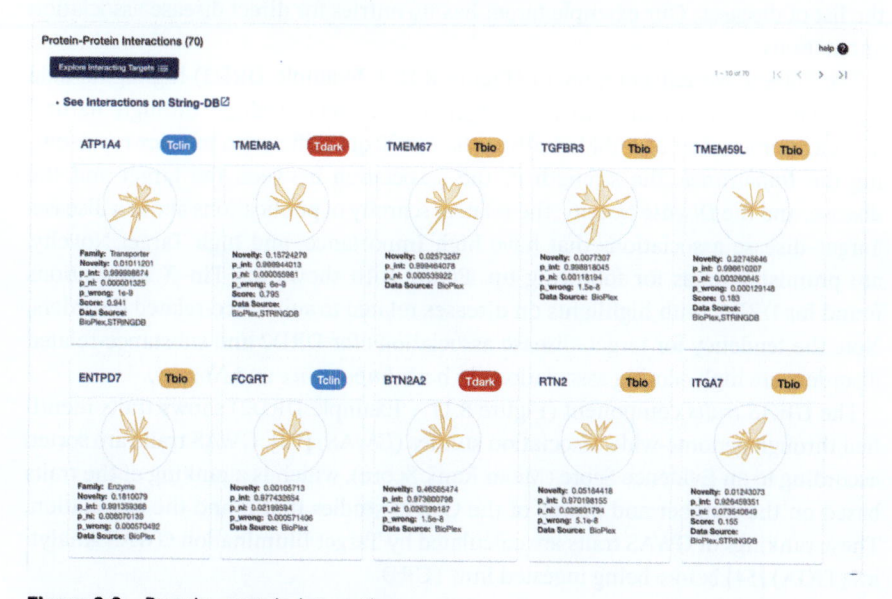

Figure 8.8 Protein–protein interactions.

- A pageable table of targets that interact with the current target. The radar plot of each target is rendered, as well as some details about the target and the measured interaction.
- The Explore Interacting Targets button will take the user to a target list page for this set of targets, for further analysis.

are 70 targets with documented physical interaction or text-mined interaction. These 70 targets will be the basis of the target list analysis presented in Section 8.3.1.2.

For the *Pathways* component, data are aggregated from five data sources: Reactome [45], KEGG [47], PathwayCommons [48], UniProt [19], and WikiPathways [49]. The Reactome Pathway tab includes an interactive widget showing a graphical representation of each annotated pathway, which highlights other targets in the pathways according to their TDL. All pathway annotations can be used as a starting point to generate a target list page that includes all the targets in each pathway. With pathway data users can generate a target list page of similar targets, a list of all targets that share any pathway annotation with the chosen target, sorted by the degree of overlap in their pathway annotations. Details on that calculation are in Section 8.2.4.3.

Phenotypic Data

Gene Ontology (GO) [50, 51] defines terms for Molecular Functions, Biological Processes, and Cellular Components that represent the normal function of gene products. From the *Gene Ontology Terms* component, Pharos shows each annotation that has been assigned to the target and can generate filtered lists of targets for any annotation.

The *Disease Associations* component (Figure 8.9 – Example GPR68) includes data from eight sources, including CTD [14], DisGeNET [15], DrugCentral [9], eRam [16], Expression Atlas [17], JensenLab [7], Monarch [18], and UniProt [19]. Users can pivot from a target details page showing a list of associated diseases to a disease list page where there are more analysis capabilities and visualizations for the list of diseases. Our example target has no entries for direct disease association annotations.

The *Disease Novelty* component (Figure 8.10 – Example DRD2) highlights data from Tin-X [52] which discovers target–disease relationships through natural language processing of PubMed abstracts. Tin-X quantifies two metrics representing the *Importance*, the strength of the association between the target and the disease, and the *Disease Novelty*, the relative scarcity of publications about a disease. Target–disease associations that have high Importance, and high Target Novelty, are promising areas for following up. Figure 8.10 shows the Tin–X associations found for DRD2, with highlights on diseases related to substance-related disorders. Note the tendency for target–disease associations for DRD2 and substance-related disorders are high-scoring associations in both *Importance* and *Novelty*.

The *GWAS traits* component (Figure 8.11 – Example DRD2) shows traits identified through genome-wide association studies (GWAS) [53]. GWAS traits are sorted according to an Evidence Score (Mean Rank Score), which is a ranking of the traits based on the number and power of the GWAS studies that found the association. These rankings of GWAS traits are calculated by Target Illumination GWAS Analytics (TIGA) [54] before being ingested into TCRD.

Similar to the Pathways data, a list of Similar Targets can be generated based on GO Terms, Associated Diseases, or GWAS Traits, as well as many other data points from this section. For example, a user could generate a target list that shares any of the associated diseases as the target of interest. Presenting the list in order of the

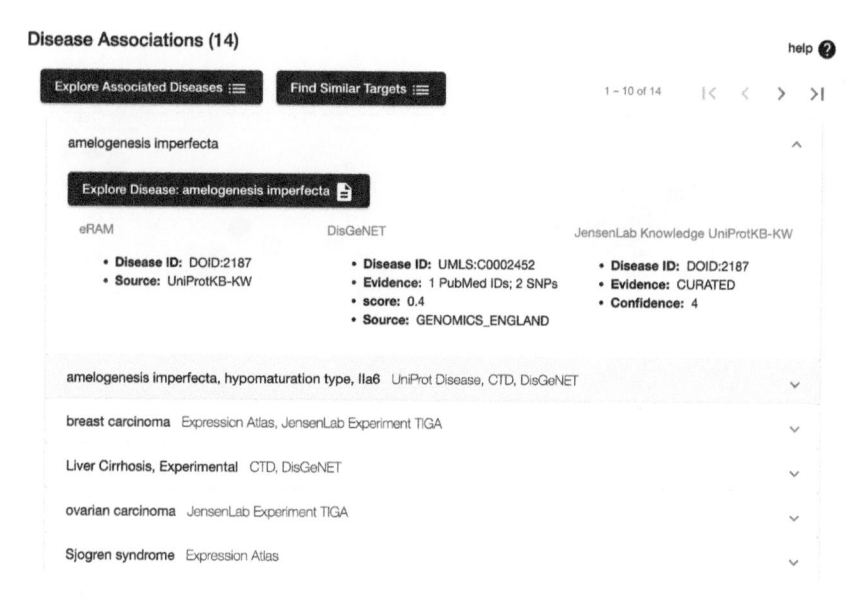

Figure 8.9 Associated diseases.

- A pageable table of associated diseases for the current target. Entries are expandable to show details of the association from each data source.
- Users can navigate to the disease details page through the Explore Disease button.
- The Explore Associated Diseases button will transfer the diseases in this table to a disease list page where further analysis can be done.
- The Find Similar Targets button will construct a target list that shares any associated diseases with the target of interest, and sort them by the degree of overlap in the sets of diseases, as described in Section 8.2.4.3.

degree of overlap allows them to easily find other targets that have the most similar sets of those associated diseases, or whichever data field the similarity calculation was based on.

Resources and Publications

Researchers can learn which typical experimental models (17 species supported) have orthologous versions of the target. Additionally, resources, such as genetic constructs, cells, mice, chemical tools, or data resources, generated by IDG grant awardees may be possible to acquire for research. The last section of the target details pages contains temporal plots of bibliometric scores [7, 55] and patent counts that inform users about the popularity of research into a particular target. Text-mined references from JensenLab, and manually curated GeneRIFs (https://www.ncbi.nlm.nih.gov/gene/about-generif) are available to review.

8.3.1.2 List Analysis

So far in this use case, as a researcher investigating the role of the dark target ATP1B4, we learned that there is some data for the target, but notably no known associated diseases. Next, we will continue our search for possible disease associations by expanding the search to related targets. One promising idea is to

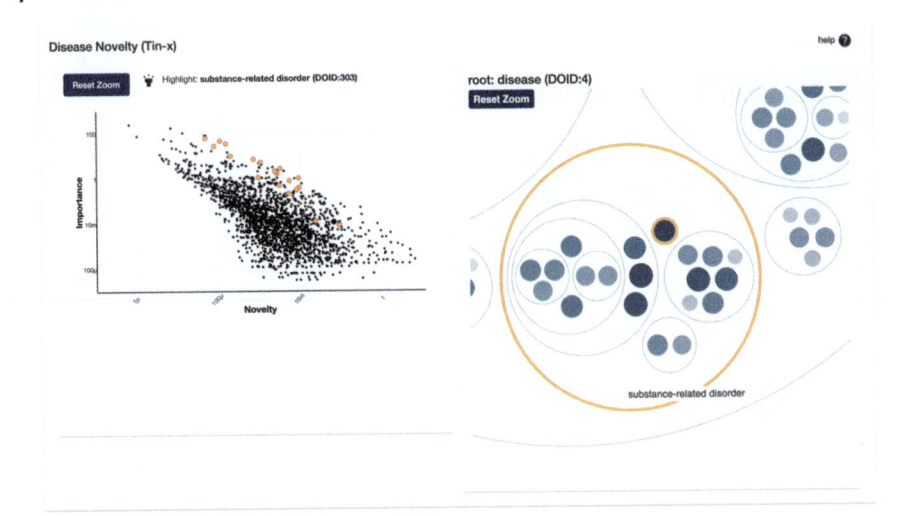

Figure 8.10 Disease novelty.

- This component highlights data from Tin-X [52] which discovers target–disease relationships through natural language processing of PubMed abstracts.
- Left shows a scatterplot of the *Importance*, the strength of the association between the target and the disease, versus the *Disease Novelty*, and the relative scarcity of publications about a disease.
- Right shows a circle-pack plot of the Importance metric for each disease association. Selecting different regions within the disease hierarchy highlights points on the scatterplot, and vice-versa.
- Target–disease associations that have high Importance, and high Target Novelty, are promising areas for following up.

look for consistent documentation for the 70 documented protein–protein interactions mentioned in section "Behavioral Data". The *Protein–Protein Interactions* component (Figure 8.8) presents a link to "Explore Interacting Targets," which takes the user to a list of 71 targets, including the 70 interacting targets plus ATP1B4 (the target of interest).

Filter Value Enrichment
As introduced in Section 8.2.3.1, the filters in the filter panel (Figure 8.2 panel E) will tell us how many of the targets in the list have each filter value. Since ATP1B4 did not have any direct disease associations, we used the *Associated Disease* filter to discover, which diseases may be associated with the set of interacting targets.

Figure 8.12 top-right shows the counts of targets in this list that are associated with each disease. At first glance, it might seem significant that 35 of the 71 (49%) targets in the list are associated with ovarian cancer, but knowing that ovarian cancer and many other cancers are associated with changes in the function and expression of many targets should lead us to be skeptical. In fact, in the unfiltered target list (Figure 8.12 top-left), 8589 of the 20,412 (42%) targets in TCRD have a documented association with ovarian cancer, meaning that even a randomly chosen

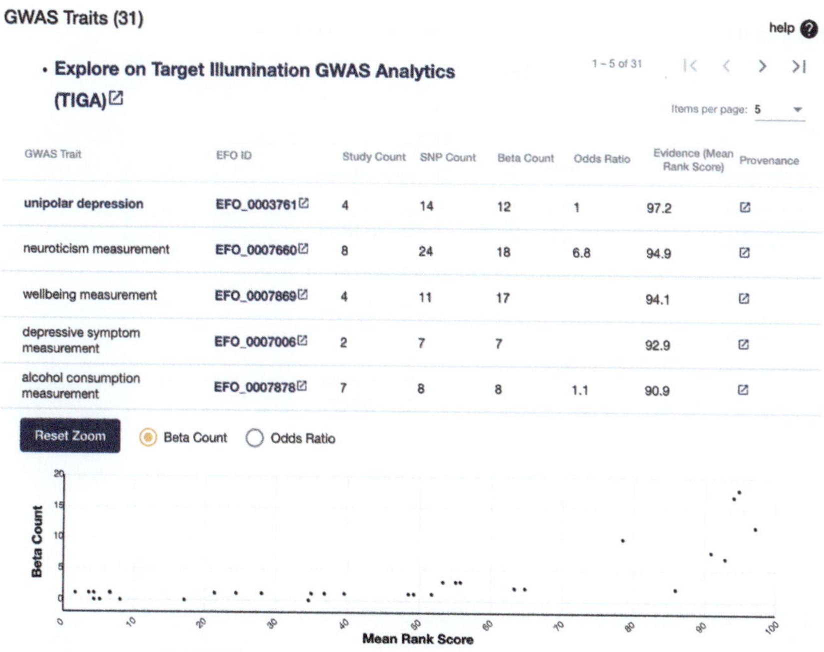

GWAS Traits (31)

- Explore on Target Illumination GWAS Analytics (TIGA)

GWAS Trait	EFO ID	Study Count	SNP Count	Beta Count	Odds Ratio	Evidence (Mean Rank Score)	Provenance
unipolar depression	EFO_0003761	4	14	12	1	97.2	
neuroticism measurement	EFO_0007660	8	24	18	6.8	94.9	
wellbeing measurement	EFO_0007869	4	11	17		94.1	
depressive symptom measurement	EFO_0007006	2	7	7		92.9	
alcohol consumption measurement	EFO_0007878	7	8	8	1.1	90.9	

Figure 8.11 GWAS traits.

- A pageable table of GWAS traits for a given target. The listing is sorted based on the Evidence Score, as calculated by the TIGA algorithm described in Section 8.3.1.4.
- The lower panel shows a plot of the Mean Rank Score vs. Beta Count. The most reliable traits would be found in the upper right of this plot.

list of proteins would include a large number of targets associated with ovarian cancer.

Pharos allows users to calculate enrichment scores using Fisher's Exact Test [31] (Section 8.2.4.5), to determine the significance of finding a given count of filter values in a filtered list. In our example, Fisher's Exact Test calculates a p-value of 0.13, which can be interpreted as the probability of finding 35 (or more) targets associated with ovarian cancer in a randomly selected list of 71 targets. The implication is that finding so many targets associated with ovarian cancer in this list is not very surprising. Calculating the enrichment scores for the entire list (Figure 8.12 bottom) reveals, which diseases are significantly overrepresented in the filtered list. The top values in this sorted list would be more promising for further investigation, especially since three out of the top four overrepresented diseases are forms of heart failure.

A similar example is given on Pharos in the "Filter Value Enrichment" tutorial. In that example, enrichment scores are calculated for the list of interacting targets for a very well-understood target, the D(2) dopamine receptor (DRD2). In that example, the enrichment scores reveal many neurological and substance-related diseases that are commonly known to be associated with DRD2. That proof of

Associated Disease

Search

☐ ovarian cancer		8589
☐ osteosarcoma		7972
☐ medulloblastoma		7142
☐ psoriasis		6906
☐ large cell medulloblastoma		6269
☐ glioblastoma		6034
☐ malignant ependymoma		5607
☐ atypical teratoid rhabdoid tumor		5491
☐ malignant glioma		4999

Associated Disease (6.11s)

Search

☐ medulloblastoma		38
☐ large cell medulloblastoma		37
☐ ovarian cancer		35
☐ glioblastoma		34
☐ psoriasis		32
☐ atypical teratoid rhabdoid tumor		31
☐ malignant glioma		29
☐ osteosarcoma		29

Filter Value Enrichment

Instructions

Filter value counts, as reported on the left panel, show which filter values are the most common for targets in the list. These raw counts are sometimes dominated by filter values that are much more likely to be found than others. This tool calculates which filter values are enriched, or over-represented, in the current list. The odds ratio of observing a given count of values is presented, as is as the p-value using Fisher's Exact test. Significance is determined according to the adjusted p-value, using the Benjamini-Hochberg procedure to limit the False Discovery Rate to α = 0.05.

Potential Use Cases

- For a list of interacting proteins to a target of interest (click 'Explore Interacting Targets' from a target details page), what values for 'Associated Disease' are overrepresented in the list?
- For a list of targets generated from your RNA-SEQ experiment, and uploaded to your profile as a custom target list (see the tutorial 'Uploading a Custom Target List' for a walkthrough), what 'Reactome Pathways' are overrepresented?
- For a list of ligands that are structurally similar to a compound of interest (see the tutorial 'Searching by Chemical Structure' for a walkthrough), what Targets have activity against those ligands?

Select a filter
Associated Disease ▼

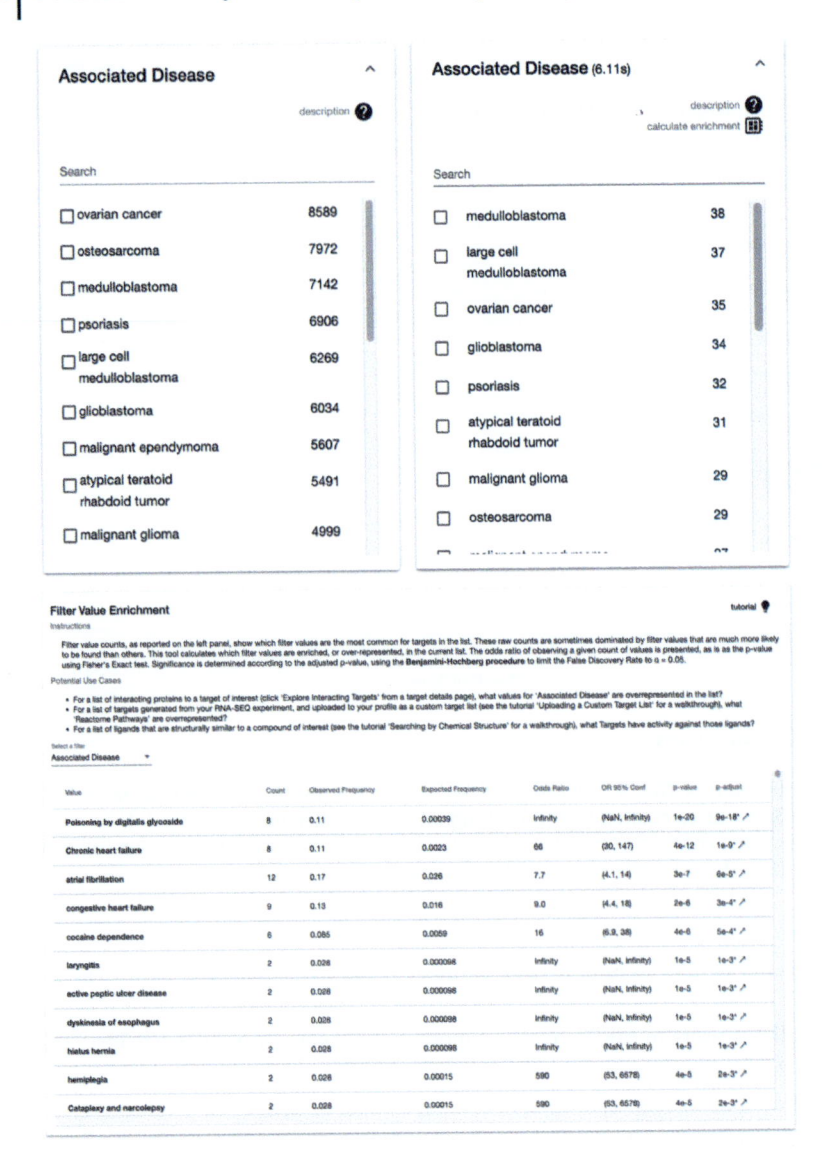

Value	Count	Observed Frequency	Expected Frequency	Odds Ratio	OR 95% Conf	p-value	p-adjust
Poisoning by digitalis glycoside	8	0.11	0.00039	Infinity	(NaN, Infinity)	1e-20	9e-18
Chronic heart failure	8	0.11	0.0023	66	(30, 147)	4e-12	1e-9
atrial fibrillation	12	0.17	0.026	7.7	(4.1, 14)	3e-7	6e-5
congestive heart failure	9	0.13	0.016	9.0	(4.4, 18)	2e-6	3e-4
cocaine dependence	6	0.085	0.0059	16	(6.3, 38)	4e-6	5e-4
laryngitis	2	0.028	0.000098	Infinity	(NaN, Infinity)	1e-5	1e-3
active peptic ulcer disease	2	0.028	0.000098	Infinity	(NaN, Infinity)	1e-5	1e-3
dyskinesia of esophagus	2	0.028	0.000098	Infinity	(NaN, Infinity)	1e-5	1e-3
hiatus hernia	2	0.028	0.000098	Infinity	(NaN, Infinity)	1e-5	1e-3
hemiplegia	2	0.028	0.00015	590	(53, 6578)	4e-5	2e-3
Cataplexy and narcolepsy	2	0.028	0.00015	590	(53, 6578)	4e-5	2e-3

Figure 8.12 Filter value enrichment.

- Top left: In a target list, the filters show the counts of targets that have each annotation. In this example, the counts of targets associated with each disease are shown for the complete unfiltered target list. Some diseases are associated with a very large number of targets.
- Top right: In a filtered list, these value counts are often affected by this bias in the data toward heavily documented filter values. In this example, this list is filtered to targets that interact with ATP1B4. Many of the top diseases in this filtered list are the same diseases as top diseases in the unfiltered list. The "calculate enrichment" button here will calculate the probability that the measured counts are explainable by random chance.
- Bottom: Results of an enrichment calculation for targets that interact with ATP1B4. Chronic heart failure is associated with 11% of the targets in the list (Count: 8 targets, Observed Frequency: 0.11). The Expected Frequency, based on the full dataset, is 0.23%. Based on Fisher's Exact Test, the probability of finding that many targets by random chance is 4e-12. p-adjust is calculated based on an adjustment for performing a large number of tests, controlling the False Discovery Rate to 0.05.

concept helps validate the method and lends credence to the idea of discovering relevant annotations for less well-studied targets.

8.3.1.3 Downloading Data

Easy data extraction is a key requirement for many researchers. Researchers studying ATP1B4 may build a download query and select the "Associated Disease" fields to download all the associated disease data for targets in the list. Users wanting to compile a list of approved drugs or active ligands for targets in the list would select the "Drugs and Ligands" fields. Heat maps and the *Sequence Alignment* component also contain shortcuts for initiating a data download with the appropriate fields.

8.3.1.4 Variations on this Use Case

Other Ways to Expand the Dataset

The path chosen in this use case was to expand the search for documentation from one dark target to a list of related targets by compiling a list of interacting targets via the "Explore Interacting Targets" button in the *Protein–Protein Interactions* component of the target details page.

Another way to expand the dataset would be to compile a list of targets that share one or more of the annotations that exist on this sparsely documented target. Beyond simply clicking what annotations are there (i.e. PANTHER Class for cation transporter) to generate a list of targets, users can also compile lists of targets based on having any overlap in documentation through the "Find Similar Targets" buttons (Section 8.2.4.3) that are available on a number of components including GO Terms and Pathways.

Alternatively, the *Protein Sequence and Structure* component allows users to easily initiate a search for targets with a homologous protein sequence (Section 8.2.4.2). A Sequence search can also be initiated from a target list page via a button highlighted in Figure 8.2 panel J. Figure 8.13 shows the resulting Sequence Alignment component on the resulting List Analysis page that illustrates, which regions of the sequence are matching in each entry in the target list.

It should also be noted that these expansions can be compounded, for example by finding a list of targets with a homologous sequence, and then filtering that list by PANTHER Class or GO term, thereby finding targets with multiple points of similarity.

Other Filters to use for Enrichment Calculation

In addition to looking for Associated Diseases that are enriched in the target list, other interesting filters to try might be IDG Family, PANTHER Class, DTO Class, Pathways, GO Functions, or GO Processes. There are no restrictions on which filters are available to calculate enrichment, beyond the requirement that the filter is categorical (i.e. not numerical).

8.3.2 Characterizing a Novel Chemical Compound

This use case is for a researcher who would like to explore the potential effects of a novel chemical compound. For the sake of the example, we will use a "novel"

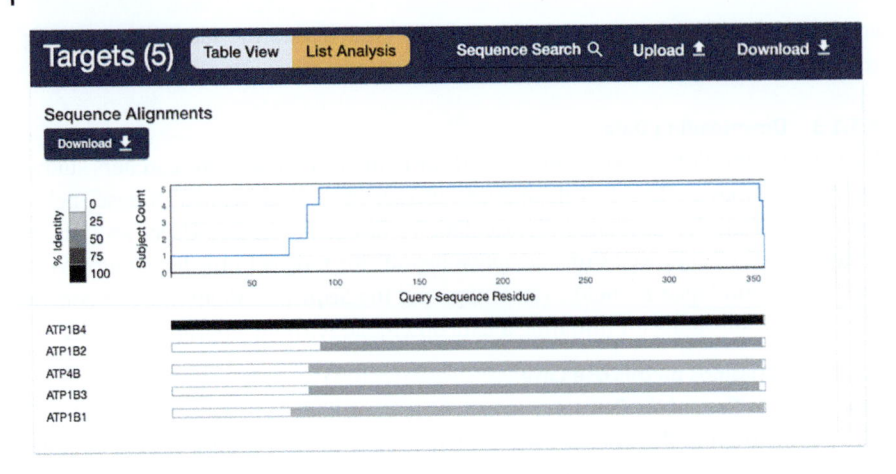

Figure 8.13 Sequence search.

- Sequence Search Results in the List Analysis tab of the resulting target list. The top plot is a density plot of aligned residues for all the aligning sequences. Below is a representation of each matching target's region of alignment, color-coded by the percent identity of the alignment.

compound represented by the following SMILES: CC1CC(O)(CCN1CCCC(=O)C1=CC=C(F)C=C1)C1=CC=C(Cl)C=C1. Note that this is a slightly modified version of haloperidol that is just for the purposes of this example, to help illustrate the concepts. Our researcher has two main questions: What targets might be affected by this compound? What effects might it have on the human body?

8.3.2.1 Finding Predicted Targets

Since this is a novel chemical compound, there would be no primary documentation to review, as was the case with the dark target in Section 8.3.1. The researcher would begin on the ligand list page, and follow the link for "Structure Search" or navigate to https://pharos.nih.gov/structure. Starting on the Structure Search page (Figure 8.14), the user can paste in the SMILES to attempt to resolve the structure to a known compound and render the compound in the MarvinJS widget.

Following the search link in the "Find Predicted Targets" card will fetch the list of targets from NCATS Predictor [30] as described in Section 8.2.4.4. The ensuing target list (Figure 8.15) is a compilation of proteins predicted as targets of the query structure, and the targets that have a known activity to the compound in the database if a matching compound was found. Since our example is a novel compound, only predicted data are available. Predicted data are highlighted in the Target Card, and in the filter panel with a shaded background.

Details about the prediction are shown in the Table View of the list pages, which includes the predicted activity, the activity for the nearest compound from the model training set, and a measure of the Applicability Domain. Prediction applicability is quantified by the Tanimoto similarity between the query structure and the nearest

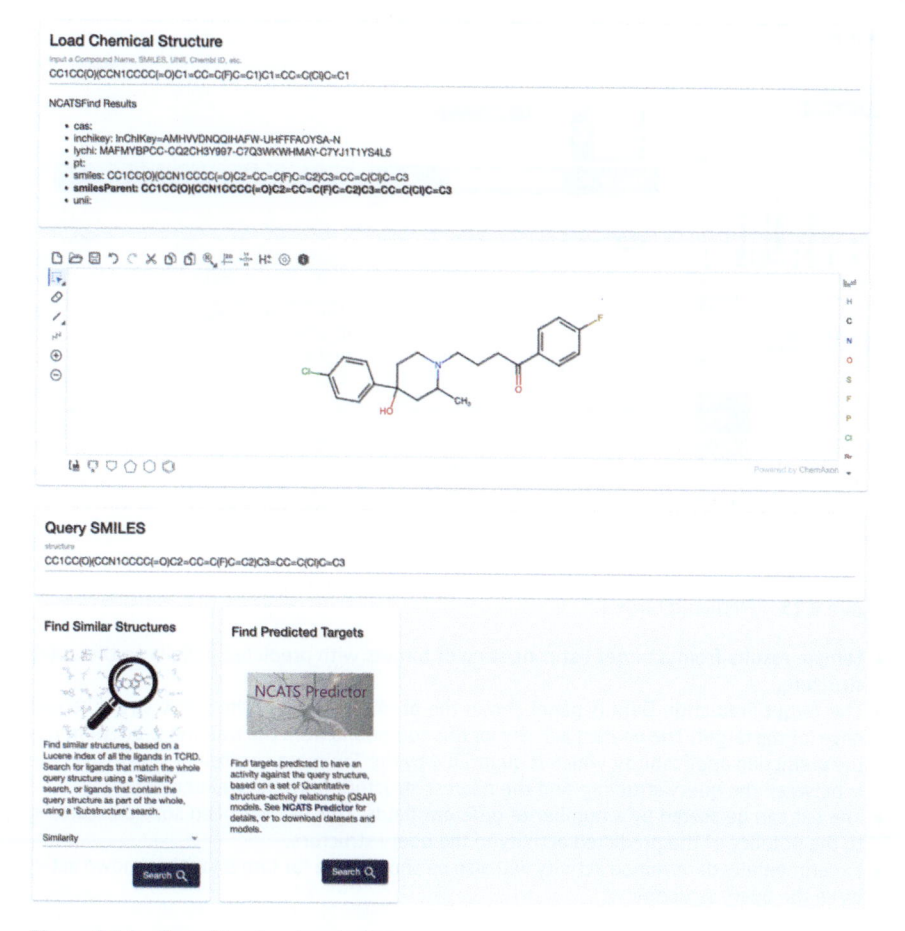

Figure 8.14 Searching by chemical structure.

- Pharos' Structure Search page allows users to initiate a search based on any chemical structure. Many types of inputs are used to resolve into a SMILES string to load into the Marvin JS Sketcher. The Sketcher can then be used to edit the query structure, upload a file, or draw a compound from scratch.
- Options are available to find similar ligands to the query structure or find targets predicted to interact with the query structure.

compound from the training set. Users can filter the list based on the numeric filter for prediction applicability, or based on the numeric filter for the predicted activity.

For our example compound, NCATS Predictor found 25 targets with predicted activity. There are several target filters to consider when the list consists of targets with activity against a given compound. Calculating filter value enrichment, as described in more detail in section "Filter Value Enrichment", yields some interesting results. Figure 8.16 shows the top five GO Functions, and the top five Associated Diseases, for this list of predicted targets. The presence of serotonin-related GO Terms, and depression-related diseases, are what we should expect from this "novel" compound that is so closely related to haloperidol.

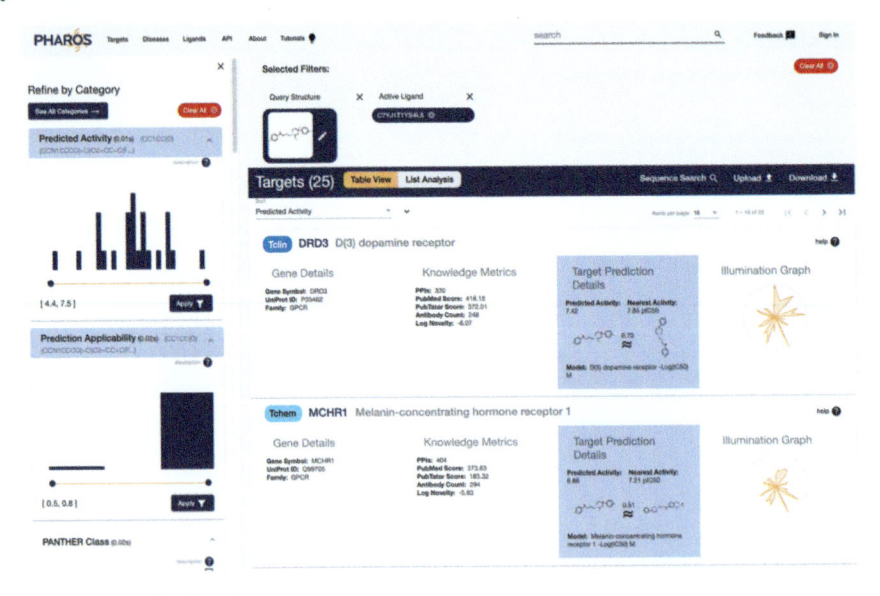

Figure 8.15 Predicted targets.

- Sample results from a target list consisting of targets with predicted activity to the query structure.
- The Target Prediction Details panel shows the predicted activity the query structure will have for the target. The nearest activity for this compound from the training set determines the prediction applicability, which is quantified by the Tanimoto coefficient shown over the ≈ between the query structure and the nearest structure from the training set.
- The list can be sorted by a number of different fields. This list has been sorted according to the potency of the predicted activity to the query structure.
- Experimentally determined activity will also be shown here for targets with a known activity to the query structure.

8.3.2.2 Analyzing Similar Ligands

Another method of investigating the potential targets or target families for a novel compound is in the analysis of the effects of a set of similar compounds. As in the previous search for predicted targets, a Similarity Search is initiated from the Structure Search page (Figure 8.14 bottom). Section 8.2.4.1 describes how this functionality works.

Pharos will display a list of all compounds from TCRD that are structurally similar to the query structure (Figure 8.17). In the Table View of the ligand list, the 2D structures are presented in order of decreasing similarity for users to browse and choose the best similarity cutoff. A Tanimoto coefficient of 0.6 is by default used to cast a wide net for matching compounds. It is usually prudent to restrict the similarity further using the numeric filter for the similarity score. Figure 8.17 shows the resulting ligand list page after searching for similar compounds to our query structure, and subsequently filtering the result list to those ligands with a Structure Similarity (i.e. Tanimoto coefficient on molecular fingerprints) greater than 0.8. This results in a list of 66 ligands from TCRD.

8.3 Use Cases

Select a filter: GO Function

Value	Count	Observed Frequency	Expected Frequency	Odds Ratio	OR 95% Conf	p-value	p-adjust
G protein-coupled serotonin receptor activity	8	0.32	0.0017	369	(146, 929)	3e-17	2e-15* ↗
neurotransmitter receptor activity	8	0.32	0.0018	342	(137, 857)	4e-17	2e-15* ↗
serotonin binding	5	0.20	0.00049	1019	(274, 3795)	5e-13	1e-11* ↗
adrenergic receptor activity	5	0.20	0.00083	424	(137, 1316)	1e-11	3e-10* ↗
drug binding	6	0.24	0.0029	119	(46, 309)	8e-11	2e-9* ↗

Select a filter: Associated Disease

Value	Count	Observed Frequency	Expected Frequency	Odds Ratio	OR 95% Conf	p-value	p-adjust
depressive disorder	15	0.60	0.015	106	(47, 238)	7e-22	5e-19* ↗
Nasal congestion	9	0.36	0.0013	674	(262, 1734)	4e-21	1e-18* ↗
Mental Depression	14	0.56	0.013	105	(47, 234)	7e-21	2e-18* ↗
Nasal discharge	9	0.36	0.0014	603	(237, 1532)	8e-21	2e-18* ↗
Mood Disorders	10	0.40	0.0090	78	(35, 176)	8e-15	1e-12* ↗

Figure 8.16 Enriched filter values in a list of predicted targets.

- Top: The top five GO Functions that are overrepresented in a list of predicted targets.
- Bottom: The top five Associated Diseases that are overrepresented in a list of predicted targets.

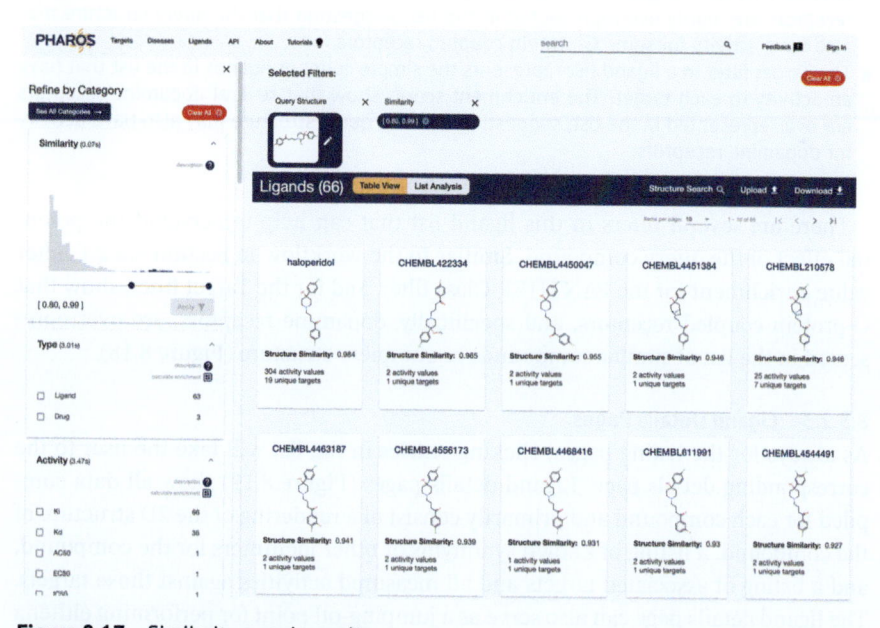

Figure 8.17 Similarity search results.

- Similarity search results for a sample query structure that was the methylated analog of haloperidol.
- The list shown here is filtered to ligands with a Structure Similarity (i.e. Tanimoto coefficient on molecular fingerprints) greater than 0.8.

Select a filter								
PANTHER Class ▼								
Value	Count	Observed Frequency	Expected Frequency	Odds Ratio	OR 95% Conf	p-value	p-adjust	
G-protein coupled receptor	64	0.97	0.19	133	(33, 544)	3e-43	4e-42* ↗	
receptor	64	0.97	0.24	101	(25, 412)	3e-37	2e-36* ↗	
isomerase	2	0.030	0.0016	20	(4.8, 81)	5e-3	0.02* ↗	
histone	1	0.015	0.00020	78	(11, 569)	0.01	0.04* ↗	
aspartic protease	2	0.030	0.025	1.2	(0.29, 4.9)	0.50	1.00	

Select a filter								
Target ▼								
Value	Count	Observed Frequency	Expected Frequency	Odds Ratio	OR 95% Conf	p-value	p-adjust	
D(2) dopamine receptor (P14416)	64	0.97	0.0092	3526	(863, 14413)	5e-128	1e-126* ↗	
D(3) dopamine receptor (P35462)	22	0.33	0.0094	53	(32, 89)	3e-28	4e-27* ↗	
D(4) dopamine receptor (P21917)	17	0.26	0.0044	80	(46, 138)	2e-25	1e-24* ↗	
Sigma non-opioid intracellular receptor 1 (Q99720)	6	0.091	0.0062	16	(6.9, 37)	4e-6	3e-5* ↗	
3-beta-hydroxysteroid-Delta(8),Delta(7)-isomerase (Q15125)	2	0.030	0.00011	294	(69, 1248)	3e-5	1e-4* ↗	

Figure 8.18 Enriched filter values in a list of similar compounds.

- In a list of compounds found through a Similarity Search to a methylated analog of haloperidol, filter value enrichment is calculated for the PANTHER Class filter and the Target filter.
- The PANTHER Class filter in a ligand list represents the count of ligands in the list that have activity for a target in each class. The enrichment scores show that G-protein coupled receptors are highly overrepresented in the list, suggesting that the query structure may also have activity for some G-protein coupled receptors.
- The Target filter in a ligand list represents the simple count of ligands in the list that have an activity to each target. The enrichment scores show that several dopamine receptors are overrepresented in the list, suggesting that the query structure may also have activity for dopamine receptors.

There are several filters in this ligand list that can help understand the potential effect of the query compound. Similar to the workflow in Section 8.3.2.1, filter value enrichment for the PANTHER Class filter, and for the Target filter, show that G-protein coupled receptors, and specifically, dopamine receptors, are overrepresented in the list of similar compounds to our query structure (Figure 8.18).

8.3.2.3 Ligand Details Pages

As always for the listing pages, clicking entries in the list will take the user to the corresponding details page. Ligand details pages (Figure 8.19) show all data compiled for each compound and primarily consist of a rendering of the 2D structure of the compound, a listing of known synonyms or other identifiers for the compound, and a listing of associated targets and all measured activities against those targets. The ligand details page can also serve as a jumping-off point for performing either a Substructure Search, a Similarity Search for other compounds in TCRD, or Exploring the targets in a target list page.

A table of target activities is displayed (Figure 8.19 bottom), along with a button to translate the list of targets into a more interactive target list page. That list page will also include predicted activities, based on functionality described in Section 8.2.4.4.

8.3 Use Cases

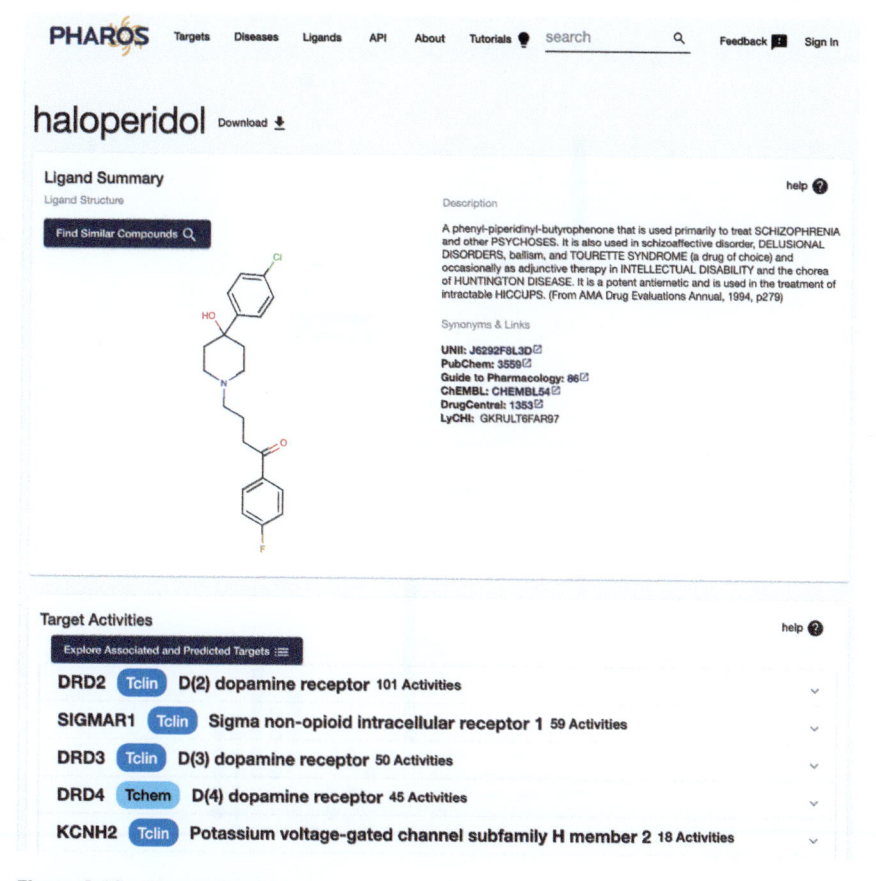

Figure 8.19 Ligand details.

- Top, Ligand Summary – This component shows the 2D structure and equivalent IDs. A button allows users to initiate either a Similarity Search or a Substructure Search, of the database based on the current ligand as a starting point.
- Bottom, Target Activities – All experimentally determined target activities are shown here. A button allows users to translate this view into a target list page, which will include targets this compound that is predicted to have activity for.

8.3.2.4 Variations on this Use Case
Other Ligand List filters

Ligand lists have filters that can help users find compounds that meet their requirements. Some of those filters were introduced in Section 8.3.2.2. Additionally, Figure 8.17 includes the Type filter, which reports whether or not the compounds have achieved FDA approval. In this example, three compounds are approved drugs, while 63 are other active ligands.

The number of targets each compound has an activity for, a measure of target specificity, is reflected in the Target Count filter (Figure 8.20). This can be used to filter the list based on how selective the compounds are.

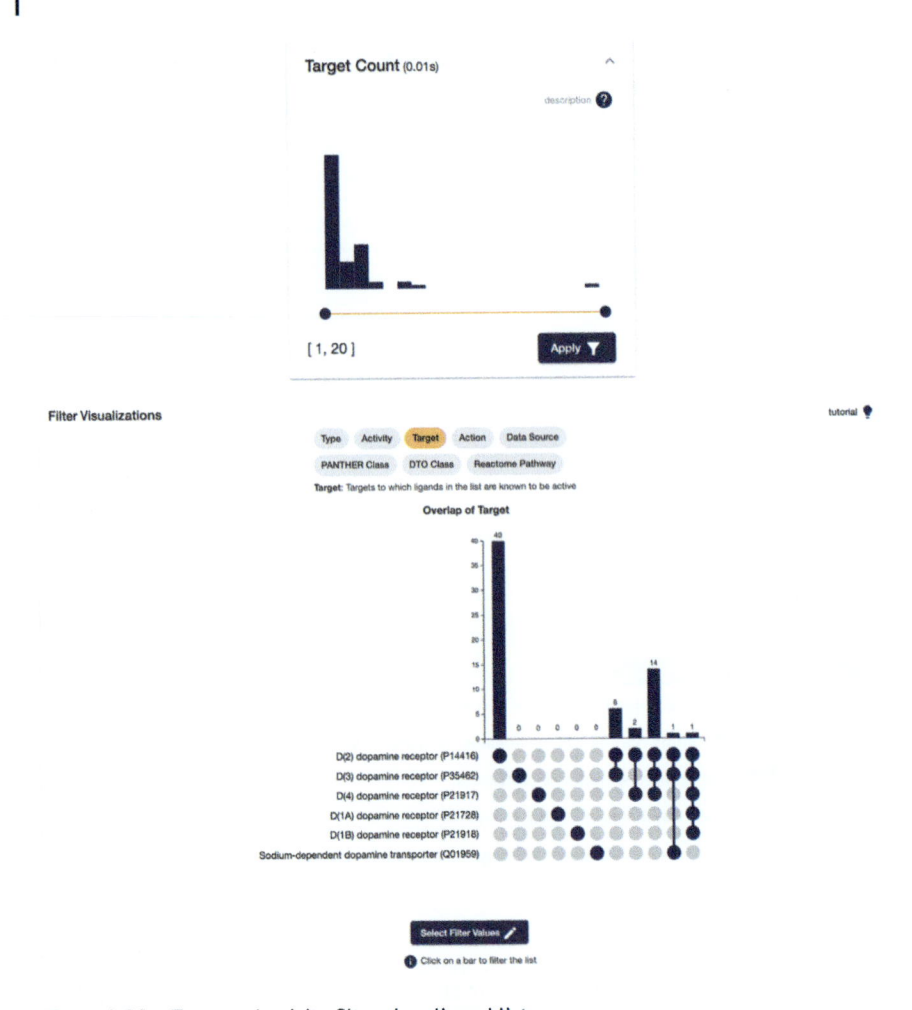

Figure 8.20 Target selectivity filters in a ligand list.

- Top: The Target Count filter in a ligand list represents the number of ligands in the list that have documented activity to different numbers of targets. Compounds with a high number are more promiscuous, while compounds with only one or two known target activities may be selective or less well-studied. The sliders at the bottom of the histogram can be used to filter the ligand list to only compounds that meet the requirements the user sets.
- Bottom: An UpSet Chart is constructed for the Target filter on a ligand list. The counts of compounds in the list with each combination of active targets are represented. Clicking on the bars or circles will filter the list to only those compounds that have the required combination of active targets.

Using the UpSet Plots

Another useful method to dive into the specificity is to build an UpSet plot [56] for the Target filter. On the List Analysis tab of the list pages, the Filter Visualizations component shows Donut Charts and UpSet Charts for the different filters, depending on how many values an entry in the list can have for that filter. If an entry can have multiple values (e.g. one compound can have activity for multiple targets), an

UpSet plot is shown to help the user understand the overlap of different filter values present in the list.

Figure 8.20 bottom shows an UpSet plot for the Target filter in this ligand list. This was constructed by selecting the Target filter from the list of buttons along the top, then selecting the targets that correspond to dopamine receptors using the "Select Filter Values" button, appearing below the first generated graph (for all targets). Interpreting the UpSet chart tells us how many compounds in the list have activity for each combination of filter values. For example, Figure 8.20 tells us there are fourteen compounds that have activity for the D2, D3, and D4 dopamine receptors, and not D1A, D1B, or the dopamine transporter. Furthermore, clicking the appropriate bar on the graph can filter the list to those fourteen compounds for follow-up.

Using the Heat Maps

The List Analysis tab will also display buttons to create heat maps (Figure 8.21). Target list pages can construct heat maps of targets in the list vs. their associated diseases, active ligands, or protein–protein interacting partners. Disease and ligand list pages can construct heat maps of the elements in the list vs. their associated targets. Heat maps are interactive in their sorting and can be used to drill down into the details of each cell in the heat map. Figure 8.21 shows the heat map of the average reported activities between compounds in the list and the associated targets for the current use case. A Details View is shown as would appear when the user clicks a cell of the heat map. Links within the Details View will navigate to the appropriate details pages for the corresponding clicked cell of the heat map.

Generating a Ligand List Based on a Target

The target details pages have Drugs and Ligands components (See Sections 8.2.3.2 and "Behavioral Data") that display all the active compounds that TCRD has for a given target. Those components have a link to explore the list of compounds on a ligand list page (See Figure 8.7). Ligand lists based on a target are an obvious use case for finding selective compounds, using the Target Count filter (see section "Other Ligand List filters"), or using the UpSet plot (see section "Using the UpSet Plots"). A special feature of ligand lists based on an associated target is the potency filter that becomes available. Figure 8.22 shows how the Target Count filter and the Potency filter can be used together to filter the list to only compounds with the required specificity and potency for the given target.

Uploading a Custom Ligand List

The functionality provided by a ligand list page can be used to explore commonalities among a set of ligands identified to be active against a target in a biological assay. From a ligand list page, the Upload button (Figure 8.2) can be used to resolve compounds by a number of chemical identifiers (see Section 8.2.4.1), and the List Analysis features such as filter value enrichment, and heat maps are useful for this task as well.

Given a chemist who has screened thousands of compounds in a cell-based phenotypic assay, the resulting hit list would be loaded into Pharos. The workflows

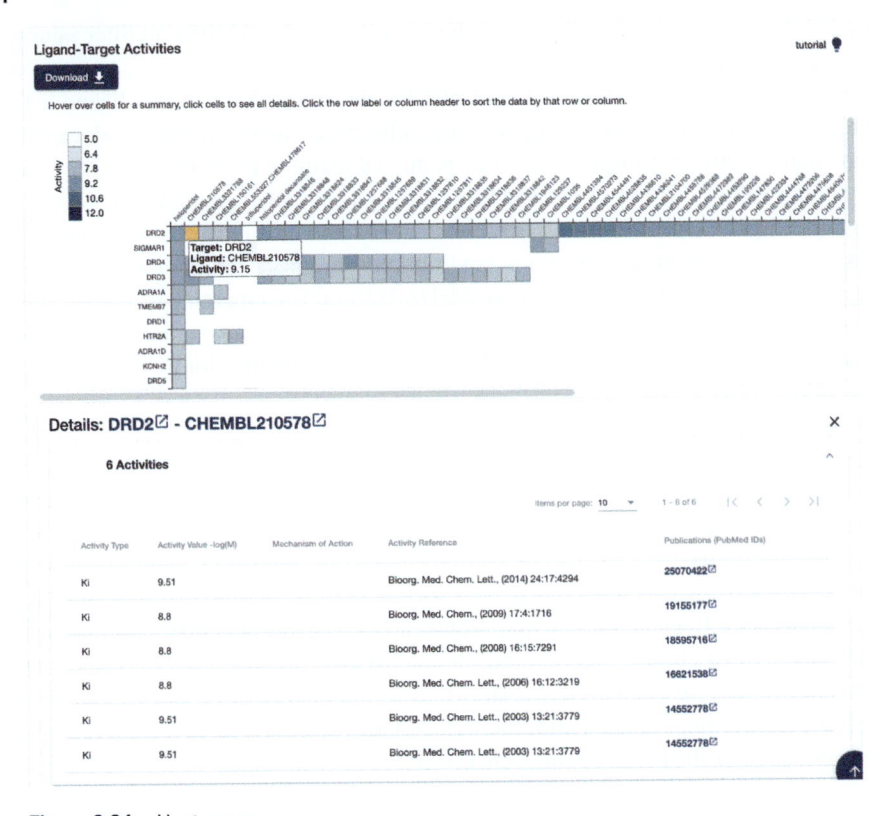

Figure 8.21 Heat maps.

- Top: A heat map showing the common targets that are associated with each compound in the list. Shading on the heat maps is informative in different ways depending on the heat map created. For ligand–target activities, the shading corresponds to the reported average potency of the measured activities.
- Downloading the data for the heat map can be initiated with the corresponding button.
- Bottom: The Details View of one cell of the heat map, opened by clicking on the cells.

described in Sections 8.3.2.2 and 8.3.2.4 show how the Target filter, PANTHER Class filter, and DTO Class filter, can help understand the roles of the targets that are at work in the screening assay. Similarly, the Target Count (Figure 8.20 left) filter and the Target filter UpSet plot (see section "Using the UpSet Plots") can help understand the selectivity profile of the ligands in the list as well.

8.3.3 Investigating Diseases

The same types of analyses that are possible for targets and ligands are available for diseases. This includes filtering a disease list based on values in the filter panel (Section 8.2.3.1), calculating filter value enrichment (see section "Filter Value Enrichment"), and generating UpSet plots (see section "Using the UpSet Plots") and heat maps (see section "Using the Heat Maps").

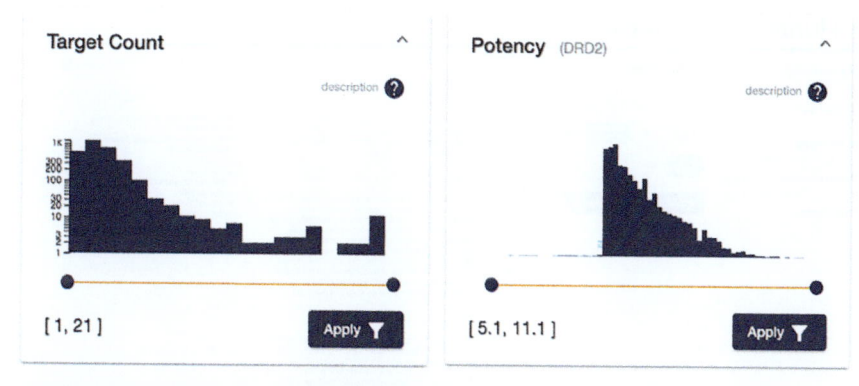

Figure 8.22 Finding appropriate ligands.

- Left: Target Count filter for a ligand list based on a target with many active compounds.
- Right: EC50 filter for the same ligand list.
- Filtering the list using these two filters can help find a compound with the required specificity (using the Target Count filter) and potency (using the EC50 filter).
- Note that the potency filters (like EC50 and IC50) are only available (and only make sense) on ligand lists based on a single target.

One thing to highlight is that disease lists can be constructed based on association with a given target. As pictured in Figure 8.9, the *Disease Association* component on target details pages has a link to generate that list. From there, the Disease Ancestry filter presents a listing of the common nodes in the disease hierarchy, for which enrichment scores can be calculated, as in section "Filter Value Enrichment".

Disease details pages are constructed for all MONDO disease terms and any disease name that could not be resolved to a standardized MONDO term. Basic descriptions from MONDO, DO, and UniProt are shown in the summary panel, as are the equivalent IDs from other ontologies (Figure 8.23). When data are available, results of GWAS studies, sorted and ranked by the TIGA algorithm, as described above, are shown for all targets associated with the disease.

The MONDO disease ontology is also informative in the hierarchical structure in which diseases are defined. This hierarchy is captured in TCRD and leveraged in Pharos. For example, asthma is a parent term for allergic and intrinsic asthma. A Pharos user browsing the disease details page for asthma can navigate up and down the hierarchy to the related disease details pages (Figure 8.24). Furthermore, when a user clicks the "Explore Associated Targets" button on each disease details page, the resulting list of targets associated with asthma will include targets with a documented association to the child terms and all descendent terms.

Lastly, the disease details pages show a plot of two bibliometric scores from TIN-X [52], analogous to the disease association data on a target details page (Figure 8.10). As described in section "Phenotypic Data", the *Importance* captures the strength of an association between a target and a disease. The *Novelty* metric measures the scarcity of publications about a target. Targets that score highly on the *Importance* metric, and at the same time, remain relatively novel, such as targets above the noise on both axes, are more likely to play a role in the disease.

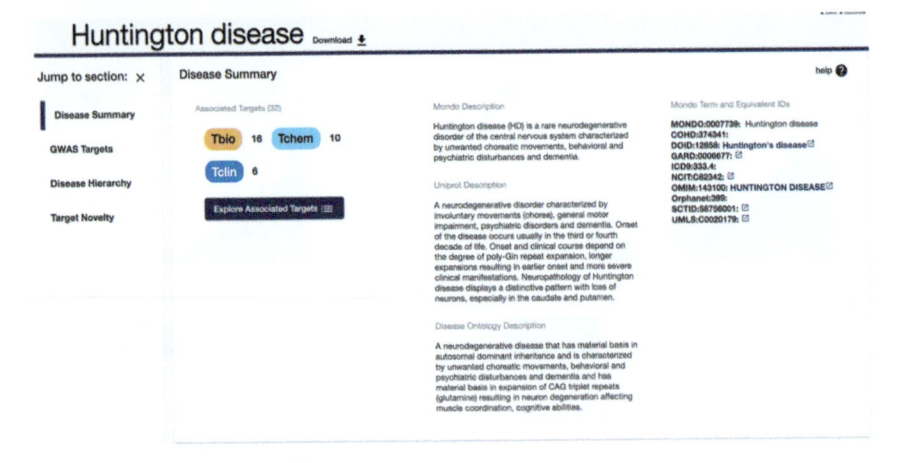

Figure 8.23 Disease summary.

- An example Disease Summary component based on Huntington Disease. This component highlights basic disease definitions from different ontologies, and a listing of equivalent disease IDs, based on the MONDO disease mappings.
- The count of targets associated with a disease and all descendent terms is displayed along with a button to navigate to a target list page of the associated targets, for further inquiry.

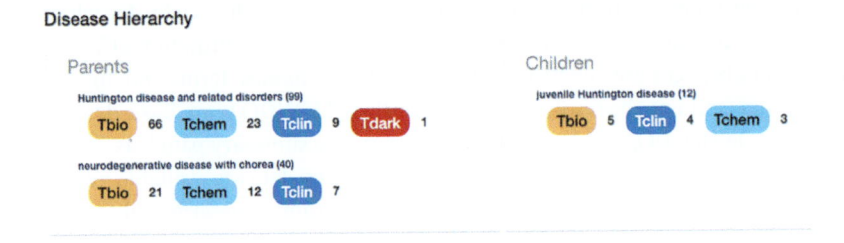

Figure 8.24 Disease hierarchy.

- Users can navigate related disease details pages by traversing the parent and child terms hierarchy. Parent terms are more general, while child terms are more specific versions of the current disease.

8.4 Discussion

Aggregating and displaying data from multiple locations is useful in its own right, as it allows for easier access to a wide range of knowledge. We note that Pharos as a data aggregation tool was successfully leveraged in drug discovery research to prioritize potential biomarkers using the novelty and protein class data within Pharos [57]. The TDL levels within Pharos are often used to prioritize druggable targets that do not have known active ligands (Tdark and Tbio) [58] or those that do have active [59]. The CSV download functionality is often used to easily download a specific type of data for a list of targets [60]. Generally, it is standard practice to allow a user to search for an entity, present matches in a list format, and subsequently, allow users to dive into details about entries in the list. As such, most database browsing websites will have an equivalent of a listing page and a set of details pages.

The power of Pharos' list pages lies in the interesting ways in which the lists can be generated, and the visualization and analysis options available. As an example, any target list page will display the counts of targets in the list that match in a Reactome Pathway, such as "Interferon Gamma Signaling." When the target list has been generated based on an association with a rare disease, having a number of those targets be a part of the same Reactome Pathway could be enlightening. Enrichment analysis for those Reactome Pathways can reveal the degree to which those hits can be explained by random chance. Similarly, generating a target list based on sequence alignment or protein–protein interactions enables a degree of illumination for dark targets based on population analysis of the group of similar, or related targets.

Behind the scenes, Pharos is written in a modular fashion allowing developers to readily expand or modify features related to fetching or processing data without affecting the rest of the functionality. As a result, the same code is used to calculate the top filter values for all filters in all models (targets, diseases, and ligands). The only difference between filters is the table and column of the data being processed. Furthermore, when new data processing functionality is added, such as the UpSet Plots [56] (see section "Using the UpSet Plots") starting from Pharos version 3.7, the plots were available for all categorical filters at once. This allows the user to generate UpSet Plots for specific use cases like viewing targets overlapping in different pathways. At the same time, less obvious use cases are also supported, such as examining target overlap from each Data Source, or the overlap of targets in the different IDG target lists. A user may want to know, which targets were found in the ProKinO [61] dataset, AND NOT the Dark Kinome Knowledgebase [62], and could use the UpSet plot for the Data Source filter for that. Similarly, a user may be interested in which targets were highlighted in the 2020 IDG target list but was removed from the 2022 IDG target list. The modular nature of the codebase supports these unexpected use cases, which might satisfy questions from a program officer, or someone thinking about quality control of different data sources, rather than a typical biologist or chemist.

In a similar way, when support for calculating Filter Value Enrichment was added in Pharos version 3.9, calculating enrichment became possible for all filters, not just for "traditional" filters like pathways. The guiding principle at work here is to develop functionality in a general way that applies to all data annotations, so as not to restrict researchers to use cases that were planned for in advance.

In the future, TCRD will continue expanding to include new and interesting datasets, while pruning some less useful, outdated ones. Additionally, efforts will be made to automate the TCRD generation and harmonization scripts. Pharos is looking toward developing a framework to easily incorporate new predictions, such as predicted effects of inhibiting kinases on cancers [63], or predicted off-target effects for ligands [64]. Incorporating more single-cell data, and developing informative visualizations to help users understand patterns in the data is another promising area of development.

Funding

National Institutes of Health Knowledge Management Center for Illuminating the Druggable Genome (ZIA TR000057-08, U24 CA224370, U24 TR002278)

References

1 Edwards, A.M., Isserlin, R., Bader, G.D. et al. (2011). Too many roads not taken. *Nature* 163–165. https://doi.org/10.1038/470163a.
2 Oprea, T.I., Bologa, C.G., Brunak, S. et al. (2018). Unexplored therapeutic opportunities in the human genome. *Nature Reviews. Drug Discovery* 17: 317–332.
3 Stoeger, T., Gerlach, M., Morimoto, R.I., and Nunes Amaral, L.A. (2018). Large-scale investigation of the reasons why potentially important genes are ignored. *PLoS Biology* 16: e2006643.
4 Illuminating the druggable genome. 9 Jul 2013 [cited 29 Aug 2022]. https://commonfund.nih.gov/idg.
5 Lin, Y., Mehta, S., Küçük-McGinty, H. et al. (2017). Drug target ontology to classify and integrate drug discovery data. *Journal of Biomedical Semantics* 8: 50.
6 Nguyen, D.-T., Mathias, S., Bologa, C. et al. (2017). Pharos: collating protein information to shed light on the druggable genome. *Nucleic Acids Research* 45: D995–D1002.
7 Pletscher-Frankild, S., Pallejà, A., Tsafou, K. et al. (2015). DISEASES: text mining and data integration of disease–gene associations. *Methods* 74: 83–89.
8 Gaulton, A., Hersey, A., Nowotka, M. et al. (2017). The ChEMBL database in 2017. *Nucleic Acids Research* D945–D954. https://doi.org/10.1093/nar/gkw1074.
9 Ursu, O., Holmes, J., Bologa, C.G. et al. (2019). DrugCentral 2018: an update. *Nucleic Acids Research* 47: D963–D970.
10 Sheils, T.K., Mathias, S.L., Kelleher, K.J. et al. (2021). TCRD and Pharos 2021: mining the human proteome for disease biology. *Nucleic Acids Research* 49: D1334–D1346.
11 Carvalho-Silva, D., Pierleoni, A., Pignatelli, M. et al. (2019). Open targets platform: new developments and updates two years on. *Nucleic Acids Research* 47: D1056–D1065.
12 Safran, M., Rosen, N., Twik, M. et al. (2021). The GeneCards suite. In: *Practical Guide to Life Science Databases* (ed. I. Abugessaisa and T. Kasukawa), 27–56. Singapore: Springer Nature Singapore.
13 UniProt Consortium (2021). UniProt: the universal protein knowledgebase in 2021. *Nucleic Acids Research* 49: D480–D489.
14 Davis, A.P., Grondin, C.J., Johnson, R.J. et al. (2021). Comparative Toxicogenomics Database (CTD): update 2021. *Nucleic Acids Research* 49: D1138–D1143.

15 Piñero, J., Ramírez-Anguita, J.M., Saüch-Pitarch, J. et al. (2020). The DisGeNET knowledge platform for disease genomics: 2019 update. *Nucleic Acids Research* 48: D845–D855.

16 Jia, J., An, Z., Ming, Y. et al. (2018). eRAM: encyclopedia of rare disease annotations for precision medicine. *Nucleic Acids Research* 46: D937–D943.

17 Papatheodorou, I., Moreno, P., Manning, J. et al. (2020). Expression Atlas update: from tissues to single cells. *Nucleic Acids Research* 48: D77–D83.

18 Mungall, C.J., McMurry, J.A., Köhler, S. et al. (2017). The Monarch Initiative: an integrative data and analytic platform connecting phenotypes to genotypes across species. *Nucleic Acids Research* 45: D712–D722.

19 UniProt Consortium (2019). UniProt: a worldwide hub of protein knowledge. *Nucleic Acids Research* 47: D506–D515.

20 Nastou, K.C., Nasi, G.I., Tsiolaki, P.L. et al. (2019). AmyCo: the amyloidoses collection. *Amyloid* 26: 112–117.

21 Schriml, L.M., Mitraka, E., Munro, J. et al. (2018). Update: classification, content and workflow expansion. *Nucleic Acids Research* 2019: D955–D962. https://doi.org/10.1093/nar/gky1032.

22 McKusick, V.A. (1998). *Mendelian Inheritance in Man: A Catalog of Human Genes and Genetic Disorders*. JHU Press.

23 Bodenreider, O. (2004). The Unified Medical Language System (UMLS): integrating biomedical terminology. *Nucleic Acids Research* 32: D267–D270.

24 Medical subject headings – home page. 2020 [cited 26 Aug 2022]. https://www.nlm.nih.gov/mesh/meshhome.html.

25 Weinreich, S.S., Mangon, R., Sikkens, J.J. et al. (2008). Orphanet: a European database for rare diseases. *Nederlands Tijdschrift voor Geneeskunde* 152: 518–519.

26 Harding, S.D., Armstrong, J.F., Faccenda, E. et al. The IUPHAR/BPS guide to PHARMACOLOGY in 2022: curating pharmacology for COVID-19, malaria and antibacterials. *Nucleic Acids Research* 2022: D1282–D1294. https://doi.org/10.1093/nar/gkab1010.

27 Bajusz, D., Rácz, A., and Héberger, K. (2015). Why is Tanimoto index an appropriate choice for fingerprint-based similarity calculations? *Journal of Cheminformatics* 7: 20.

28 Altschul, S.F., Gish, W., Miller, W. et al. (1990). Basic local alignment search tool. *Journal of Molecular Biology* 215: 403–410.

29 Levandowsky, M. and Winter, D. (1971). Distance between sets. *Nature* 234: 34–35.

30 Zakharov, A.V., Zhao, T., Nguyen, D.-T. et al. (2019). Novel consensus architecture to improve performance of large-scale multitask deep learning QSAR models. *Journal of Chemical Information and Modeling* 59: 4613–4624.

31 Fisher, R.A. (1992). Statistical methods for research workers. In: *Breakthroughs in Statistics: Methodology and Distribution* (ed. S. Kotz and N.L. Johnson), 66–70. New York, NY: Springer New York.

32 Yekutieli, D. and Benjamini, Y. (1999). Resampling-based false discovery rate controlling multiple test procedures for correlated test statistics. *Journal of Statistical Planning and Inference* 82: 171–196.

33 Rouillard, A.D., Gundersen, G.W., Fernandez, N.F. et al. (2016). The harmonizome: a collection of processed datasets gathered to serve and mine knowledge about genes and proteins. *Database* 2016: https://doi.org/10.1093/database/baw100.

34 Thomas, P.D., Campbell, M.J., Kejariwal, A. et al. (2003). PANTHER: a library of protein families and subfamilies indexed by function. *Genome Research* 13: 2129–2141.

35 Carithers, L.J., Ardlie, K., Barcus, M. et al. (2015). A novel approach to high-quality postmortem tissue procurement: the GTEx project. *Biopreservation and Biobanking* 13: 311–319.

36 Thul, P.J. and Lindskog, C. (2018). The human protein atlas: a spatial map of the human proteome. *Protein Science* 27: 233–244.

37 Kim, M.-S., Pinto, S.M., Getnet, D. et al. (2014). A draft map of the human proteome. *Nature* 509: 575–581.

38 Palasca, O., Santos, A., Stolte, C. et al. (2018). TISSUES 2.0: an integrative web resource on mammalian tissue expression. *Database* 2018: https://doi.org/10.1093/database/bay003.

39 Mungall, C.J., Torniai, C., Gkoutos, G.V. et al. (2012). Uberon, an integrative multi-species anatomy ontology. *Genome Biology* 13: R5.

40 Watkins X, Garcia LJ, Pundir S, Martin MJ, UniProt Consortium (2017). ProtVista: visualization of protein sequence annotations. *Bioinformatics* 33: 2040–2041.

41 Berman, H.M., Westbrook, J., Feng, Z. et al. (2000). The Protein Data Bank. *Nucleic Acids Research* 28: 235–242.

42 Jumper, J., Evans, R., Pritzel, A. et al. (2021). Highly accurate protein structure prediction with AlphaFold. *Nature* 596: 583–589.

43 Varadi, M., Anyango, S., Deshpande, M. et al. (2022). AlphaFold Protein Structure Database: massively expanding the structural coverage of protein-sequence space with high-accuracy models. *Nucleic Acids Research* 50: D439–D444.

44 Szklarczyk, D., Gable, A.L., Nastou, K.C. et al. (2020). The STRING database in 2021: customizable protein–protein networks, and functional characterization of user-uploaded gene/measurement sets. *Nucleic Acids Research* 49: D605–D612.

45 Fabregat, A., Jupe, S., Matthews, L. et al. (2018). The Reactome Pathway Knowledgebase. *Nucleic Acids Research* 46: D649–D655.

46 Huttlin, E.L., Bruckner, R.J., Navarrete-Perea, J. et al. (2021). Dual proteome-scale networks reveal cell-specific remodeling of the human interactome. *Cell* 184: 3022–3040.e28.

47 Kanehisa, M. and Goto, S. (2000). KEGG: kyoto encyclopedia of genes and genomes. *Nucleic Acids Research* 28: 27–30.

48 Cerami, E.G., Gross, B.E., Demir, E. et al. (2011). Pathway Commons, a web resource for biological pathway data. *Nucleic Acids Research* 39: D685–D690.

49 Martens, M., Ammar, A., Riutta, A. et al. (2021). WikiPathways: connecting communities. *Nucleic Acids Research* 49: D613–D621.

50 Ashburner, M., Ball, C.A., Blake, J.A. et al. (2000). Gene ontology: tool for the unification of biology. *The Gene Ontology Consortium. Nature Genetics* 25: 25–29.

51 Gene Ontology Consortium (2021). The Gene Ontology resource: enriching a GOld mine. *Nucleic Acids Research* 49: D325–D334.
52 Cannon, D.C., Yang, J.J., Mathias, S.L. et al. (2017). TIN-X: target importance and novelty explorer. *Bioinformatics* 33: 2601–2603.
53 Buniello, A., MacArthur, J.A.L., Cerezo, M. et al. (2019). The NHGRI-EBI GWAS Catalog of published genome-wide association studies, targeted arrays and summary statistics 2019. *Nucleic Acids Research* 47: D1005–D1012.
54 Yang, J.J., Grissa, D., Lambert, C.G. et al. (2021). TIGA: target illumination GWAS analytics. *Bioinformatics*, https://doi.org/10.1093/bioinformatics/btab427.
55 Wei, C.-H., Kao, H.-Y., and Lu, Z. (2013). PubTator: a web-based text mining tool for assisting biocuration. *Nucleic Acids Research* 41: W518–W522.
56 Lex, A., Gehlenborg, N., Strobelt, H. et al. (2014). UpSet: visualization of intersecting sets. *IEEE Transactions on Visualization and Computer Graphics* 20: 1983–1992.
57 Tawa, G.J., Braisted, J., Gerhold, D. et al. (2021). Transcriptomic profiling in canines and humans reveals cancer specific gene modules and biological mechanisms common to both species. *PLoS Computational Biology* 17: e1009450.
58 Marazzi, L., Shah, M., Balakrishnan, S. et al. (2022). NETISCE: a network-based tool for cell fate reprogramming. *npj Systems Biology and Applications* 8 (1): 21. https://doi.org/10.1038/s41540-022-00231-y.
59 Korrapati, S., Taukulis, I., Olszewski, R. et al. (2019). Single cell and single nucleus RNA-Seq reveal cellular heterogeneity and homeostatic regulatory networks in adult mouse stria vascularis. *Frontiers in Molecular Neuroscience* 12: 316. https://doi.org/10.3389/fnmol.2019.00316. PMID: 31920542; PMCID: PMC6933021.
60 Federico, A., Pavel, A., Moebus, L. et al. (2021). The integration of large-scale public data and network analysis uncovers molecular characteristics of. *bioRxiv* https://doi.org/10.1101/2021.05.10.443441.
61 Gosal, G., Kochut, K.J., and Kannan, N. (2011). ProKinO: an ontology for integrative analysis of protein kinases in cancer. *PLoS One* 6: e28782.
62 Berginski, M.E., Moret, N., Liu, C. et al. (2021). The Dark Kinase Knowledgebase: an online compendium of knowledge and experimental results of understudied kinases. *Nucleic Acids Research* 49: D529–D535.
63 Ravanmehr, V., Blau, H., Cappelletti, L. et al. (2021). Supervised learning with word embeddings derived from PubMed captures latent knowledge about protein kinases and cancer. *NAR Genomics and Bioinformatics* 3: lqab113.
64 Keiser, M.J., Roth, B.L., Armbruster, B.N. et al. (2007). Relating protein pharmacology by ligand chemistry. *Nature Biotechnology* 25: 197–206.

Part III

Users' Points of View

9

Mining for Bioactive Molecules in Open Databases

Guillem Macip, Júlia Mestres-Truyol, Pol Garcia-Segura, Bryan Saldivar-Espinoza, Santiago Garcia-Vallvé, and Gerard Pujadas

Departament de Bioquímica i Biotecnologia, Carrer Marcel·lí Domingo 1, Universitat Rovira i Virgili, Research group in Cheminformatics & Nutrition, 43007 Tarragona, Catalonia, Spain

9.1 Introduction

An important goal of drug-discovery researchers is to determine which molecules in chemical compound databases have a specific bioactivity. This goal can be achieved either by experimentally testing compound libraries to find molecules that show the desired bioactivity (a process known as high-throughput screening; HTS) [1, 2] or by computationally predicting the bioactivity of interest in files containing the structure of hundreds of thousands, or even millions, of chemical compounds encoded in the form of electronic archives (a process known as virtual screening; VS) [3, 4]. In VS, the researcher does not need to physically have the chemical compounds since their description in electronic format is sufficient. The cost of VS is therefore much lower than the cost of HTS, where the bioactivity of a large number of compounds is measured experimentally.

Like all screening techniques, VS is sometimes compared to looking for a needle in a haystack. However, using VS to find molecules that exhibit the desired activity is much easier than finding the needle since VS is a targeted search (unlike searching for a needle, where there is no privileged direction and all search directions are equally possible). This targeted search can be guided by the characteristics of existing drugs for the same target or by the structure of the macromolecular target itself.

Figure 9.1 shows an example of a typical VS workflow that is frequently used in our laboratory [5–7] (other VS pipelines may also be successfully employed [8, 9]). This VS workflow consists of several sequential filters (i.e. ADMET/PAINS, protein–ligand docking, pharmacophore, and shape/electrostatic) where the output molecules of one filter are the input molecules of the next filter, and so on. The inverted pyramid shape in Figure 9.1 also shows that, as the VS progresses, the number of available molecules decreases since molecules that do not pass a filter are discarded and not evaluated by the remaining filters. If the VS is designed correctly, it is expected that, as the molecules pass through the various filters, the resulting

Open Access Databases and Datasets for Drug Discovery, First Edition.
Edited by Antoine Daina, Michael Przewosny, and Vincent Zoete.
© 2024 WILEY-VCH GmbH. Published 2024 by WILEY-VCH GmbH.

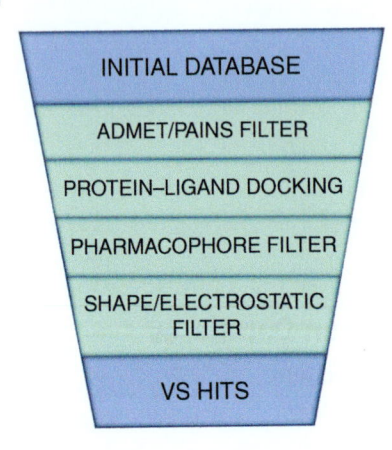

Figure 9.1 Overview of a typical virtual screening (VS) workflow previously used in our laboratory. The shape of the funnel is related to the number of molecules evaluated at each stage of the VS. Since these are elimination stages in which compounds that do not pass a filter are discarded and therefore not evaluated by the subsequent filters, the number of available molecules becomes smaller and smaller.

[Funnel diagram with layers from top to bottom: INITIAL DATABASE, ADMET/PAINS FILTER, PROTEIN–LIGAND DOCKING, PHARMACOPHORE FILTER, SHAPE/ELECTROSTATIC FILTER, VS HITS]

molecular sample will be enriched in compounds with the desired bioactivity. In other words, the probability that a randomly chosen molecule is an active one must be lower in the starting database than at the end of the VS.

In this chapter, we describe the main methods used during a VS, determine which open databases are useful during this process, and explain how to validate the accuracy of the bioactivity predictions made by the VS. All the resources mentioned in this chapter are listed in Table 9.1, which also contains information on how to access them.

9.2 Main Tools for Virtual Screening

VS have traditionally been classified as either Ligand-Based VS (LBVS) or Structure-Based VS (SBVS) depending on whether the 3D structure of the target is used (SBVS) or not used (LBVS) during the VS workflow [3]. However, ligand- and structure-based methods can also appear combined in the same VS pipeline [10–12]. Interestingly, if the experimental 3D structure of the target is unavailable but the structure from a homologous protein is known, then a homology model of the target can be built and SBVS methods can be used to find new active compounds in chemical databases [5, 13]. With the AlphaFold program, [14–16] it is currently possible to predict the structure of almost any protein (even if no experimental 3D structure of homologous proteins of the target of interest is known) with a high degree of accuracy. This means that almost all the technologies used in the VS (SBVS or LBVS) are applicable to any target (though the application of AlphaFold results in the field of drug discovery is still at a very early stage and rather uncertain [17–19]). The following sections describe the filters in Figure 9.1.

9.2.1 ADMET and PAINS Filtering

To be effective as a drug, a bioactive molecule must be able not only to reach its target in the organism at a sufficient concentration but also to remain there in bioactive form long enough for the expected biological events to occur [20]. ADME, the

Table 9.1 Resources mentioned in this chapter.

Main tools for virtual screening
ADMET and PAINS filtering
SwissADME (http://www.swissadme.ch/)
FAF-Drugs4 (https://fafdrugs4.rpbs.univ-paris-diderot.fr/)
Protein–ligand docking
Rigid protein–ligand docking
AutoDock Vina (https://vina.scripps.edu/)
Induced fit protein–ligand docking
SLIDE (https://github.com/psa-lab/SLIDE)
PELE Web server (https://pele.bsc.es/pele.wt)
Ensemble protein–ligand docking
DINC-COVID (http://dinc-covid.kavrakilab.org/)
Edock-ML (http://edock-ml.umsl.edu/)
Pharmacophore search
Structure-based pharmacophore
Pharmit (http://pharmit.csb.pitt.edu)
ZINCPharmer (http://zincpharmer.csb.pitt.edu/)
Ligand-based pharmacophore
PharmaGist (http://bioinfo3d.cs.tau.ac.il/PharmaGist/)
Shape/electrostatic similarity
ESP-Sim (https://github.com/hesther/espsim)
ElectroShape (https://ub.cbm.uam.es/chemogenomics/)
Protein-structure databases
PDB (https://www.rcsb.org/)
PDB-REDO Databank (https://pdb-redo.eu/)
SWISS-MODEL Repository (https://swissmodel.expasy.org/repository)
AlphaFold Protein Structure Database (https://alphafold.ebi.ac.uk/)
Validating binding site and ligand coordinates in three-dimensional protein complexes
VHELIBS (https://github.com/URVquimioinformatica-COS/VHELIBS)
Databases for searching new drugs
COCONUT (https://coconut.naturalproducts.net/)
GDBs (https://gdb.unibe.ch/downloads/)
ZINC20 (https://zinc20.docking.org/)
Databases of active molecules
The Binding Database (https://www.bindingdb.org/)
ChEMBL Database (https://www.ebi.ac.uk/chembl/)
PubChem (https://pubchem.ncbi.nlm.nih.gov/)

(continued)

Table 9.1 (Continued)

Databases of decoy molecules
DUD-E (http://dude.docking.org/)
DEKOIS (http://www.pharmchem.uni-tuebingen.de/dekois/)
VDS (http://compbio.cs.toronto.edu/VDS/)
Tools for building custom-based decoy sets
DUD-E tool (http://dude.docking.org/generate)
DecoyFinder (https://github.com/URVquimioinformatica-COS/DecoyFinder)
Format descriptions
SDF (https://depth-first.com/articles/2020/07/13/the-sdfile-format/)
SMILES (https://www.daylight.com/dayhtml/doc/theory/theory.smiles.html)
PDB file format (http://www.wwpdb.org/documentation/file-format-content/format33/v3.3.html)

acronym for absorption, distribution, metabolism, and excretion [21], describes how pharmacokinetic behavior is simplified into discrete parameters to be addressed in the drug discovery/preclinical phases. All four criteria influence the levels and kinetics of drug exposure to tissues and thus the performance and pharmacological activity of the compound as a drug. When, in addition to ADME properties, the potential or actual toxicity of the compound is taken into account, the acronym ADME-Tox, ADME/T, or ADMET is used instead [22]. PAINS, the acronym for Pan Assay Interference Compounds, on the other hand, refers to compounds that interfere with assay read-out or that can also react nonspecifically with numerous targets in such a way that they often generate false positives [23].

Filters to remove from the initial database those molecules that are predicted to be PAINS or that have unfavorable ADMET properties are not part of the VS workflow itself but part of the initial pretreatment phase of the molecules on which the screening of bioactive compounds will be performed (being a PAINS or having unfavorable ADMET properties is an intrinsic characteristic of the molecule itself and independent of the target against which the VS will be performed). Open access servers such as SwissADME [20, 24] and FAFDrugs4 [22, 25] can predict which input molecules (in SMILES format for SwissADME and SDF/SMILES format for FAFDrugs4 [26, 27]) may be PAINS or have bad ADMET properties.

9.2.2 Protein–Ligand Docking

Protein–ligand docking predicts the coordinates of the complex between a protein and a drug from their individual structures [28]. During this process, the protein structure is usually considered rigid (or small conformational changes are allowed in a very localized part of its structure), while the small molecule is considered able to change its initial conformation to adapt to the protein-binding site. However, since some targets show significant flexibility in their binding site, considering them as rigid during protein–ligand docking is a too strict approach. To overcome this limitation, several strategies have been developed, including induced fit docking [29–33] and ensemble docking [34, 35]. The most important difference between these two approaches is that, while induced docking attempts to directly simulate the coupled motion of the receptor and ligand, ensemble docking uses a set of different target structures (either experimental or from molecular dynamics simulations) to perform calculations. AutoDock Vina [36, 37] is often used for protein–ligand rigid docking whereas SLIDE [32] and Edock-ML [35] are examples of induced fit and ensemble protein–ligand docking, respectively.

9.2.3 Pharmacophore Search

A pharmacophore is a 3D abstract description of molecular features (i.e. pharmacophoric sites) that are necessary for molecular recognition and biological activity of a ligand by its target. A pharmacophore may also contain exclusion volumes that indicate the positions of the binding site that the ligand cannot fill because they are already occupied by the atoms of the target itself [3].

The simplest way to obtain a pharmacophore is from the three-dimensional (3D) structure of a complex between the target of interest and a drug that has the desired activity on this target (referred to as a structure-based pharmacophore).

When several drugs are known to be bioactive with respect to the same target but the 3D structure of the target is not known, a ligand-based pharmacophore can be obtained (assuming that all these ligands also share the target binding site and the binding mode). Here, it is assumed that the combination of conformers (one per ligand) with the maximum number of common pharmacophoric sites corresponds to the way all these ligands bind to the 3D structure of the target (the common sites are also assumed to represent the intermolecular interactions responsible for their recognition and bioactivity with respect to the target). If inactive compounds are also known, they can be used to add exclusion volumes to the ligand-based pharmacophore.

Once a pharmacophore has been obtained, it can be used to search for small molecules that occupy the maximum number of pharmacophore sites and at the same time do not occupy exclusion volumes. Molecules that fit the pharmacophore will be candidates for having the same bioactivity for the target as the molecule (or molecules) from which the pharmacophore was obtained.

PharmaGist [38, 39] is a free resource for constructing ligand-based pharmacophores, while Pharmit (see Figure 9.2) [41–43] and ZINCPharmer [44, 45] are free resources for building structure-based pharmacophores. Moreover, all three resources can be used to screen small molecule databases.

Pharmacophores can also be used to examine the poses resulting from a previous protein–ligand docking step. In this way, it is possible to assess whether the ligands, once oriented within the target binding site, are able to establish the intermolecular interactions needed to show high activity toward the drug target. In fact, this is another way to exploit the main strength of protein–ligand docking algorithms (i.e. their ability to find the bioactive pose) and obviate their main weakness

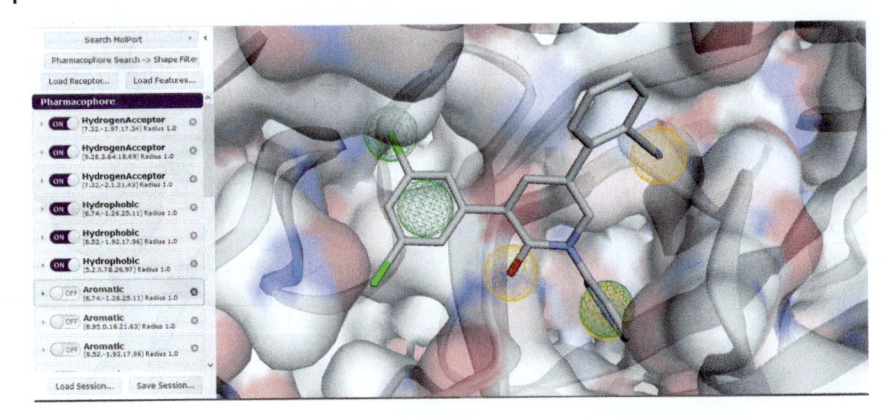

Figure 9.2 The Pharmit web interface for a pharmacophore search. A pharmacophore query for SARS-CoV-2 M-pro in complex with a perampanel derivative (PDB 7L10 [40]) is shown on the Pharmit web interface [41].

(i.e. their inability to correctly calculate the affinity of each pose for the target). To do this, one would only need to make sure that, for each ligand, the output of the docking program provides a sufficient number of poses to ensure that the correct one is among them (regardless of whether the scoring function places it at the top of the predicted affinity ranking for the target). This strategy has been successfully used to identify bioactive compounds for different targets [10, 11] and is similar to using constraints during protein–ligand docking (though, in our opinion, using pharmacophores allows greater flexibility in the VS strategy than using these constraints because, among other things, pharmacophore site types are more diverse than protein–ligand docking constraints).

9.2.4 Shape/Electrostatic Similarity

Two molecules that, upon binding to a given target, share a 3D shape and an electrostatic charge distribution on their surface (even though they have a different chemical structure) may have similar bioactivity for that target [46, 47]. It is therefore possible to compare the shape and electrostatic surface area of the poses that have passed through the previous filters (these would be the pharmacophore-compliant docking poses; see Figure 9.1) with the experimental poses of drugs that are cocrystallized with the target of interest. However, care must first be taken to superimpose the structure of all these complexes onto the structure of the target used to obtain the docking poses and the pharmacophore. Only in this way can it be guaranteed that the comparison is made between molecules with the same relative orientation in the target binding site. Moreover, if more than one complex between a highly active drug and the target of interest is available, each docking pose must be compared with each experimental pose, and the highest similarity must be chosen. Then, if more than one docking pose is available for the same ligand, only the one that shows the greatest similarity to one of the experimental poses to which it is compared will be kept (while the rest will be discarded) [6, 7, 11]. Finally, poses with a similarity

	H11 at 3BYZ	ZINC03851930
2D chemical structure		
Shape similarity (ET_shape= 0.560)		
Electrostatic surface similarity (ET_pb = 0.640)		

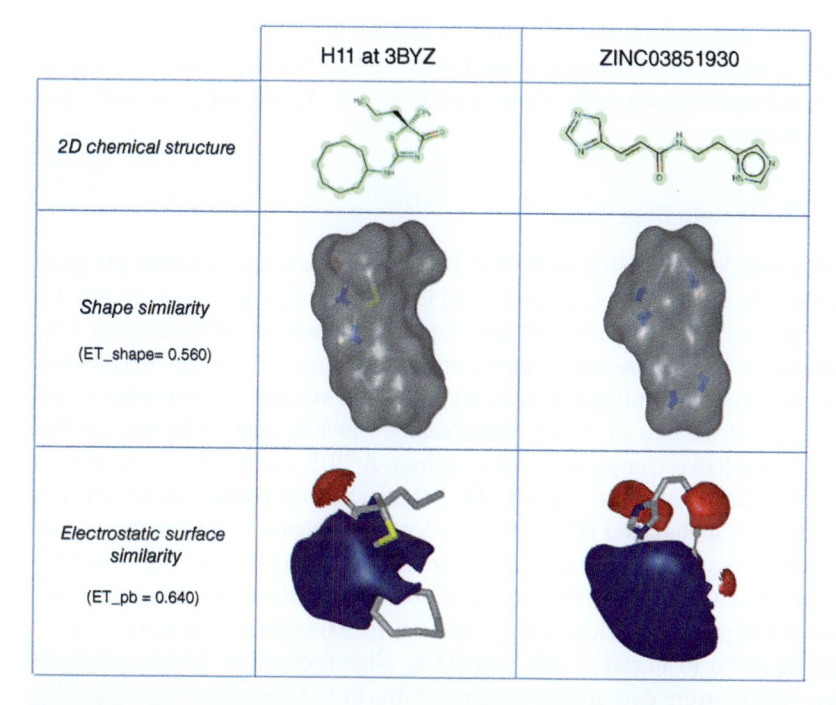

Figure 9.3 Shape and electrostatic similarity. Shape and electrostatic comparison between the experimental pose of the H11 ligand in the PDB entry 3BYZ [48] and the docked pose of the ZINC03851930 ligand in the 3BYZ binding site.

below a certain threshold will be discarded. This threshold must be selective enough to reduce, as much as possible, the number of false positives during VS validation (even if this means increasing the number of false negatives) [11].

Figure 9.3 shows the comparison between two poses, one of which is experimental (corresponding to the H11 ligand in the 3BYZ structure [48]), and the other corresponds to the docking pose of the ZINC03851930 ligand in the same structure. The shape similarity between the two poses is 0.560 (where 1.0 corresponds to a perfect overlap, i.e. the same shape), and the Poisson–Boltzmann electrostatic similarity is 0.640 (where 1.0 corresponds to an identical electrostatic potential overlap).

ESP-Sim [49] and ElectroShape [47] are examples of free resources for shape/electrostatic similarity searches.

9.2.5 Protein-Structure Databases

Many tools used during a VS require the 3D structure of the target to which the drug is to bind. These 3D structures may have been obtained experimentally (using techniques such as X-ray diffraction, nuclear magnetic resonance [NMR], or electron microscopy) or may result from predictions obtained directly from their sequence (using techniques such as homology modeling or protein threading). Several public databases exist from which these 3D structures can be obtained. The most important ones are the Protein Data Bank (PDB) [50] and the PDB-REDO Databank [51] for experimentally obtained structures and the SWISS-MODEL Repository [52] and the AlphaFold Protein Structure Database (AlphaFold DB) [15] for computationally predicted structures.

9.2.6 The Protein Data Bank

The PDB, which was created in 1971 at Brookhaven National Laboratory (Upton, NY), originally contained seven structures [53]. Its purpose was to act as an international repository in which to deposit the coordinates of proteins determined by X-ray diffraction and make these data available on request. Since then, it has also included protein structures determined by other techniques (NMR and electron microscopy) and the 3D structures of other biomolecules (nucleic acids, oligosaccharides, and their respective complexes with proteins). A PDB entry, which contains all the information relating to a particular 3D structure deposited in the PDB, is designated by a 4-character alphanumeric identifier called a PDB identifier or PDB ID, which always begins with a number from 1 to 9 (e.g. 6LU7). There are currently over 193,000 entries in the PDB, of which 168,000 correspond to proteins, 10,600 correspond to protein–nucleic acid complexes, 10,200 to protein–oligosaccharides complexes, 3900 to nucleic acids, and 22 to oligosaccharides. Of these 193,000 entries, 167,000 were determined by X-ray diffraction, 13,700 were determined by NMR, and 12,000 were determined by electron microscopy [54]. The coordinates of the PDB structures are contained in text-only files (one file for each PDB entry) in a PDB-specific format [55] that is soon to be replaced by the mmCIF format [56]. All PDB files can be downloaded without restriction from the PDB or PDBe websites [57, 58].

9.2.7 The PDB-REDO Databank

The PDB-REDO databank [59] contains optimized versions of existing PDB entries that simultaneously satisfy two criteria: (i) the entry has been obtained by X-ray diffraction; and (ii) the author deposited the corresponding structure factor files along with the coordinates. All PDB entries that satisfy both criteria are treated with a consistent protocol that reduces effects due to differences in age, software, and depositor, thus making PDB-REDO a great dataset for large-scale structure analysis studies [51, 60]. For example, an evaluation of the goodness of fit of the coordinates of 39,820 protein/ligand complexes to the electron density map using the VHELIBS program showed that both binding-site and ligand coordinates were much more reliable if they were obtained from PDB-REDO than if they were obtained from PDB [61]. Specifically, while VHELIBS rated 14,304 binding sites and 25,350 ligands obtained from PDB-REDO as "Good" (the other categories were "Dubious" and "Bad"), these values decreased by 50% when the data were obtained from PDB [62] and EDS [63] (7671 and 12,419, respectively). It is therefore recommended that, whenever possible, priority should be given to working with structures obtained from PDB-REDO rather than those obtained directly from PDB.

9.2.8 The SWISS-MODEL Repository

The purpose of the SWISS-MODEL Repository is to provide access to an up-to-date collection of annotated 3D protein models generated for all UniProtKB sequences [64] for which no experimental structures are available [52]. Since the structures in this repository were obtained by homology modeling (and these types of models can only be obtained by the automated SWISS-MODEL pipeline for those proteins that have a minimum of 30% sequence identity with at least one protein of known 3D structure that acts as a template during model construction), this repository contains only structural models for a fraction of the UniProtKB proteins. Interestingly, in cases where templates corresponding to the same sequence segment exhibit significant conformational differences, several models are generated to reflect structural diversity.

To inform users about the expected local accuracy, the quality of the various models is evaluated and annotated using the QMEAN tool (only high-quality models – i.e. those with an overall QMEANDisCo score above 0.5 – are imported into the SWISS-MODEL repository) [65]. If the homology-modeled structure for a sequence is unavailable, the user can build it interactively through the SWISS-MODEL workspace [66, 67]. Currently, the repository contains 2,258,794 homology models that can be freely downloaded [68].

9.2.9 The AlphaFold Protein Structure Database

AlphaFold DB was released in July 2021 [15, 69]. This database contains the 3D structures predicted by the AlphaFold program (CASP14 winner) for proteins of experimentally unknown 3D structure [16]. Since, unlike the SWISS-Model, AlphaFold does not need homologous protein structures to make its predictions [14], AlphaFold DB contains structural models of proteins that are not in the SWISS-Model Repository. The first release of this database covered the human proteome and the proteomes of 20 other key organisms (e.g. *Arabidopsis thaliana*, *Escherichia coli*, and *Oryza sativa*), while the second release added the majority of manually curated UniProt entries (e.g. Swiss-Prot) [70]. AlphaFold DB currently contains over 200 million entries that include the human proteome and the proteomes of 47 other key organisms that are important in research and global health [69].

Regarding the quality of the predicted 3D structures, AlphaFold produces a per-residue estimate of their confidence on a scale from 0 to 100. This confidence estimate, called pLDDT, corresponds to the score predicted by the model on the lDDT-Cα metric. This value is stored in the B-factor fields of the AlphaFold database files in PDB format, but, unlike the B-factor, the higher the value of pLDDT, the better the quality of the prediction. Regions with pLDDT > 90 are thus expected to be modeled with high accuracy, while those with pLDDT between 70 and 90 are expected to be modeled well, and those with pLDDT between 50 and 70 are of low confidence and should be treated with caution.

In theory, it would be advisable to use only AlphaFold DB structures during drug discovery or development if their binding sites have a pLDDT value between

90 and 100. In general, however, the current version of AlphaFold is considered not yet sufficiently accurate for its models to be used in drug discovery or design [17–19]. It has been argued, for example, that the current AlphaFold implementation cannot predict all the relevant conformations of a target because its main assumption is that, based on the sequence alone, a unique 3D structure of a protein can be described (whereas proteins can exist in multiple conformations that are all relevant for their functional role) [17]. This inability to control the output conformation of the predicted 3D structure (which, for instance, can be controlled if the predicted 3D structure is obtained via homology modeling by selecting the appropriate template structure) is therefore an important limitation when using these predicted protein structures for drug discovery and design.

All data provided by AlphaFold DB are freely available for academic and commercial use under Creative Commons Attribution 4.0 license terms.

9.3 Validating Binding Site and Ligand Coordinates in Three-Dimensional Protein Complexes

One could assume that all PDB files corresponding to experimentally known structures are of high quality. However, we should not forget that these models are derived from the interpretation of experimental data and that the accuracy of atom coordinates is not homogeneous between different PDB entries or even within the same PDB entry [71]. Before using a PDB file for drug discovery and design, therefore, the accuracy of the drug binding site coordinates should be validated because, for example, they are crucial for the proper behavior of protein–ligand docking programs. With proteins obtained by X-ray diffraction (the method of choice for studying the structure of macromolecules complexed with small molecular ligands [18]), this can be done simply by using the Validation HElper for LIgands and Binding Sites (VHELIBS) program [61, 72]. VHELIBS is a software that facilitates the validation of binding site and ligand coordinates for users of protein structures with little or no knowledge of crystallography. Using a graphical user interface for PDB entries (see Figure 9.4), VHELIBS checks how well the ligand and binding-site coordinates match the electron density map. The user can thus specify threshold values for numerous properties related to the fit of the coordinates to the electron density (*Real Space R, Real Space Correlation Coefficient,* and *average occupancy* are used by default), and the program will automatically classify residues and ligands as "Good," "Dubious," or "Bad" based on the specified limits. The default values used for the parameters have been carefully chosen (and are valid for most situations) but advanced users can easily adjust them if necessary. VHELIBS takes as input a user-supplied list of PDB or UniProtKB codes (which are mapped to their corresponding PDB codes) that can be entered directly from the GUI or provided in a text file. Finally, once the automatic classification is finished, the user can also visually check the quality of the fit of the residues and ligands to the electron density map and reclassify them if necessary (see Figure 9.4).

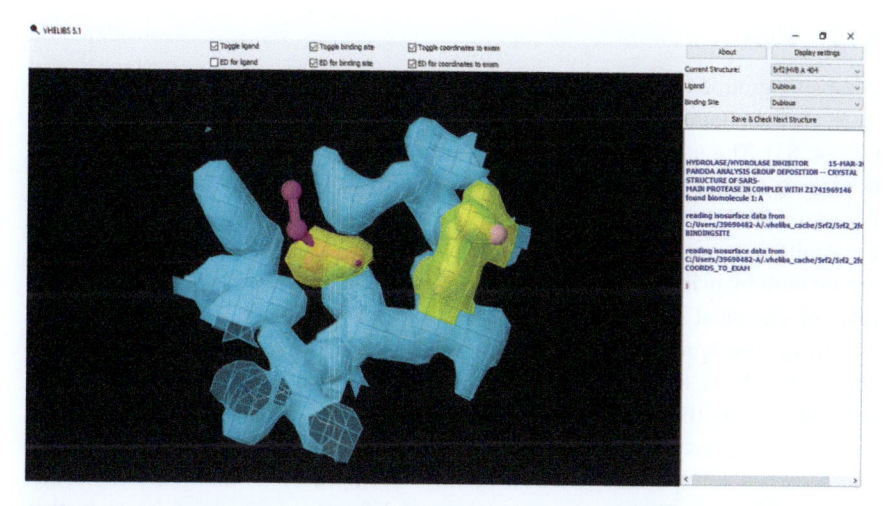

Figure 9.4 VHELIBS results display screen. Display screen of the VHELIBS results in which the coordinates of the HVB ligand and its binding site to the 5RF2 structure [73] are compared with its corresponding electron density map. The yellow electron density corresponds to the dubious part of the structure whose reliability must be visually verified.

9.4 Databases for Searching New Drugs

Three main types of databases can be used to screen for new drugs using VS: (i) those containing molecules that are either physically available in a commercial catalog or can be isolated from a natural source; (ii) those containing "virtual" molecules; and (iii) those containing molecules that are either physically available or available on-demand. An example of the first group is the COlleCtion of Open Natural ProdUcTs (COCONUT) [74] while GDB-11 [75] is an example of the second, and ZINC20 [76] is an example of the third.

9.4.1 COCONUT

COCONUT is a good example of a database containing molecules that can be isolated from natural sources [74]. COCONUT is a generalistic natural products database that gathers data from over 50 open natural product resources (e.g. AfroDB [77], Marine Natural Products [78], NPAtlas [79], Super Natural II [80], TCMDB@Taiwan [81], and UNPD [82]). As well as the molecular structure, each entry in the database is associated, if available, with its known stereochemical forms, literature, organisms that produce them, and natural geographical occurrence. The latest version of COCONUT (January 2022) contains 407,270 different molecules that can be downloaded free of charge, without restriction, and in several formats that are ready for use in VS pipelines [83].

9.4.2 GDBs

Databases grouped under the acronym Generated DataBases (GDBs) aim to populate all the chemical space that molecules known so far have not yet occupied [75, 84, 85]. The authors have therefore assembled various databases while establishing an upper limit on the number of nonhydrogen atoms they can contain. For example, the GDB-11 database contains the 26.4 million molecules (including 110.9 million stereoisomers, three- and four-membered rings and triple bonds) that can be built by using a maximum of 11 C, N, O, and F atoms and following simple rules of chemical stability and synthetic feasibility [75]. The GBD-13 database, which was constructed in a similar manner to GBD-11 but uses a maximum of 13 atoms of C, N, O, S, and Cl, contains 977,468,314 small drug-like molecules [84]. GBD-17, on the other hand, was constructed using a maximum of 17 atoms of C, N, O, S, and halogens and contains 166.4 billion molecules [85]. Unlike known drugs and bioactive compounds, GDBs contain a plethora of nonaromatic molecules with a 3D shape. These are extremely useful for drug discovery because they generally have more desirable ADMET properties than the mostly aromatic and planar structures of known drug molecules [86]. Using GDB-17 as raw material, the same research group also obtained GDBMedChem [87]. This is a collection of 10 million small molecules from GDB-17 that were selected by applying rules inspired by medicinal chemistry to exclude problematic functional groups and complex molecules and further sampling the resulting subset uniformly in terms of molecular size, stereochemistry, and polarity. GDBMedChem molecules, which are more diverse and very different from known molecules in terms of substructures, represent an excellent source of diversity for drug discovery. The GDB and GDBMedChem databases can be downloaded free of charge in several formats suitable for use in a VS (however, GDBs should not be used as part of or in patents, and large sections of them should not be redistributed without the express written permission from the authors) [88].

9.4.3 ZINC20

ZINC20 is a free database containing over 230 million purchasable compounds (as well as nonpurchasable ones) in ready-to-dock, 3D formats sourced from 310 catalogs from 150 companies/institutions [76]. The database is organized in such a way the molecules from some or all of these catalogs (and also for specific subsets of them [89]) can be downloaded for local use. For example, anyone interested in doing a VS of natural molecules can select the biogenic subset that contains all the molecules of natural origin dispersed in these 310 catalogs [90]. The current number of molecules available for download in the biogenic subset is 135,335, of which 61,592 are commercially available [89].

9.5 Databases of Bioactive Molecules

Collections of bioactive small molecules that exhibit the desired activity against a target are important for discovering new bioactive molecules that share the same activity against the same target. For example, the characteristics of these already-known bioactive small molecules can be used to guide the search at some stages of a VS. However, another important application of these collections of bioactive molecules is that they facilitate validation (from a theoretical point of view) of the extent to which the designed VS strategy is able to identify them when they are mixed with other molecules that do not show bioactivity for their target. Fortunately, several open access databases, such as BindingDB [91, 92], PubChem [93, 94], and ChEMBL [95, 96], contain these collections.

9.5.1 The BindingDB Database

BindingDB, which has been operating since 2001, is a public, online database of binding affinities focused primarily on the interactions of proteins considered to be drug targets with drug-like small molecules [91, 92]. It includes data extracted from the literature and selected confirmatory bioassays from PubChem and ChEMBL entries for which a well-defined protein target is provided. BindingDB contains 2.5 million binding data for 1.1 million compounds and 8821 protein targets [91]. To search for compounds that show activity against a certain target, several search methods are available. First, the sequence or name of the target can be used. Much more complex requests can also be performed via the advanced search, which not only includes the identity of the target (via its accession code in UniprotKB) but also filters the results using, for example, bioactivity ranges or the article or patent where the bioactivities have been published. Small molecules that satisfy the search criteria can easily be compiled in 2D or 3D SDF format [27] for download and local use. In addition, BindingDB has a Chrome/Firefox extension (*i.e.* BDBFind) that, once installed, enables users to know automatically when BindingDB has the data for an article, PubMed entry, or US patent they are searching for online. Moreover, BDBFind provides direct links to enable users to view or download these data. Data curated by BindingDB are made available under a Creative Commons Attribution License [97] as long as BindingDB is cited [98].

9.5.2 PubChem

PubChem is a chemical database of the National Institute of Health (NIH). Launched in 2004, it contains mainly small molecules (as well as larger molecules such as nucleotides, carbohydrates, lipids, peptides, and chemically modified macromolecules). For all these molecules, PubChem collects information on their chemical structure, chemical and physical properties, biological activities, patents, health, safety, toxicity data, etc. [93, 94]. PubChem contains 293 million bioactivities for 110 million compounds and 184,481 protein targets. To search for compounds that show activity against a given protein target, PubChem has a simple search tool on its home page from which, based on the target's UniProtKB access code, users can access different pages with full information about it (this information can also be accessed from https://pubchem.ncbi.nlm.nih.gov/protein/

XXX, where XXX should be replaced by the above-mentioned UniProtKB access code). Specifically, information about all compounds whose activity has been measured with respect to the target of interest can be found in the "Chemicals and bioactivities" section of these pages. This information can be exported in different file formats for local use. The simple CSV format shows the PubChem code (*i.e.* CID) but not the structure of the various compounds (e.g. in SMILES format [26]) to which each experimental bioactivity corresponds. XML and JSON formats include more identification types like IUPAC and common chemical names. An external tool such as ChemmineR [99] can then be used to obtain the structures from the corresponding CIDs or chemical names. As well as for recruiting compounds with bioactivity against a specific target, PubChem can be used for other chemoinformatics-related tasks such as developing bioactivity and toxicity prediction models, discovering polypharmacological (multi-target) ligands, or identifying new targets (for drug repurposing or predicting off-target side effects) [100]. PubChem is an open access database from which most data can be downloaded free of charge, though exceptions may exist when the licensing agreements of the original sources of the information collected prevent the bulk downloading of certain datasets.

9.5.3 ChEMBL

ChEMBL is a manually curated database of bioactive molecules with drug-like properties. It is obtained, for example, from the primary scientific literature and public screening campaigns and is hosted at the European Bioinformatics Institute (EBI). For each molecule in the database, ChEMBL contains data such as: (i) its two-dimensional (2D) structure; (ii) calculated properties (e.g. logP, molecular weight, Lipinski parameters, etc.); and (iii) various measures of its bioactivity (e.g. binding constants, pharmacology data, and ADMET) [95, 96]. The ChEMBL v31 contains 19.7 million bioactivities for 2.3 million compounds and 15,072 targets. The best way to search for compounds that show activity against a given protein target is to use the target's UniProtID with the *Simple Search* tool and identify the ChEMBL ID for that target (e.g. CHEMBL2842 for human mTOR). The *Target Report Card* will then show which drug-like molecules have measured experimental bioactivity data for it. The bioactivity information on that report card contains data for: (i) drugs and clinical candidates; (ii) activity charts (how available activity data are distributed among the various ways of measuring it; e.g. IC_{50}, K_i, or K_d); (iii) the distribution of associated bioassays (i.e. binding, functional or ADME); (iv) the ligand efficiency distribution (*i.e.* a plot of the binding efficiency index relative to the surface efficiency index); and (v) drug-like molecules with experimental bioactivity for that target and distributed according to their molecular weight (where the 2D SDF file of each set of molecules can be easily downloaded). Interestingly, molecules with quantitative bioactivity in a specific range can also be downloaded in several formats for each molecular weight range. ChEMBL data are made available under a Creative Commons Attribution-Share Alike 3.0 Unported License [101].

9.6 Databases of Inactive/Decoy Molecules

When theoretically validating a VS, as well as having molecules with the desired bioactivity, it is essential to have molecules that are known (or presumed) not to be active with respect to the target of interest. This will make it possible to evaluate whether the VS is capable of distinguishing active compounds from inactive ones when they are mixed (a situation that is similar to what occurs when we apply the VS to a database of chemical compounds to search for new active molecules).

9.6.1 Collecting Experimentally Inactive Compounds from PubChem

Some bioactivity compound databases (especially PubChem) are a good place to find compounds with no activity for a specific target. In many cases, these inactive compounds come from HTS assays. One way to obtain these inactive compounds from PubChem is to use the PubChem BioAssay Advanced Search Builder and search for the UniProtKB code of the target (UniProt Accession field) with the word "Inactive" in all fields [102]. For example, the search for human mTOR inhibitors (accession number P42345 in UniProtKB) yields 15 results. The first is entitled "InCell qHTS Assay for Inhibitors of the mTORC1 Signaling Pathway in WT MEF Cells: Hit Validation." Accessing the main page of this assay shows that of the 796 compounds tested for mTOR inhibitor activity, 516 are inactive [103]. Finally, after viewing the data table of the 796 compounds, the section of the data table corresponding to the inactive compounds can be exported for local use (and the structures of those compounds can be obtained from their CID by using tools such as ChemmineR [99] or by translating common/IUPAC names into structures).

9.6.2 Collecting Presumed Inactive Compounds from Decoy Databases

If it is impossible to obtain compounds that have been experimentally shown to be inactive against a given target (or few are available with these characteristics), decoys can be used. Decoys are molecules that are assumed to be inactive against a target (i.e. they are unlikely to bind to the target) [104]. In addition, the physical properties of the decoys must be sufficiently similar to those of the active compounds so that enrichment during VS validation is not simply a matter of separation by trivial physical characteristics leading to artificial enrichment [105, 106]. Some databases contain sets of decoys for certain selected targets. The most widely used decoy database is DUD-E [107, 108] (though others such as DEKOIS [109, 110] and VDS [111, 112] are also used for benchmarking/validation studies).

The Directory of Useful Decoys Enhanced (DUD-E) contains sets of actives and decoys for 102 protein targets [107, 108]. For each active molecule, DUD-E provides 50 decoys that, relative to it, have (i) similar physical properties (*i.e.* molecular weight, calculated logP, number of rotatable bonds, net molecular charge, and hydrogen bond donors and acceptors); and (ii) a different topology (i.e. 2D fingerprints were used to minimize the topological similarity between the decoys and its corresponding active). DUD-E also tries to: (i) avoid potential false decoys (i.e. hidden actives) by using a stringent topological dissimilarity filter; and (ii) include, when possible, experimentally inactive molecules in the corresponding DUD-E decoy-target sets.

9.6.3 Building Custom-Based Decoy Sets

If there are no inactive compounds for the target of interest or there are no decoys for that target of interest in any of the databases mentioned above [105, 107, 109], programs exist that enable users to obtain them from a set of known actives of the target [104, 113]. The tool that enables decoys to be generated using the selection criteria employed by DUD-E, which is available on DUD-E's own website, obtains the decoys from the purchasable subset of the ZINC database [113].

DecoyFinder is a graphical tool that helps users to find sets of decoy molecules for a given group of active ligands [104]. To do so, it uses one of two methods: (i) the fast method (the default method used by the current version of the program), which finds decoys with similar molecular weights to those of the corresponding target active set; or (ii) the slow method, which searches for decoy molecules that physically resemble the active set of the target (i.e. have a similar number of rotational bonds, hydrogen bond acceptors and donors, logP value, and molecular weight) but are chemically different from the active one (defined by a Tanimoto coefficient threshold between the MACCS fingerprints of the active ligand and the decoy molecule). Optionally, with the latter method a Tanimoto coefficient threshold can be set between decoys to ensure chemical diversity in the decoy set.

9.7 Main Metrics for Evaluating the Success of a Virtual Screening

Clearly, the best way to evaluate the success of a VS is to evaluate biological activity in vitro, in cellulo, or in vivo [3]. However, this is not always possible. A computational validation, which can be performed during the development of the VS process to set up various parameters, is always useful. This essentially involves applying the VS process to a set of molecules (active molecules) with the activity we are looking for and that are mixed with inactive molecules (or decoys) for the same target. The VS is then expected to selectively predict the active molecules.

Several metrics can be used to quantify the success of the validation of a VS. These can be applied to the entire VS process or to individual steps of the VS. The enrichment factor (EF) measures the fraction of active molecules that survive the VS (i.e. the ratio between the proportion of actives at the end of the VS process and their proportion in the starting database that is being screened) or one of its steps [114]. An EF > 1 indicates that we are enriching the set of compounds selected by VS (or the VS step) with active molecules while inactive molecules or decoys are being discarded. An EF of 1 indicates that the VS (or the VS step) is not enriching the dataset in active molecules. When the output of a VS step consists of a score (such as a docking score) that can be sorted, the ratio of active molecules found in a specific percentage of the validation dataset can be used. This is useful because in a VS, a key objective is to find active molecules as highly ranked as possible. For example, "EF at 1%" represents the EF within the top 1% of the molecules ranked by decreasing values of predicted affinity for the target or molecular similarity to the reference active compounds, for instance, depending on the chosen approach.

ROC curves can be used in sorted datasets to evaluate the performance of a VS or one of its steps. ROC curves represent true positive rates (active molecules) vs. false positive rates (inactive molecules or decoys predicted as active molecules), while the area under the ROC curve (AUC), which measures the ability of a classifier to distinguish between classes, is used as a summary of the ROC curve. AUC values, which range from 0 to 1, represent the probability that a random active molecule is ranked higher than a random inactive molecule or decoy. An AUC value of 1 is obtained if all active molecules are ranked higher than inactive ones (for example, when the docking scores of all active molecules are more negative than any inactive molecule or decoy). An AUC value of 0.5 means that the VS approach is not better at identifying active molecules than random selection. However, identical AUC values for two different VS steps do not mean that they have the same performance (see Figure 9.5). One VS step may find an inactive molecule in the initial part of the ranking, while the other may find some active molecules in the lower part. To prioritize performances in which active molecules are found first, the Boltzmann-Enhanced Discrimination of ROC (BEDROC) [115] metric can be used. BEDROC assigns more weight to early-ranked molecules. However, datasets with different ratios of active/inactive molecules cannot be compared directly with this metric.

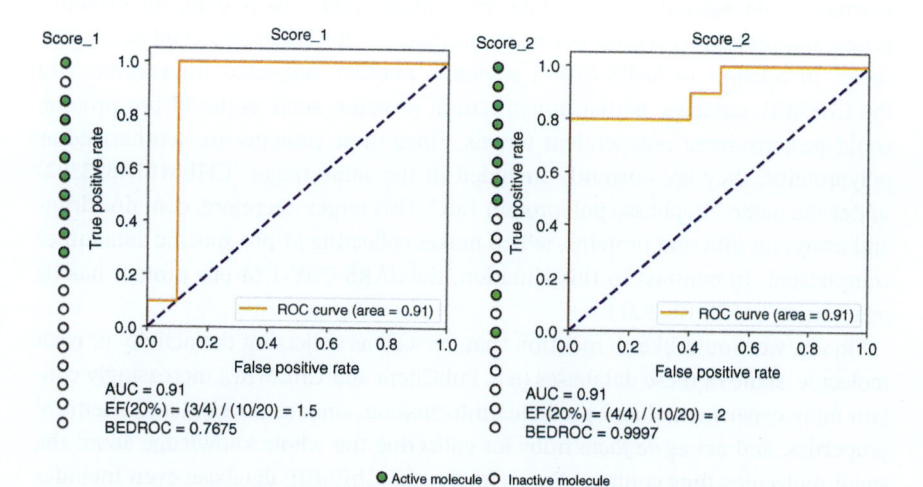

Figure 9.5 Scores are sorted in descending order for two steps of a VS (*Score_1* and *Score_2*). The data set consists of 10 active and 10 inactive molecules. The AUC for both steps of the VS is 0.91, but the values of EF (20%) and BEDROC differ.

9.8 Concluding Remarks

Open databases containing the bioactivity data of small molecules have become an essential part of any VS project because, as well as guiding the construction of the VS workflow itself (e.g. establishing pharmacophores based on how they interact – or are supposed to interact – with the target), they can also be used to validate it. However, the enormous amount of bioactivity data in these databases also has its downside: different assays and experimental conditions may provide different values of measured activities for a given compound, and this must be taken into account when using these data. Bioassay results in these databases also provide information on molecules that are not very potent or are even inactive. Inactive molecules do not usually appear in publications, but, as mentioned above, they are important for validating a VS process. In addition, including inactive data in machine learning methods produces models with higher predictive capacity for bioactivity [116]. Interestingly, programmatic access to these databases through an API allows easy remote access to all these bioactivity data as well as the development of data processing workflows [117–119].

One clear area for improvement in these bioactivity databases is the time it takes from when an article describing the activity of a compound is published until its data appear in one of these databases. Our recent experience in collecting SARS-CoV-2 M-pro inhibitors from the literature [120, 121] has shown us that sometimes it is not easy to know which compound an article refers to. Sometimes only a 2D representation, an abbreviation, or a number is available. Ideally, each compound should be accompanied by a notation describing its structure, such as SMILES, which also includes its stereochemistry. Also, authors could submit compounds and their bioactivities directly to the appropriate open databases, or journals could require all such data to be made public, as is done for proteins, genes, and protein structures before the authors submit the manuscript describing them. In relation to SARS-CoV-2 research, another suggested improvement of the ChEMBL database is that nonstructural proteins, such as the M-pro protein, could be considered independent targets. Since these proteins are synthesized as polyproteins, they are currently included in the same target (CHEMBL4523582) under the name "Replicase polyprotein 1ab." This target, therefore, contains drugs and assays for different proteins, which makes collecting M-pro-specific data rather complicated. In contrast to this situation, the SARS-CoV-1 M-pro protein has its own target (CHEMBL3927).

Finally, we would like to mention that, as well as collecting the activity of each molecule, some of these databases (e.g. PubChem and ChEMBL) increasingly contain more experimental and predicted information, such as physical and chemical properties, and act as *de facto* hubs for collecting the whole knowledge about the small molecules they contain. For example, the ChEMBL database even includes a target prediction, at three different confidence levels, and shows the ChEMBL targets that are predicted to interact with each compound in the database [122]. Including a section in these databases dedicated to the targets and integrating information from bioassay databases makes it easy to compile all the information available for a given target.

References

1. Giri, A.K. and Ianevski, A. (2022). High-throughput screening for drug discovery targeting the cancer cell-microenvironment interactions in hematological cancers. *Expert Opinion on Drug Discovery* 17: 181–190. https://doi.org/10.1080/17460441.2022.1991306.
2. Xu, T., Zheng, W., and Huang, R. (2021). High-throughput screening assays for SARS-CoV-2 drug development: Current status and future directions. *Drug Discovery Today* 26: 2439–2444. https://doi.org/10.1016/J.DRUDIS.2021.05.012.
3. Gimeno, A.; Ojeda-Montes, M.J.; Tomás-Hernández, S.; Cereto-Massagué, A.; Beltrán-Debón, R.; Mulero, M.; Pujadas, G.; Garcia-Vallvé, S. The light and dark sides of virtual screening: what is there to know? *International Journal of Molecular Sciences* 2019, 20, 1375. https://doi.org/10.3390/ijms20061375.
4. da Silva Rocha, S.F.L., Olanda, C.G., Fokoue, H.H., and Sant'Anna, C.M.R. (2019). Virtual screening techniques in drug discovery: review and recent applications. *Current Topics in Medicinal Chemistry* 19: 1751–1767. https://doi.org/10.2174/1568026619666190816101948.
5. Sala, E., Guasch, L., Iwaszkiewicz, J. et al. (2011). Identification of human IKK-2 inhibitors of natural origin (Part I): modeling of the IKK-2 kinase domain, virtual screening and activity assays. *PLoS One* 6: e16903. https://doi.org/10.1371/journal.pone.0016903.
6. Guasch, L., Ojeda, M.J., González-Abuín, N. et al. (2012). Identification of novel human dipeptidyl peptidase-IV inhibitors of natural origin (part I): virtual screening and activity assays. *PLoS One* 7: e44971. https://doi.org/10.1371/journal.pone.0044971.
7. Guasch, L., Sala, E., Castell-Auví, A. et al. (2012). Identification of PPARgamma partial agonists of natural origin (I): development of a virtual screening Procedure and in vitro validation. *PLoS One* 7: e50816. https://doi.org/10.1371/journal.pone.0050816.
8. Gimeno, A., Mestres-Truyol, J., Ojeda-Montes, M.J. et al. (2020). Prediction of novel inhibitors of the main protease (M-pro) of SARS-CoV-2 through consensus docking and drug reposition. *International Journal of Molecular Sciences* 21: 1–30. https://doi.org/10.3390/ijms21113793.
9. Ibrahim, I.M., Elfiky, A.A., Fathy, M.M. et al. (2022). Targeting SARS-CoV-2 endoribonuclease: a structure-based virtual screening supported by in vitro analysis. *Scientific Reports* 12: 13337. https://doi.org/10.1038/S41598-022-17573-6.
10. Ojeda-Montes, M.J., Casanova-Martí, À., Gimeno, A. et al. (2019). Mining large databases to find new leads with low similarity to known actives: application to find new DPP-IV inhibitors. *Future Medicinal Chemistry* 11: 1387–1401. https://doi.org/10.4155/fmc-2018-0597.

11 Gimeno, A., Cuffaro, D., Nuti, E. et al. (2021). Identification of broad-spectrum MMP inhibitors by virtual screening. *Molecules* 26: https://doi.org/10.3390/molecules26154553.

12 Gimeno, A., Ardid-Ruiz, A., Ojeda-Montes, M.J. et al. (2018). Combined ligand- and receptor-based virtual screening methodology to identify structurally diverse protein tyrosine phosphatase 1B inhibitors. *ChemMedChem* 13: 1939–1948. https://doi.org/10.1002/cmdc.201800267.

13 Sala, E., Guasch, L., Iwaszkiewicz, J. et al. (2011). Identification of human IKK-2 inhibitors of natural origin (part II): in Silico prediction of IKK-2 inhibitors in natural extracts with known anti-inflammatory activity. *European Journal of Medicinal Chemistry* 46: 6098–6103. https://doi.org/10.1016/j.ejmech.2011.09.022.

14 Jumper, J. and Hassabis, D. (2022). Protein structure predictions to atomic accuracy with AlphaFold. *Nature Methods* 19: 11–12. https://doi.org/10.1038/s41592-021-01362-6.

15 Varadi, M., Anyango, S., Deshpande, M. et al. (2022). AlphaFold protein structure database: massively expanding the structural coverage of protein-sequence space with high-accuracy models. *Nucleic Acids Research* 50: D439–D444. https://doi.org/10.1093/nar/gkab1061.

16 Jumper, J., Evans, R., Pritzel, A. et al. (2021). Highly accurate protein structure prediction with AlphaFold. *Nature* 596: 583–589. https://doi.org/10.1038/s41586-021-03819-2.

17 Schauperl, M. and Denny, R.A. (2022). AI-based protein structure prediction in drug discovery: impacts and challenges. *Journal of Chemical Information and Modeling* 62: 3142–3156. https://doi.org/10.1021/ACS.JCIM.2C00026.

18 Perrakis, A. and Sixma, T.K. (2021). AI revolutions in biology: the joys and perils of AlphaFold. *EMBO Reports* 22: e54046. https://doi.org/10.15252/embr.202154046.

19 He, X., You, C., Jiang, H. et al. (2022). AlphaFold2 versus experimental structures: evaluation on G protein-coupled receptors. *Acta Pharmacologica Sinica* 44: 1–7. https://doi.org/10.1038/S41401-022-00938-Y.

20 Daina, A., Michielin, O., and Zoete, V. (2017). SwissADME: a free web tool to evaluate pharmacokinetics, drug-likeness and medicinal chemistry friendliness of small molecules. *Scientific Reports* 7: 42717. https://doi.org/10.1038/srep42717.

21 Doogue, M.P. and Polasek, T.M. (2013). The ABCD of clinical pharmacokinetics. *Therapeutic Advances in Drug Safety* 4: 5–7. https://doi.org/10.1177/2042098612469335.

22 Lagorce, D., Bouslama, L., Becot, J. et al. (2017). FAF-Drugs4: free ADME-tox filtering computations for chemical biology and early stages drug discovery. *Bioinformatics* 33: 3658–3660. https://doi.org/10.1093/bioinformatics/btx491.

23 Baell, J.B. and Nissink, J.W.M. (2018). Seven year itch: pan-assay interference compounds (PAINS) in 2017-utility and limitations. *ACS Chemical Biology* 13: 36–44. https://doi.org/10.1021/ACSCHEMBIO.7B00903.

24 SwissADME. Available online: http://www.swissadme.ch/ (accessed on Aug 19, 2022).

25 FAFDrugs4 Home. Available online: https://fafdrugs4.rpbs.univ-paris-diderot.fr/ (accessed 19 August 2022).

26 Daylight Theory: SMILES. Available online: https://www.daylight.com/dayhtml/doc/theory/theory.smiles.html (accessed 19 August 2022).

27 The SDfile Format. Available online: https://depth-first.com/articles/2020/07/13/the-sdfile-format/ (accessed 19 August 2022).

28 Pujadas, G., Vaque, M., Ardevol, A. et al. (2008). Protein-ligand docking: a review of recent advances and future perspectives. *Current Pharmaceutical Analysis* 4: 1–19. https://doi.org/10.2174/157341208783497597.

29 Miller, E.B., Murphy, R.B., Sindhikara, D. et al. (2021). Reliable and accurate solution to the induced fit docking problem for protein-ligand binding. *Journal of Chemical Theory and Computation* 17: 2630–2639. https://doi.org/10.1021/acs.jctc.1c00136.

30 Paul, D.S. and Gautham, N. (2017). iMOLSDOCK: induced-fit docking using mutually orthogonal Latin squares (MOLS). *Journal of Molecular Graphics & Modelling* 74: 89–99. https://doi.org/10.1016/j.jmgm.2017.03.008.

31 Bolia, A. and Ozkan, S.B. (2016). Adaptive BP-dock: an induced fit docking approach for full receptor flexibility. *Journal of Chemical Information and Modeling* 56: 734–746. https://doi.org/10.1021/acs.jcim.5b00587.

32 Zavodszky, M.I., Lei, M., Thorpe, M.F. et al. (2004). Modeling correlated main-chain motions in proteins for flexible molecular recognition. *Proteins* 57: 243–261. https://doi.org/10.1002/prot.20179.

33 Madadkar-Sobhani, A. and Guallar, V. (2013). PELE web server: atomistic study of biomolecular systems at your fingertips. *Nucleic Acids Research* 41: W322–W328. https://doi.org/10.1093/nar/gkt454.

34 Hall-Swan, S., Devaurs, D., Rigo, M.M. et al. (2021). DINC-COVID: a webserver for ensemble docking with flexible SARS-CoV-2 proteins. *Computers in Biology and Medicine* 139: 104943. https://doi.org/10.1016/j.compbiomed.2021.104943.

35 Chandak, T. and Wong, C.F. (2021). EDock-ML: a web server for using ensemble docking with machine learning to aid drug discovery. *Protein Science* 30: 1087–1097. https://doi.org/10.1002/pro.4065.

36 Trott, O. and Olson, A.J. (2010). AutoDock Vina: improving the speed and accuracy of docking with a new scoring function, efficient optimization, and multithreading. *Journal of Computational Chemistry* 31: 455–461. https://doi.org/10.1002/jcc.21334.

37 AutoDock Vina Available online: https://vina.scripps.edu/ (accessed 19 August 2022).

38 Schneidman-Duhovny, D., Dror, O., Inbar, Y. et al. (2008). PharmaGist: a webserver for ligand-based pharmacophore detection. *Nucleic Acids Research* 36: W223–W228. https://doi.org/10.1093/nar/gkn187.

39 PharmaGist Webserver. Available online: http://bioinfo3d.cs.tau.ac.il/pharma/index.html (accessed 19 August 2022).

40 Deshmukh, M.G., Ippolito, J.A., Zhang, C.-H. et al. (2021). Structure-guided design of a perampanel-derived pharmacophore targeting the SARS-CoV-2 main protease. *Structure* 29: 1–11. https://doi.org/10.1016/j.str.2021.06.002.

41 Pharmit: interactive exploration of chemical space. Available online: http://pharmit.csb.pitt.edu (accessed 19 August 2022).

42 Sunseri, J. and Koes, D.R. (2016). Pharmit: interactive exploration of chemical space. *Nucleic Acids Research* 44: W442–W448. https://doi.org/10.1093/nar/gkw287.

43 Koes, D.R. (2018). The pharmit backend: a computer systems approach to enabling interactive online drug discovery. *IBM Journal of Research and Development* 62: 1–6. https://doi.org/10.1147/jrd.2018.2883977.

44 Koes, D.R. and Camacho, C.J. (2012). ZINCPharmer: pharmacophore search of the ZINC database. *Nucleic Acids Research* 40: W409–W414. https://doi.org/10.1093/nar/gks378.

45 ZINCPharmer website. Available online: http://zincpharmer.csb.pitt.edu/ (accessed 19 August 2022).

46 Kumar, A. and Zhang, K.Y.J. (2018). Advances in the development of shape similarity methods and their application in drug discovery. *Frontiers in Chemistry* 6: 315. https://doi.org/10.3389/fchem.2018.00315.

47 Armstrong, M.S., Morris, G.M., Finn, P.W. et al. (2010). ElectroShape: fast molecular similarity calculations incorporating shape, chirality and electrostatics. *Journal of Computer-Aided Molecular Design* 24: 789–801. https://doi.org/10.1007/s10822-010-9374-0.

48 Johansson, L., Fotsch, C., Bartberger, M.D. et al. (2008). 2-amino-1,3-thiazol-4(5H)-ones as potent and selective 11beta-hydroxysteroid dehydrogenase type 1 inhibitors: enzyme-ligand co-crystal structure and demonstration of pharmacodynamic effects in C57Bl/6 mice. *Journal of Medicinal Chemistry* 51: 2933–2943. https://doi.org/10.1021/jm701551j.

49 Bolcato, G., Heid, E., and Boström, J. (2022). On the value of using 3D shape and electrostatic similarities in deep generative methods. *Journal of Chemical Information and Modeling* 62: 1388–1398. https://doi.org/10.1021/ACS.JCIM.1C01535/SUPPL_FILE/CI1C01535_SI_001.PDF.

50 Burley, S.K., Bhikadiya, C., Bi, C. et al. (2021). RCSB Protein Data Bank: powerful new tools for exploring 3D structures of biological macromolecules for basic and applied research and education in fundamental biology, biomedicine, biotechnology, bioengineering and energy sciences. *Nucleic Acids Research* 49: D437–D451. https://doi.org/10.1093/nar/gkaa1038.

51 Joosten, R.P., Long, F., Murshudov, G.N., and Perrakis, A. (2014). The PDB_REDO server for macromolecular structure model optimization. *IUCrJ* 1: 213–220. https://doi.org/10.1107/S2052252514009324.

52 Bienert, S., Waterhouse, A., de Beer, T.A.P. et al. (2017). The SWISS-MODEL Repository-new features and functionality. *Nucleic Acids Research* 45: D313–D319. https://doi.org/10.1093/nar/gkw1132.

53 (1971). Crystallography: protein data bank. *Nature: New Biology* 233: 223–223. https://doi.org/10.1038/newbio233223b0.

54 PDB Data Distribution by Experimental Method and Molecular Type. Available online: https://www.rcsb.org/stats/summary (accessed 19 August 2022).
55 PDB file format version 3.3. Available online: http://www.wwpdb.org/documentation/file-format-content/format33/v3.3.html (accessed 19 August 2022).
56 PDBx/mmCIF Dictionary Resources Available online: https://mmcif.wwpdb.org/ (accessed 19 August 2022).
57 RCSB Protein Data Bank Homepage. Available online: https://www.rcsb.org/ (accessed 19 August 2022).
58 Armstrong, D.R., Berrisford, J.M., Conroy, M.J. et al. (2020). PDBe: improved findability of macromolecular structure data in the PDB. *Nucleic Acids Research* 48: D335–D343. https://doi.org/10.1093/NAR/GKZ990.
59 The PDB-REDO server for macromolecular structure model optimization. Available online: https://pdb-redo.eu/ (accessed 19 August 2022).
60 Joosten, R.P., Salzemann, J., Bloch, V. et al. (2009). PDB_REDO: automated re-refinement of X-ray structure models in the PDB. *Journal of Applied Crystallography* 42: 376–384. https://doi.org/10.1107/S0021889809008784.
61 Cereto-Massagué, A., Ojeda, M.J., Joosten, R.P. et al. (2013). The good, the bad and the dubious: VHELIBS, a validation helper for ligands and binding sites. *Journal of Cheminformatics* 5: 36. https://doi.org/10.1186/1758-2946-5-36.
62 Berman, H.M., Battistuz, T., Bhat, T.N. et al. (2002). The protein data bank. *Acta Crystallographica. Section D, Biological Crystallography* 58: 899–907.
63 Kleywegt, G.J., Harris, M.R., Zou, J.Y. et al. (2004). The uppsala electron-density server. *Acta Crystallographica, Section D: Biological Crystallography* 60: 2240–2249. https://doi.org/10.1107/S0907444904013253.
64 Boutet, E., Lieberherr, D., Tognolli, M. et al. (2016). UniProtKB/Swiss-Prot, the manually annotated section of the UniProt knowledgeBase: how to use the entry view. *Methods in Molecular Biology* 1374: 23–54. https://doi.org/10.1007/978-1-4939-3167-5_2.
65 Benkert, P., Biasini, M., and Schwede, T. (2011). Toward the estimation of the absolute quality of individual protein structure models. *Bioinformatics* 27: 343–350. https://doi.org/10.1093/bioinformatics/btq662.
66 Waterhouse, A., Bertoni, M., Bienert, S. et al. (2018). SWISS-MODEL: homology modelling of protein structures and complexes. *Nucleic Acids Research* 46: W296–W303. https://doi.org/10.1093/nar/gky427.
67 SWISS-MODEL Available online: https://swissmodel.expasy.org/ (accessed 19 August 2022).
68 The SWISS-MODEL Repository Available online: https://swissmodel.expasy.org/repository (accessed 19 August 2022).
69 AlphaFold Protein Structure Database. Available online: https://alphafold.ebi.ac.uk/ (accessed 19 August 2022).
70 AlphaFold Protein Structure Database. Download page Available online: https://alphafold.ebi.ac.uk/download (accessed 19 August 2022).
71 Rhodes, G. (2006). *Crystallography made crystal clear : a guide for users of macromolecular models*. Elsevier/Academic Press ISBN 9780125870733.

72 VHELIBS by URVnutrigenomica-CTNS. Available from: https://github.com/URVquimioinformatica-COS/VHELIBS.

73 Douangamath, A., Fearon, D., Gehrtz, P. et al. (2020). Crystallographic and electrophilic fragment screening of the SARS-CoV-2 main protease. *Nature Communications* 11: 1–11. https://doi.org/10.1038/s41467-020-18709-w.

74 Sorokina, M., Merseburger, P., Rajan, K. et al. (2021). COCONUT online: collection of open natural products database. *Journal of Cheminformatics* 13: 2. https://doi.org/10.1186/s13321-020-00478-9.

75 Fink, T. and Reymond, J.-L. (2007). Virtual exploration of the chemical universe up to 11 atoms of C, N, O, F: assembly of 26.4 million structures (110.9 million stereoisomers) and analysis for new ring systems, stereochemistry, physicochemical properties, compound classes, and drug discovery. *Journal of Chemical Information and Modeling* 47: 342–353. https://doi.org/10.1021/ci600423u.

76 Irwin, J.J., Tang, K.G., Young, J. et al. (2020). ZINC20-A free ultralarge-scale chemical database for ligand discovery. *Journal of Chemical Information and Modeling* 60: 6065–6073. https://doi.org/10.1021/acs.jcim.0c00675.

77 Ntie-Kang, F., Zofou, D., Babiaka, S.B. et al. (2013). AfroDb: a select highly potent and diverse natural product library from African medicinal plants. *PLoS One* 8: e78085. https://doi.org/10.1371/journal.pone.0078085.

78 Gentile, D., Patamia, V., Scala, A. et al. (2020). Putative inhibitors of SARS-CoV-2 main protease from a library of marine natural products: a virtual screening and molecular modeling study. *Marine Drugs* 18: 225. https://doi.org/10.3390/md18040225.

79 van Santen, J.A., Jacob, G., Singh, A.L. et al. (2019). The natural products atlas: an open access knowledge base for microbial natural products discovery. *ACS Central Science* 5: 1824–1833. https://doi.org/10.1021/acscentsci.9b00806.

80 Banerjee, P., Erehman, J., Gohlke, B.-O. et al. (2015). Super Natural II – a database of natural products. *Nucleic Acids Research* 43: D935–D939. https://doi.org/10.1093/nar/gku886.

81 Chen, C.Y.-C. (2011). TCM Database@Taiwan: the world's largest traditional Chinese medicine database for drug screening in silico. *PLoS One* 6: e15939. https://doi.org/10.1371/journal.pone.0015939.

82 Gu, J., Gui, Y., Chen, L. et al. (2013). Use of natural products as chemical library for drug discovery and network pharmacology. *PLoS One* 8: e62839. https://doi.org/10.1371/journal.pone.0062839.

83 COCONUT database download page. Available online: https://coconut.naturalproducts.net/download (accessed 19 August 2022).

84 Blum, L.C. and Reymond, J.-L. (2009). 970 million druglike small molecules for virtual screening in the chemical universe database GDB-13. *Journal of the American Chemical Society* 131: 8732–8733. https://doi.org/10.1021/ja902302h.

85 Ruddigkeit, L., van Deursen, R., Blum, L.C., and Reymond, J.-L. (2012). Enumeration of 166 billion organic small molecules in the chemical universe database GDB-17. *Journal of Chemical Information and Modeling* 52: 2864–2875. https://doi.org/10.1021/ci300415d.

86 Meier, K., Bühlmann, S., Arús-Pous, J., and Reymond, J.-L. (2020). The generated databases (GDBs) as a source of 3D-shaped building blocks for use in medicinal chemistry and drug discovery. *Chimia (Aarau).* 74: 241–246. https://doi.org/10.2533/chimia.2020.241.

87 Awale, M., Sirockin, F., Stiefl, N., and Reymond, J.-L. (2019). Medicinal chemistry aware database GDBMedChem. *Molecular Informatics* 38: e1900031. https://doi.org/10.1002/minf.201900031.

88 GDB databases download page. Available online: https://gdb.unibe.ch/downloads/ (accessed 19 August 2022).

89 Molecules contributing to the biogenic subset in ZINC20. Available online: https://zinc20.docking.org/substances/subsets/biogenic/ (accessed 19 August 2022).

90 Catalogs contributing to the biogenic subset in ZINC20. Available online: https://zinc20.docking.org/catalogs/subsets/biogenic/ (accessed 19 August 2022).

91 The Binding Database Available online: https://www.bindingdb.org/ (accessed 19 August 2022).

92 Chen, X., Liu, M., and Gilson, M.K. (2001). BindingDB: a web-accessible molecular recognition database. *Combinatorial Chemistry & High Throughput Screening* 4: 719–725. https://doi.org/10.2174/1386207013330670.

93 Kim, S., Chen, J., Cheng, T. et al. (2021). PubChem in 2021: new data content and improved web interfaces. *Nucleic Acids Research* 49: D1388–D1395. https://doi.org/10.1093/nar/gkaa971.

94 PubChem Available online: https://pubchem.ncbi.nlm.nih.gov/ (accessed 19 August 2022).

95 ChEMBL Database Available online: https://www.ebi.ac.uk/chembl/ (accessed 19 August 2022).

96 Gaulton, A., Hersey, A., Nowotka, M. et al. (2017). The ChEMBL database in 2017. *Nucleic Acids Research* 45: D945–D954. https://doi.org/10.1093/nar/gkw1074.

97 Creative Commons Attribution License Available online: https://creativecommons.org/licenses/by/3.0/us/ (accessed 19 August 2022).

98 Gilson, M.K., Liu, T., Baitaluk, M. et al. (2016). BindingDB in 2015: a public database for medicinal chemistry, computational chemistry and systems pharmacology. *Nucleic Acids Research* 44: D1045–D1053. https://doi.org/10.1093/nar/gkv1072.

99 Cao, Y., Charisi, A., Cheng, L.-C. et al. (2008). ChemmineR: a compound mining framework for R. *Bioinformatics* 24: 1733–1734. https://doi.org/10.1093/bioinformatics/btn307.

100 Kim, S. (2016). Getting the most out of PubChem for virtual screening. *Expert Opinion on Drug Discovery* 11: 843–855. https://doi.org/10.1080/17460441.2016.1216967.

101 Creative Commons Attribution-Share Alike 3.0 Unported License. Available online: https://creativecommons.org/licenses/by-sa/3.0/ (accessed 19 August 2022).

102 The PubChem BioAssay Advanced Search Builder Available online: https://www.ncbi.nlm.nih.gov/pcassay/advanced (accessed 19 August 2022).

103 InCell qHTS Assay for Inhibitors of the mTORC1 Signaling Pathway in WT MEF Cells: Hit Validation. Available online: https://pubchem.ncbi.nlm.nih.gov/bioassay/651793 (accessed 19 August 2022).

104 Cereto-Massagué, A., Guasch, L., Valls, C. et al. (2012). DecoyFinder: an easy-to-use python GUI application for building target-specific decoy sets. *Bioinformatics* 28: 1661–1662. https://doi.org/10.1093/bioinformatics/bts249.

105 Huang, N., Shoichet, B.K., and Irwin, J.J. (2006). Benchmarking sets for molecular docking. *Journal of Medicinal Chemistry* 49: 6789–6801. https://doi.org/10.1021/jm0608356.

106 Bender, A. and Glen, R.C. (2005). A discussion of measures of enrichment in virtual screening: comparing the information content of descriptors with increasing levels of sophistication. *Journal of Chemical Information and Modeling* 45: 1369–1375. https://doi.org/10.1021/ci0500177.

107 Mysinger, M.M., Carchia, M., Irwin, J.J., and Shoichet, B.K. (2012). Directory of useful decoys, enhanced (DUD-E): better ligands and decoys for better benchmarking. *Journal of Medicinal Chemistry* 55: 6582–6594. https://doi.org/10.1021/jm300687e.

108 DUD-E: A Database of Useful (Docking) Decoys - Enhanced. Available online: http://dude.docking.org/ (accessed 19 August 2022).

109 Bauer, M.R., Ibrahim, T.M., Vogel, S.M., and Boeckler, F.M. (2013). Evaluation and optimization of virtual screening workflows with DEKOIS 2.0 – a public library of challenging docking benchmark sets. *Journal of Chemical Information and Modeling* 53: 1447–1462. https://doi.org/10.1021/ci400115b.

110 DEKOIS: Demanding Evaluation Kits for Objective In silico Screening. Available online: http://www.pharmchem.uni-tuebingen.de/dekois/ (accessed 19 August 2022).

111 Wallach, I. and Lilien, R. (2011). Virtual decoy sets for molecular docking benchmarks. *Journal of Chemical Information and Modeling* 51: 196–202. https://doi.org/10.1021/ci100374f.

112 Virtual Decoy Sets. Available online: http://compbio.cs.toronto.edu/VDS/ (accessed 16 January 2022).

113 Make Decoys for your own ligands. Available online: http://dude.docking.org/generate (accessed 19 August 2022).

114 Pearlman, D.A. and Charifson, P.S. (2001). Improved scoring of ligand-protein interactions using OWFEG free energy grids. *Journal of Medicinal Chemistry* 44: 502–511. https://doi.org/10.1021/jm000375v.

115 Truchon, J.-F. and Bayly, C.I. (2007). Evaluating virtual screening methods: good and bad metrics for the "early recognition" problem. *Journal of Chemical Information and Modeling* 47: 488–508. https://doi.org/10.1021/ci600426e.

116 Mervin, L.H., Afzal, A.M., Drakakis, G. et al. (2015). Target prediction utilising negative bioactivity data covering large chemical space. *Journal of Cheminformatics* 7: 51. https://doi.org/10.1186/s13321-015-0098-y.

117 (2018). NCBI resource coordinators database resources of the national center for biotechnology information. *Nucleic Acids Research* 46: D8–D13. https://doi.org/10.1093/nar/gkx1095.

118 Davies, M., Nowotka, M., Papadatos, G. et al. (2015). ChEMBL web services: streamlining access to drug discovery data and utilities. *Nucleic Acids Research* 43: W612–W620. https://doi.org/10.1093/nar/gkv352.

119 Nowotka, M.M., Gaulton, A., Mendez, D. et al. (2017). Using ChEMBL web services for building applications and data processing workflows relevant to drug discovery. *Expert Opinion on Drug Discovery* 12: 757–767. https://doi.org/10.1080/17460441.2017.1339032.

120 Macip, G., Garcia-Segura, P., Mestres-Truyol, J. et al. (2021). Haste makes waste: a critical review of docking-based virtual screening in drug repurposing for SARS-CoV-2 main protease (M-pro) inhibition. *Medicinal Research Reviews* 42: 744–769. https://doi.org/10.1002/med.21862.

121 Macip, G.; Garcia-Segura, P.; Mestres-Truyol, J.; Saldivar-Espinoza, B.; Pujadas, G.; Garcia-Vallvé, S. A review of the current landscape of SARS-CoV-2 main protease inhibitors: have we hit the bullseye yet? *International Journal of Molecular Sciences* 2021, 23, 259. https://doi.org/10.3390/ijms23010259.

122 Bosc, N., Atkinson, F., Felix, E. et al. (2019). Large scale comparison of QSAR and conformal prediction methods and their applications in drug discovery. *Journal of Cheminformatics* 11: 4. https://doi.org/10.1186/s13321-018-0325-4.

10

Open Access Databases – An Industrial View
Michael Przewosny

Borngasse 43, D-52064 Aachen, Germany

10.1 Academic vs. Industrial Research

Since the spread of the Internet, extensive changes have taken place in many areas, both professionally and private. Modernization took place in many areas of the economy, new branches of the economy emerged, and communication behavior and the use of the media changed.

This also led to enormous changes in technical and scientific fields. Until the mid-1990s, this accumulated knowledge was only available in printed form, mostly freely accessible in university libraries. Digitization was pushed by institutions and publishers, not only for commercial purposes but also to create worldwide access to data and information. Not only are journals and books now available online, but the inclusion of this content in searchable databases has also been accomplished.

Before these online databases were established, the life of scientists was characterized by time-consuming research in bound data collections. For chemists who were preparing a research project or a doctoral thesis, it meant disappearing into libraries for several days to evaluate the current state of knowledge and defining this as the starting point for their scientific work. The best-known data collections were the Gmelin for inorganic chemistry and the Beilstein for organic chemistry, in which structured research was possible [1, 2]. Chemical Abstracts (CA) was also available across disciplines, provided by the Chemical Abstracts Service (CAS), a subdivision of the American Chemical Society (ACS) established in 1907. The aim was to bring together and index all chemistry-related information (journals, books, patents, dissertations, congresses, etc.) in order to make them available [3, 4].

The result of digitization is the commercial online databases Reaxys and SciFinder.

Reaxys (https://www.elsevier.com/solutions/reaxys) is the successor to Crossfire, which provided access to the Beilstein, Gmelin, and Patent Chemistry databases until 2010. The Windows-based version since then has access to the three databases and allows all chemistry-related searches for structures, substructures, reactions, and synthesis planning based on journals and patents. Provider is the publishing house Elsevier (Table 10.1).

Open Access Databases and Datasets for Drug Discovery, First Edition.
Edited by Antoine Daina, Michael Przewosny, and Vincent Zoete.
© 2024 WILEY-VCH GmbH. Published 2024 by WILEY-VCH GmbH.

Table 10.1 Available databases for virtual screening.

Database	Number of Compounds	URL
Asinex	91,473	http://www.asinex.com/
BindingDB	520,000	http://bindingdb.org
ChemBridge	1.3 million	https://www.chembridge.com/
COCONUT	407,270[a]	https://coconut.naturalproducts.net/
PubChem	11 million	https://pubchem.ncbi.nlm.nih.gov/
Zinc15	230 million[b]	https://zinc15.docking.org/

a) Natural products.
b) Purchasable compounds.

SciFinder (https://www.cas.org/solutions/cas-scifinder-discovery-platform/cas-scifinder) is a database developed by the CAS in which not only chemical but also biological information can be searched [5, 6].

Reaxys and SciFinder are established for data analysis in academic and industrial research because of the amount of data and the clear search and filter options as well as the export of search results in form of Excel lists and chemical structure lists as sdf-files (structure data file).

Academic and industrial research differ fundamentally in their focus. Research at universities is free, deals primarily with basic research, and is financed by state funding or industrial cooperation. Industrial research, e.g. materials science, pharmaceutical research, and others, have the goal of developing new materials, drugs or dosage forms and bringing them to the market as commercially viable products and being refinanced through a life cycle process.

In the pharmaceutical industry, the development of a new active ingredient involves an extensive, time-consuming, and costly process. Not only the indication but also the selection of a possible chemical or biological agent and its formulation must be carefully evaluated.

The development of a possible new active ingredient is divided into several development phases (Scheme 10.1):

Much information on the individual development steps can be researched in commercial and publicly accessible databases and collections.

At the beginning of a project in pharmaceutical research, there is an assessment of both the indication and the possible target. In this Target Assessment (TA), a team of chemists, biologists, biochemists, and pharmacologists is formed, which, based on the results of research, decides whether it makes sense to deal with a target or an indication. A large number of scientific sources are available for obtaining this information; in addition to journals and patents, databases are the most important resource. The topicality of the information sought is of great relevance in industry because of its financial interests and requires both scientific and economically reliable data, which is a big difference from university research. In addition, strategic aspects such as contract research organizations (CROs), contract development,

10.1 Academic vs. Industrial Research

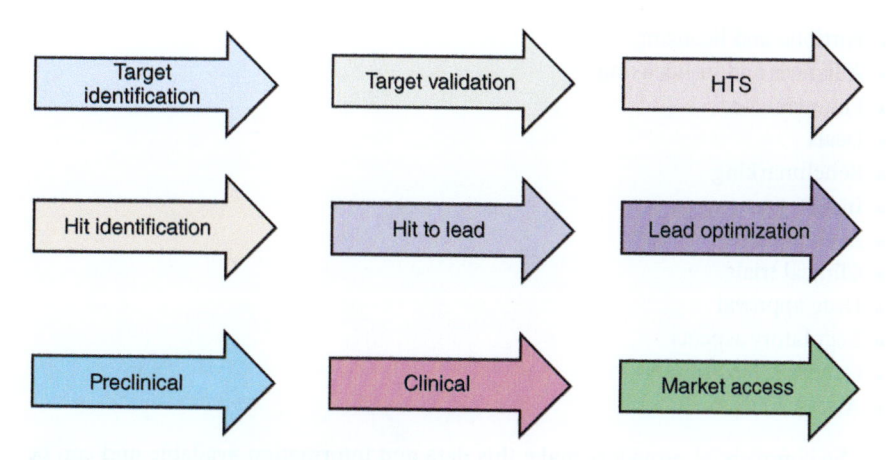

Scheme 10.1 Overview of the R&D process.

production, manufacturing organizations (CDMOs), in- or out-licensing, outsourcing, offshoring, company takeovers, etc.) must be assessed.

Obtaining this necessary and up-to-date information Competitive Intelligence, (CI) is time-consuming and costly and can only be provided by the industrial side with great effort. The alternative is represented by commercial providers who search for all the necessary information from all available sources (Internet, patent services, company websites, analyst websites, regulatory institutions, authorities, etc.), compile them and save them in the form of Excel files or SD files. Make files available for analysis. The best-known and established providers are:

- Adis Insight – https://adisinsight.springer.com/
- Citeline (formerly PharmaProjects) – https://pharmaintelligence.informa.com/
- Clarivate (formerly Cortellis) – https://clarivate.com/cortellis/
- Evaluate – https://www.evaluate.com/
- GlobalData – https://www.globaldata.com/
- Integrity (Clarivate Analytics) – https://integrity.clarivate.com/integrity/xmlxsl

The information provided relates to a variety of aspects and is relevant for deciding how to proceed:

- Patent status
- Drugs and biologics
- Molecular interactions
- Pharmacology data points
- Discovery and preclinical
- Safety and pharmacovigilance
- Metabolism, pharmacokinetic (PK), and toxicology
- Competitive intelligence (CI)
- Drug reports
- Meeting reports
- Company profiles

- Portfolio and licensing
- Alliances and in-licensing
- Financial data
- Deals
- Benchmarking
- Industry news
- Drug pipeline
- Clinical trials
- Drug approval
- Regulatory aspects
- Generics, biosimilars
- Alerts

The commercial providers make this data and information available and can be downloaded as reports for any desired search term.

The problem for small and medium-sized biopharmaceutical or pharmaceutical companies is the limited financial possibilities to access this information. The establishment of databases at universities and research institutions was promoted over several years through private- and state-financed projects in order to generate and compile general and specific information and make it available for research and development.

As already mentioned, the TA is the starting point for a new project in which chemists and biologists collect a large amount of information in order to create a basis for decision-making.

It is traditionally the task of chemists to create an overview of the patent situation of biological targets, substances, or pharmaceutical dosage forms, the so-called CI. The national and international patent offices are state-financed organizations that decide on the granting of patents after an examination procedure. All information on submitted invention disclosures, processing status, and patent granting is freely accessible on the websites of the patent offices.

- Deutsches Patent- und Markenamt (DPMA) – https://www.dpma.de/
- European Patent Office (EPO) – https://www.epo.org/
- United States Patent and Trademark Office (USPTO) – https://www.uspto.gov/
- Japanese Patent Office (JPO)
- China National Intellectual Property Administration (CNIPA) – https://english.cnipa.gov.cn/
- Swiss Federal Institute of Intellectual Property (IGE-IPI) – https://www.ige.ch/en/

It is possible to research a large amount of information in the patent databases using search masks and to download patents and the associated information in pdf format for further evaluation.

The EPO website, for example, offers access to more than 130 million patent documents, an example is the advanced search *via* https://worldwide.espacenet.com/advancedSearch?locale=en_EP (Scheme 10.2). A search on the websites of the regional patent offices is similar.

```
┌─ Enter keywords ──────────────────────────────────────────────┐
│  Title: [i]                                                   │
│                                          plastic and bicycle  │
│  ┌─────────────────────────────────────────────────────────┐  │
│  └─────────────────────────────────────────────────────────┘  │
│  Title or abstract: [i]                                       │
│                                                         hair  │
│  ┌─────────────────────────────────────────────────────────┐  │
│  └─────────────────────────────────────────────────────────┘  │
└───────────────────────────────────────────────────────────────┘

┌─ Enter numbers with or without country code ─────────────────┐
│  Publication number: [i]                                      │
│                                                 WO2008014520  │
│  ┌─────────────────────────────────────────────────────────┐  │
│  └─────────────────────────────────────────────────────────┘  │
│  Application number: [i]                                      │
│                                                 DE201310112935│
│  ┌─────────────────────────────────────────────────────────┐  │
│  └─────────────────────────────────────────────────────────┘  │
│  Priority number: [i]                                         │
│                                                 WO1995US15925│
│  ┌─────────────────────────────────────────────────────────┐  │
│  └─────────────────────────────────────────────────────────┘  │
└───────────────────────────────────────────────────────────────┘

┌─ Enter one or more dates or date ranges ─────────────────────┐
│  Publication date: [i]                                        │
│                                      2014-12-31 or 20141231  │
│  ┌─────────────────────────────────────────────────────────┐  │
│  └─────────────────────────────────────────────────────────┘  │
└───────────────────────────────────────────────────────────────┘

┌─ Enter name of one or more persons/organisations ────────────┐
│  Applicant(s): [i]                                            │
│                                              Institut Pasteur │
│  ┌─────────────────────────────────────────────────────────┐  │
│  └─────────────────────────────────────────────────────────┘  │
│  Inventor(s): [i]                                             │
│                                                        Smith  │
│  ┌─────────────────────────────────────────────────────────┐  │
│  └─────────────────────────────────────────────────────────┘  │
└───────────────────────────────────────────────────────────────┘

┌─ Enter one or more classification symbols ───────────────────┐
│  CPC [i]                                                      │
│                                                    F03G7/10   │
│  ┌─────────────────────────────────────────────────────────┐  │
│  └─────────────────────────────────────────────────────────┘  │
│  IPC [i]                                                      │
│                                                    H03M1/12   │
│  ┌─────────────────────────────────────────────────────────┐  │
│  └─────────────────────────────────────────────────────────┘  │
└───────────────────────────────────────────────────────────────┘
```

Scheme 10.2 EPO search mask for an advanced search.

The disadvantage is that many patents are published in their national languages, which is a problem with Asian patents in particular. Most patents available as pdf files are scanned image files, and searching in these files is only possible after conversion to readable formats; the alternative is a paid translation. Google Patents (https://patents.google.com/ (accessed 20 April 2022)) offers a free solution whereby the patents can be downloaded not only in their national language but also in English translation as a pdf file, which gives access to the information contained in foreign patents.

The search for a new drug begins with the identification of a suitable target such as proteins, signaling pathways, genes, and nucleic acid sequences that are associated with a disease:

- G-Protein-coupled receptors (GPCRs)
- Ion channels
- Nuclear receptors
- Enzymes
- Transporters
- DNA
- RNA

In order to study the interaction of a possible active substance with a receptor, it is necessary to find the binding site of the ligand on a protein. Knowledge of the three-dimensional (3D) structure of the biological macromolecule is helpful for understanding the function of a protein. The Protein Data Bank (PDB), founded in 1971, is the largest structural database for proteins, DNA, and RNA (https://www.rcsb.org/ (accessed 24 April 2022)). The structures are determined by X-ray structure analysis and NMR spectroscopy and are freely available. The following sequences and structures of biological macromolecules can be searched [7].

The following sequences and structures of biological macromolecules can be searched:

- 189,735 protein structures
- 56,800 structures of human sequences
- 14,225 nucleic acid containing structures

Internationalization took place in 2003 with the establishment of the Worldwide Protein Data Bank (wwPDB) (http://www.wwpdb.org/ (accessed 24 April 2022) by Protein Data Bank in Europe (PDBe) (https://www.ebi.ac.uk/pdbe/ (accessed 24 April 2022)), Protein Data Bank Japan (PDBj) (https://pdbj.org/ (accessed 24 April 2022)), and Biological Magnetic Resonance Bank (BMRB) (https://bmrb.io/ (accessed 24 April 2022).

Another protein database with information on peptide sequences, protein sequences, and functions can be found in UNI-Prot (Universal Protein Resource, https://beta.uniprot.org/ (accessed 24 April 2022)) [8].

An analog database for 3D structures of nucleic acids is the Nucleic Acid Database (NDB), founded in 1992, in which sequences, structures, and functions can be searched freely (http://ndbserver.rutgers.edu/ (accessed 24 April 2022)) [9].

The development of a new database with additional information on sequences, functions, and interactions of nucleic acids was described in 2018 through a collaboration between Rutgers University NDB and Bowling Green State University (RNAhub services). The NDB is to be replaced under the name Nucleic Acid Knowledge Base (NAKB) [10].

Another source for information on nucleosides and nucleotides is the DNA Data Bank of Japan (DDBJ, https://www.ddbj.nig.ac.jp (accessed 24 April 2022)) [11].

A European archive is The European Nucleotide Archive (ENA, https://www.ebi.ac.uk/ena/ (accessed 24 April 2022)) in which data can be stored and information can be searched for [12].

An overview of all existing targets, signaling pathways and ligands can be found in the DrugBank (https://go.drugbank.com/ (accessed 24 April 2022)) [13].

Another database on binding affinities, ligand–target interactions, and pathways is the Binding Database (bindingDB, http://bindingdb.org/bind/index.jsp (accessed 24 April 2022)). BindingDB contains 249,5891 binding data for 8813 receptors and 10,711,154 small molecules [14].

Not only the structure of the receptors is relevant for development, but the structure of the ligands must also be considered. For drugs with chiral centers, knowledge of the exact structure of stereoisomers (enantiomers, diastereomers, and racemates) is extremely important for biological function. Biologically active racemates are composed of two enantiomers that can have different biological effects. The eutomer represents the active form, and the distomer represents the less active form. The absolute configuration is determined by X-ray structure analysis, and the results of these investigations are publicly available.

Established in 1965, the Cambridge Structural Database (CSD) contains over one million 3D structures of small organic and organometallic molecules determined by X-ray diffraction or neutron diffraction (https://www.ccdc.cam.ac.uk/solutions/csd-core/components/csd/ (accessed 24 April 2022)) [15]. A total of 50,000 new structures are added to CSD every year.

Another database for organic, inorganic, metal–organic compounds, and minerals is the Crystallography Open Database (COD) in which 487,565 structures of molecules are available (http://www.crystallography.net/cod/ (Accessed 24 April 2022)) [16].

After a successful target validation, it is necessary to establish an appropriate assay in order to test a large number of compounds in a high-throughput process (high-throughput screening, HTS) with the aim of identifying biologically active substances (hit-finding).

The substances that are screened in the substance libraries in the HTS consist of compounds synthesized in-house, external syntheses from cooperation with CROs, and substances purchased from commercial suppliers as listed:

- Asinex – https://www.asinex.com/screening-libraries-(all-libraries)
- Charles River – https://www.criver.com/products-services/discovery-services/screening-and-profiling-assays/screening-libraries/compound-screening-libraries?region=3696
- ChemBridge – https://www.chembridge.com/
- Enamine – https://enamine.net/compound-libraries
- Evotec – https://www.evotec.com/en/execute/drug-discovery-services/hit-identification
- I.F. Labs – https://iflab.com/
- Maybridge – https://www.thermofisher.com/de/de/home/industrial/pharma-biopharma/drug-discovery-development/screening-compounds-libraries-hit-identification.html

- SoftFocus® Libraries – https://www.criver.com/products-services/discovery-services/screening-and-profiling-assays/screening-libraries/compound-screening-libraries/softfocus-subscription-libraries?region=3696

There is a specific assay for each target to determine the inhibitory or activating properties of a substance.

The ChEMBL or ChEMBLdb database (https://www.ebi.ac.uk/chembl/ (accessed April 25 2022) provides an overview of the known and available assays. ChEMBL is a chemical database of biologically active substances with drug-like properties. Currently, 299,151 assays can be accessed and downloaded in the form of report cards, including references and patents [17].

The world's largest database of information on chemical compounds and their physical and biological properties, safety data, and toxicological data is PubChem (https://pubchem.ncbi.nlm.nih.gov/ (accessed 25 April 2022)) [18]. There are 111 million compounds, 280 million substances, and 295 million bioactivities available. Biological and toxicological data can be searched at PubChem BioAssays (https://pubchemdocs.ncbi.nlm.nih.gov/bioassays (accessed 25 April 2022)) [19].

Pharos (https://pharos.nih.gov/ (accessed 25 April 2022)) is a National Institutes of Health (NIH) sponsored Knowledge Management Center (KMC) database for Illuminating the Druggable Genome (IDG). It includes 20,412 targets, information on 13,704 diseases, and 339,220 ligands [20].

Natural products are a reliable source as lead structures for the development of new drugs. COlleCtion of Open Natural ProdUcTs (COCONUT), https://coconut.naturalproducts.net/ (accessed 25 April 2022)) is a freely accessible database on natural products [21]. The database lists 407,270 searchable natural substances, which are also available for download as sd files.

The results of an HTS run are the basis for further procedure in the projects. A precise analysis of the found active molecules (hits) such as structure, compound class, and patent status is important in order to develop lead structures. The aim of lead structure optimization is to improve the pharmacological, pharmacokinetic, and toxicological properties in order to avoid the risk of possible side effects and to improve bioavailability.

The most common reason for the occurrence of side effects is the insufficient drug metabolism, the pharmacokinetic profile (DMPK), and the formation of reactive metabolites [22]. When creating a DMPK profile, absorption, the stability and structure of formed metabolites, and inhibition or activation of cytochrome peroxidase P450 (CYP) are taken into account [23]. Furthermore, the metabolic enzymes sulfotransferases (SULTs) and UDP-glucuronosyltransferase (UGT) play an important role in the in vivo degradation of drugs. Data and information on the enzymes, metabolites involved, and their biological and toxicological data can be found in several Open-Access databases.

The Human Metabolome Database (HMDB) (https://hmdb.ca/ (accessed 25 April 2022)) was established by the Human Metabolome Project and is funded by Genome Canada [24]. HMBD contains 220,945 entries for chemical, biological, biochemical, and molecular biology data and also 8610 enzyme and transporter sequences.

In addition to chemical structures, analytical data such as NMR and MS are also available. There is a link to numerous other databases:

- KEGG: Kyoto Encyclopedia of Genes and Genomes https://www.genome.jp/kegg/
- PubChem – https://pubchem.ncbi.nlm.nih.gov/
- MetaCyc Metabolic Pathway Database – https://metacyc.org/
- ChEBI: Chemical Entities of Biological Interest – https://www.ebi.ac.uk/chebi/
- PDB: Protein Data Bank – https://www.rcsb.org/
- UniProt – https://www.ebi.ac.uk/uniprot/index
- GenBank – www.ncbi.nlm.nih.gov
- DrugBank – https://go.drugbank.com/
- T3DB: Toxin and Toxin Target Database – http://www.t3db.ca/
- SMPDB: Small Molecule Pathway Database – https://www.smpdb.ca/
- FooDB – https://foodb.ca/

The MetaCyc Metabolic Pathway Database (https://metacyc.org/ (accessed 26 April 2022)) contains a collection of 13,698 enzymes, 3006 metabolic pathways and their primary and secondary metabolites from 3295 different organisms [25].

Die Pathway Datenbank HumanCyc (https://humancyc.org/ (accessed 26 April 2022)) ist ein Archiv zu humanen metabolischen Signalwegen, menschlichen Metaboliten und dem menschlichen Genom [26].

The KEGG Pathway Database (Kyoto Encyclopedia of Genes and Genomes (accessed 26 April 2022)) is a collection of databases on biological pathways, drugs, genomes, diseases, and chemicals [27].

SMPDB (The Small Molecule Pathway Database, https://www.smpdb.ca/ (accessed 27 April 2022)) is an interactive database containing 49,827 signaling pathways, 55,734 substances, and 1576 proteins [28]. It contains more information on signaling pathways that are not searchable in other signaling pathway databases.

Additional information on ADME-Tox [29] are in the relevant databases ChEMBL (https://www.ebi.ac.uk/chembl/ (accessed 26 April 2022)), PubChem (https://pubchem.ncbi.nlm.nih.gov/ (accessed 26 April 2022)), and DrugBank (https://go.drugbank.com/ (accessed 26 April 2022)) [30].

Further information and links to signaling pathway databases can be found at Pathway (https://pathbank.org/others#metabolic (accessed 26 April 2022)).

When developing an active ingredient, the toxicological properties must also be considered. A substance can have toxic effects, but there is also the possibility that toxic metabolites are formed [31, 32].

TOXNET (TOXicology Data NETwork, https://toxnet.nlm.nih.gov/ (accessed 26 April 2022)) is a collection of databases containing information on active ingredients, chemicals, diseases, environmental data, safety, poisons, and regulations. The database is operated by the Toxicology and Environmental Health Information Program (TEHIP). TOXNET consists of several databases:

- CCRIS – Chemical Carcinogenesis Research Information System
- CPDB – Carcinogenic Potency Database
- DART® – Developmental and Reproductive Toxicology Database

- CTD – Comparative Toxicogenomics Database
- GENE-TOX – Genetic Toxicology
- HSDB® – Hazardous Substances Data Bank
- Haz-Map®
- Household Products Database
- IRIS – Integrated Risk Information System
- ITER – International Toxicity Estimates for Risk
- LactMed® – Drugs and Lactation
- TRI – Toxics Release Inventory
- TOXMAP®
- TOXLINE®

During a research and development project, it is not only important to follow the preclinical advances, but also the clinical development. After a potential drug candidate clears the hurdle into the clinic, clinical trials take place to test efficacy, improved efficacy over known therapies, side effects, and safety in humans. The clinical studies are carried out by pharmaceutical companies and commissioned study centers [33].

The US National Library of Medicine tracks and documents planned, ongoing, and completed trials that receive public or private funding (https://clinicaltrials.gov/ (accessed 26 June 2022)). To date, 419,313 studies have been documented in 220 countries. On the homepage, it is possible to perform a simple or an advanced search for tested substance, indication, therapy, and status of the study (Schemes 10.3 and 10.4).

A European database variant, the EU Clinical Trials Register (https://www.clinicaltrialsregister.eu/ (accessed 26 April 2022)) is also freely accessible. The EU Clinical Trials Register offers access to 42,312 clinical trials with a EudraCT protocol.

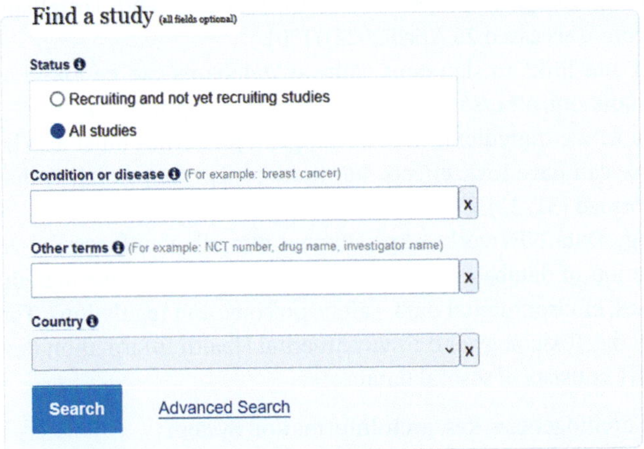

Scheme 10.3 Search mask for a simple search on https://clinicaltrials.gov/

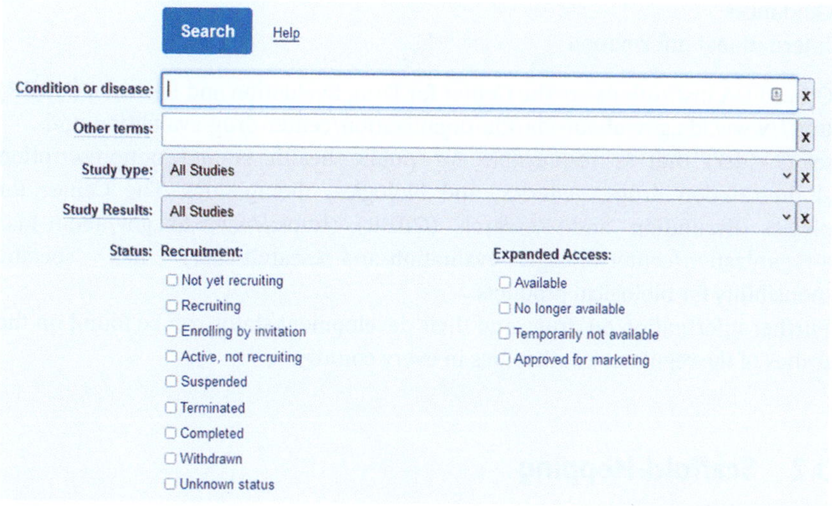

Scheme 10.4 Search mask for an advanced search pm https://clinicaltrials.gov/ct2/search/advanced?cond=&term=&cntry=&state=&city=&dist=.

EudraCT (European Union Drug Regulating Authorities Clinical Trials Database, https://eudract.ema.europa.eu/ (accessed 30 April 2022)) is the European database where all clinical trials on medicinal products authorized in the European Union are listed. This database contains information on ongoing clinical trials provided by the trial sponsors.

An overview of research activities and the development status of candidate substances from the competition is possible with a simple internet search; search terms "company name" and "pipeline" deliver current results.

Additional information on all phases and issues of drug development can be obtained from regulatory bodies, such as the European Medicines Agency (EMA), https://www.ema.europa.eu/en (accessed 26 April 2022)), located in Amsterdam (Netherlands) since 2019 (formerly in London (United Kingdom)) and the U.S. Food and Drug Administration (FDA), https://www.fda.gov/ (accessed 26 April 2022)), located in Silver Springs, Maryland (United States). Information on the following topics is available on both websites:

- Submissions
- Registration
- Recent drug approvals
- Manufacturing
- Medication Guides
- Drug applications
- Drug compounding
- Drug safety communications
- Shortages
- Warning letters
- Recalls

- Guidances
- International information

Other FDA institutions are the Center for Drug Evaluation and Research (CDER) (https://www.fda.gov/about-fda/fda-organization/center-drug-evaluation-and-research-cder) that is responsible for public health is and nonprescription and prescription drugs, generics, and biological therapeutics. The Center for Biologics Evaluation and Research (CBER) (https://www.fda.gov/about-fda/fda-organization/center-biologics-evaluation-and-research-cber) has specific responsibility for biological products.

Further information on drugs and their development status can be found on the websites of the regulatory authorities in every country.

10.2 Scaffold-Hopping

The aim of medicinal chemistry is to synthesize new active ingredients with improved properties. One method is scaffold hopping or rescaffolding, in which the basic structure of a known active ingredient is changed or replaced [34]. This method is very similar to the bioisoster approach, but instead of replacing individual atoms or functional groups, the central scaffold is replaced. Through this exchange, a higher activity toward the receptor is to be achieved, the ADME-Tox profile is to be improved in order to reduce side effects. It is also possible to circumvent existing patent protection, such as the example of the phosphodiesterase 5 (PDE5) inhibitor Sildenafil **1** from Pfizer, which was approved in 1998 under the name Viagra®. Chemically, sildenafil is a 1*H*-pyrazolo[4,3-*d*]pyrimidin-7(4*H*)-one.

In 2003, Bayer AG received approval for its PDE5 inhibitor Vardenafil, which was marketed under the name Levitra®. The new core structure is an imidazo[5,1-*f*][1,2,4]triazin-4(3*H*)-one, which allowed Bayer to circumvent patent protection on sildenafil.

Scaffold hopping can be simplified and accelerated by using computer-assisted methods. The commercial software ReCore was developed by the company BioSolveIT (https://www.biosolveit.de/ (accessed 27 April 2022)) [35].

When searching for a new scaffold, a drug molecule (e.g. COX2 inhibitor celecoxib 3) is imported into ReCore. By designating cleavage sites on the pyrazole backbone at positions **1** and **5**, the two substituents are fixed. ReCore's algorithm

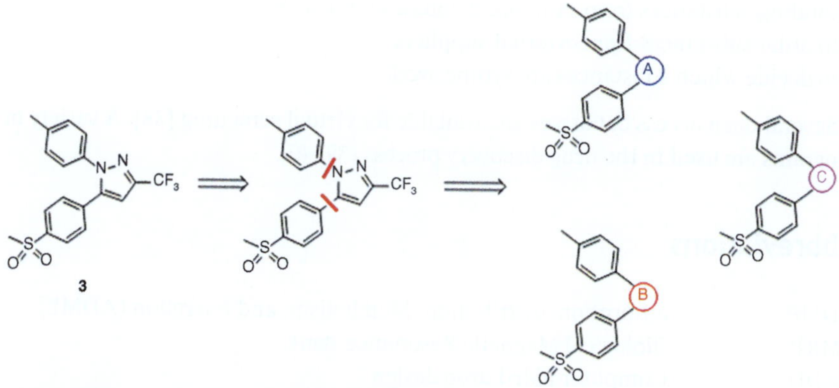

Scheme 10.5 Principle of scaffold-hopping.

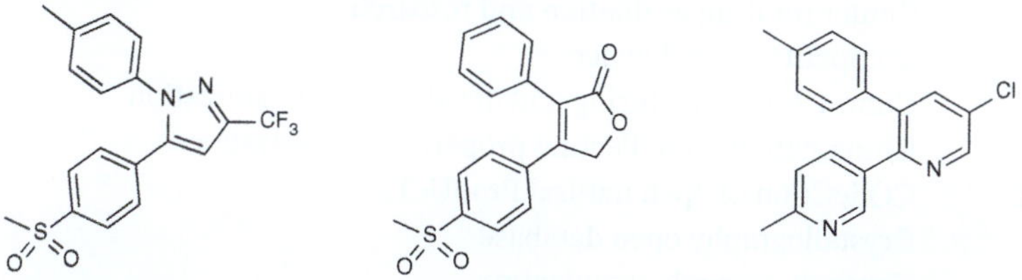

Celecoxib (Celebrex, Searle) approved 1998

Rofecoxib (Vioxx, Merck) approved 1999

Etoricoxib (Arcoxia, Merck) approved 2004

Scheme 10.6 COX2 inhibitors.

compares the unsubstituted pyrazole fragment with 3D structures from imported libraries and finds possible new scaffolds A, B, or C (Schemes 10.5 and 10.6):

Other COX2 inhibitors, such as rofecoxib and etoricoxib, were found by applying scaffold hopping.

In principle, any substance library from known online databases can be used, such as some of the listed ones:

- in-House repositories
- ZINC (https://zinc.docking.org/) – 230 million purchasable compounds
- PDB (Protein Data Bank) (https://www.rcsb.org/)
- CSD (The Cambridge Structural Database) (https://www.ccdc.cam.ac.uk/solutions/csd-core/components/csd/)

10.3 Virtual-Screening

Another method of computer-aided drug design (CADD) in the search for new active ingredients is in-silico or virtual screening (VS) [36]. In this computer-based method, compound libraries are searched to identify new structures that are suitable for further investigation and development [37]. VS is used to:

- Finding substances from in-house databases for a HTS
- to order substances from external suppliers
- to decide which substances are synthesized.

Several open access databases are available for virtual screening [38]. A variety of programs are used in the drug discovery process [39, 40].

Abbreviations

ADME	absorption, distribution, Metabolism, and Excretion (ADME)
BMRB	Biological Magnetic Resonance Bank
CADD	Computer-aided drug design
CAS	Chemical abstract service
CBER	Center for biologics evaluation and research
CDER	Center for drug evaluation and research
CI	Competitive intelligence
CMDO	Contract manufacturing and development organization
CNIPA	China national intellectual property administration
COCONUT	COlleCtion of open natural ProdUcTs
COD	Crystallography open database
CRO	Contract research organization
CSD	Cambridge structural database
CYP	Cytochrom peroxidase P450
DDBJ	DNA Data Bank of Japan
DPMA	Deutsches Patent- und Markenamt
DMPK	Drug Metabolism and Pharmacokinetic
EMA	European Medicines Agency
ENA	European Nucleotide Archive
EPO	European Patent office
FDA	U.S. Food and Drug Administration
GPCRs	G-Protein Coupled Receptors
HTS	High-Throughput Screening
IDG	Illuminating the Druggable Genome
IGE-IPI	Swiss Federal Institute of Intellectual Property
JPO	Japanese Patent Office - https://www.jpo.go.jp/e/
KMC	Knowledge Management Center
NAKB	Nucleic Acid Knowledge Base
NDB	Nuclear Database
NIH	National Institute of Health
PDB	Protein Data Bank
PDBe	Protein Data Bank in Europe
PDBj	Protein Data Bank Japan
PDE	Phosphodiesterase
PK	Pharmacokinetic
sdf	Structure Data File

SULT	Sulfotransferase
TA	Target Assessment
UGT	UDP-Glucuronosyltransferase
USPTO	United States Patent and Trademark Office
VS	Virtual Screening
wwPDB	Worldwide Protein Data Bank

References

1 Wiggins, G. (1996). Caught in a CrossFire: academic libraries and Beilstein. *Journal of Chemical Information and Modeling* 36: 746–749. https://doi.org/10.1021/ci950250c.

2 Zass, E. (1996). From handbooks to databases on the net: new solutions and old problems in information retrieval for chemists. *Journal of Chemical Information and Modeling* 36: 942–948. https://doi.org/10.1021/ci950249d.

3 The World's Largest Collection of Chemistry Insights. https://www.cas.org/about/cas-content

4 Jacobs, A., Williams, D., Hickey, K. et al. (2022). CAS common chemistry in 2021: expanding access to trusted chemical information for the scientific community. *Journal of Chemical Information and Modeling* 62: 2737–2743. https://doi.org/10.1021/acs.jcim.2c00268.

5 Ridley, D.D. (2015). *Information Retrieval: SciFinder*, 2e. Wiley.

6 Hübner, K. (2019). Chemical abstracts service - 150 millionen substanzen. *Chemie in unserer Zeit* 53: 140–147. https://doi.org/10.1002/ciuz.201980052.

7 Berman, H.M. (2008). The Protein Data Bank: a historical perspective. *Acta Crystallographica Section A* 64: 88–95. https://doi.org/10.1107/S0108767307035623.

8 The UniProt Consortium (2017). UniProt: the universal protein knowledgebase. *Nucleic Acids Research* 45 (Database Issue): D158–D169. https://doi.org/10.1093/nar/gkw1099.

9 Narayanan, B.C., Westbrook, J., Ghosh, S. et al. (2014). The nucleic acid database: new features and capabilities. *Nucleic Acids Research* 42 (Database Issue): D114–D122. https://doi.org/10.1093/nar/gkt980.

10 Berman, H.M., Lawson, C.L., and Schneider, B. (2022). Developing community resources for nucleic acid structures. *Lifestyles* 12 (4): 540. https://doi.org/10.3390/life12040540.

11 Okido, T., Kodama, Y., Mashima, J. et al. (2022). DNA Data Bank of Japan (DDBJ) update report 2021. *Nucleic Acids Research* 50 (Database Issue): D102–D105. https://doi.org/10.1093/nar/gkab995.

12 Cummins, C., Ahamed, A., Aslam, R. et al. (2022). The European nucleotide archive in 2021. *Nucleic Acids Research* 50 (Database Issue): D106–D110. https://doi.org/10.1093/nar/gkab1051.

13 Wishart, D.S., Knox, C., and Guo, A.C. (2008). DrugBank: a knowledgebase for drugs, drug actions and drug targets. *Nucleic Acids Research* 36 (Database issue): D901–D906. https://doi.org/10.1093/nar/gkm958.

14 Gilson, M.K., Liu, T., Baitaluk, M. et al. (2016). BindingDB in 2015: a public database for medicinal chemistry, computational chemistry and systems pharmacology. *Nucleic Acids Research* 44 (Database Issue): D1045–D1053. https://doi.org/10.1093/nar/gkl999.

15 Groom, C.R., Bruno, I.J., Lightfoot, M.P., and Ward, S.C. (2016). The Cambridge structural database. *Acta Crystallographica Section B* 72 (2): 171–179. https://doi.org/10.1107/S2052520616003954.

16 Gražulis, S., Daškevič, A., Merkys, A. et al. (2012). Crystallography Open Database (COD): an open-access collection of crystal structures and platform for world-wide collaboration. *Nucleic Acids Research* 40 (D1): D420–D427. https://doi.org/10.1093/nar/gkr900.

17 Davies, M., Nowotka, M., Papadatos, G. et al. (2015). ChEMBL web services: streamlining access to drug discovery data and utilities. *Nucleic Acids Research* 43 (Web Server Issue): W612–W620. https://doi.org/10.1093/nar/gkv352.

18 Kim, S., Chen, J., Cheng, T. et al. (2021). PubChem in 2021: new data content and improved web interfaces. *Nucleic Acids Research* 49 (Database Issue): D1388–D1395. https://doi.org/10.1093/nar/gkaa971.

19 Butkiewicz, M., Wang, Y., Bryant, S.H. et al. (2017). High-Throughput screening assay datasets from the PubChem database. *Chemical Informatics* 3 (1): 1–12. https://doi.org/10.21767/2470-6973.100022.

20 Nguyen, D.-T., Mathias, S., Bologa, C. et al. (2017). Pharos: collating protein information to shed light on the druggable genome. *Nucleic Acids Research* 45 (D1): D995–D1002. https://doi.org/10.1093/nar/gkw1072.

21 Sorokina, M., Merseburger, P., Rajan, K. et al. (2021). COCONUT online: collection of open natural products database. *Journal of Cheminformatics* 13: 2. https://doi.org/10.1186/s13321-020-00478-9.

22 Testa, B., Krämer, S.D., Wunderli-Allenspach, H., and Folkers, G. (ed.) (2006). *Pharmacokinetic Profiling in Drug Research - Biological, Physicochemical, and Computational Strategies*. Zürich (Switzerland): VHCA, Verlag Helvetica Chimica Acta.

23 Ortiz de Montellano, P.R. (ed.) (2015). *Cytochrome P450 - Structure, Mechanism, and Biochemistry*, 4the. Switzerland: Springer International Publishing.

24 Wishart, D.S., Djoumbou Feunang, Y., Marcu, A. et al. (2018). HMDB 4.0: the human metabolome database for 2018. *Nucleic Acids Research* 46 (Database Issue): D608–D617. https://doi.org/10.1093/nar/gkx1089.

25 Caspi, E., Billington, R., Keseler, I.M. et al. (2020). The MetaCyc database of metabolic pathways and enzymes - a 2019 update. *Nucleic Acids Research* 48 (Database Issue): D445–D453. https://doi.org/10.1093/nar/gkz862.

26 Romero, P. (ed.) (2012). The HumanCyc pathway-genome database and pathway tools software as tools for imaging and analyzing metabolomics data. In: Fan, T.M., Lane A., Higashi R. (eds) *The Handbook of Metabolomics*. Methods in Pharmacology and Toxicology. Humana Press, Totowa, NJ. https://doi.org/10.1007/978-1-61779-618-0_13.

27 Kanehisa, M., Goto, S., Sato, Y. et al. (2014). Data, information, knowledge and principle: back to metabolism in KEGG. *Nucleic Acids Research* 42 (Database Issue): D199–D205. https://doi.org/10.1093/nar/gkt1076.
28 Jewison, T., Su, Y., Disfany, F.M. et al. (2014). SMPDB 2.0: big Improvements to the small molecule pathway database. *Nucleic Acids Research* 42 (Database Issue): D478–D484. https://doi.org/10.1093/nar/gkt1067.
29 ADME = Administration, Distribution, Metabolism, Excretion.
30 Canault, B., Bourg, S., Vayer, P. et al. (2017). Comprehensive Network Map of ADME-Tox Databases. *Molecular Informatics* 36 (10): 1700029. https://doi.org/10.1002/minf.201700029.
31 Said Faqi, A. (ed.) (2017). *Comprehensive Guide to Toxicology in Nonclinical Drug Development*, 2e. Amsterdam: Elsevier Inc.
32 Will, Y., McDuffie, J.E., Olaharski, A.J., and Jeffy, J.B. (ed.) (2016). *Drug Discovery Toxicology - From Target Assessment to Translational Biomarkers*. NJ: John Wiley & Sons, Inc.
33 https://www.roche.com/innovation/process/clinical-trials/about#b74e294d-1765-419e-8b38-96aaa88d62fa (accessed 26 April 2022).
34 Brown, N. (ed.) (2014). *Scaffold Hopping in Medicinal Chemistry (Methods and Principles in Medicinal Chemistry)*, vol. 58. Weinheim, Germany: Wiley-VCH Verlag GmbH & Co. KGaA.
35 Maass, P., Schulz-Gasch, T., Stahl, M., and Rarey, M. (2007). Recore: a fast and versatile method for scaffold hopping based on small molecule crystal structure conformations. *Journal of Chemical Information and Modeling* 47 (2): 390–399. https://doi.org/10.1021/ci060094h.
36 Varnek, A. and Tropsha, A. (ed.) (2008). *Chemoinformatics Approaches to Virtual Screening*. Cambridge: Royal Society of Chemistry.
37 Murugan, N.A., Podobas, A., Gadioli, D. et al. (2022). A review on parallel virtual screening softwares for high-performance computers. *Pharmaceuticals* 15 (1): 63. https://doi.org/10.3390/ph15010063.
38 Shaker, B., Ahmad, S., Lee, Y. et al. In silico methods and tools for drug discovery. *Computers in Biology and Medicine* 137: 104851. https://doi.org/10.1016/j.compbiomed.2021.104851.
39 Maia, E.H.B., Assis, C., de Oliveira, T.A. et al. (2020). Structure-based virtual screening: from classical to artificial intelligence. *Frontiers in Chemistry* 8 (4): 343. https://doi.org/10.3389/fchem.2020.00343.
40 https://en.wikipedia.org/wiki/List_of_protein-ligand_docking_software (accessed 25 April 2022).

Index

a

academic vs. industrial research 299–310
  Binding Database 305
  Cambridge Structural Database (CSD) 305
  clinical trials 308
  Competitive Intelligence (CI) 301
  Crystallography Open Database (COD) 305
  R&D process 301
Acetaminophen 70, 71
ADME-Tox 274, 307, 310
AlphaFold Database 177, 179–180, 192, 279–280
AlphaFold program 272, 279
American Chemical Society (ACS) 299
angiotensin-converting enzyme (ACE) inhibitors 80, 82, 84
Apixaban 117
Approved Drugs component 244
artificial intelligence/machine learning (AI/ML) tools 68
Asinex 305
Assay ID (AID) 44
AutoDock Vina 275
automatic rebuilding of protein backbone and side chains 203–204

b

BCR–ABL kinase inhibitor 122, 123
Beilstein 299
BindingDB Database 283, 305
BioAssay data collections 43
BioChemGraph project 166
bioisostere 101
  classical vs. non-classical 102–105
bioisosteric replacement, in drug discovery 105–106
bioisosterism 101, 102, 105, 106
BioMagResBank (BMRB) 141
BLAST (blastp) algorithm 241
Boltzmann-Enhanced Discrimination of ROC (BEDROC) 287

c

Cambridge Structural Database (CSD) 42, 152, 305, 311
carbohydrates 149–150, 155, 204, 214
Center for Biologics Evaluation and Research (CBER) 310
Center for Drug Evaluation and Research (CDER) 310
Charles Rive 305
ChemAxon 73, 86, 240
ChEMBL 2, 4, 56, 57, 107, 109, 111, 118, 232, 234, 283, 284, 288, 306, 307
ChemBridge 305
chemical abstracts service (CAS) 45, 299
Chemical Taxonomy 73, 91
China National Intellectual Property Administration (CNIPA) 302
ciprofloxacin 118, 120
classical vs. non-classical bioisostere 102–105

Open Access Databases and Datasets for Drug Discovery, First Edition.
Edited by Antoine Daina, Michael Przewosny, and Vincent Zoete.
© 2024 WILEY-VCH GmbH. Published 2024 by WILEY-VCH GmbH.

Classification Browser 51, 52
3C-like protease (3CLpro) 94
COlleCtion of Open Natural ProdUcTs (COCONUT) 281, 306
color-Tanimoto (CT) score 46, 48
Combo-Tanimoto (ComboT) score 48
competitive intelligence (CI) 301
computer-aided drug design (CADD) 1, 2, 311
computer-aided structure-based drug design 190–191
COVID-19 94, 111, 164, 191
COVID Moonshot campaign 164
COX2 inhibitors 311
cytochrome peroxidase P450 (CYP) 306
cytochrome P450 monooxygenase enzymes 212

d

Define Secondary Structure of Proteins (DSSP) analysis 220
details pages 236
Deutsches Patent-und Markenamt (DPMA) 302
Die Pathway Datenbank HumanCyc 307
Disease Novelty component 246, 248
DrugBank 2, 68, 305
   categories section 73
   drug cards 70
   identification section 70–71
   knowledgebase 69
   overview of 68–69
   pharmacology 71–73
   properties section 73
   research using 94
   Targets, Enzymes, Carriers, and Transporters section 73–77
DrugBank Online's Advanced Search Functionality 80–83
drug metabolism and pharmacokinetic profile (DMPK) 306
drug-related non-classical bioisosteres 103
Drug Target Ontology (DTO) 242

e

EGFR 104
Electron Microscopy Data Bank (EMDB) 141
Enamine 305
enrichment factor (EF) 286
enzyme inhibitors 84, 85
Estrogen-related receptor gamma ligand-binding domain 179
EU Clinical Trials Register 308
European Nucleotide Archive (ENA) 305
European Patent Office (EPO) 302
European Union Drug Regulating Authorities Clinical Trials Database (EudraCT) 309
Evotec 305
Expression Data component 243

f

Filter Value Enrichment 248–251, 263
findability, accessibility, interoperability, and reuse (FAIR) principles 3, 141, 220, 223
Find Predicted Targets 252
fingerprint-based 2-D similarity search method 45–46, 48

g

Gaussian-shape overlay-based 3-D similarity methods 45
Gefitinib 104
GeneCards 233
Gene Ontology (GO) 52, 246
Gene, Protein, Pathway, and Taxonomy collections 43
Generated DataBases (GDBs) 282
genome-wide association studies (GWAS) 67, 246
glycoprotein structure model rebuilding 214
Gmelin 299
Google Patents 303
GWAS Traits component 246

h

high-throughput screening (HTS) 2, 41, 67, 105, 111, 271, 305
histidine flip and improved ligand parameterization 208–210
hit finding 105, 106, 108, 117, 133, 305
human B-raf protein kinase 181
Human Metabolome Database (HMDB) 306

i

Identifier Exchange Service 52
isosteres 101
isosterism 101, 102

j

Japanese Patent Office (JPO) 302

k

KEGG Pathway Database 307

l

lead compounds 105, 106, 118, 124, 129
lead optimization 105, 106, 108, 120, 133
Ligand-Based VS (LBVS) 272
Lipinski's rule of five (Ro5), for drug-likeness 55
Literature Knowledge Panels 49–50, 60

m

machine learning (ML) 1, 58, 93, 165, 166, 288
main protease protein (Mpro) 164
MarvinJS Widget 240, 252
Maybridge 305
metabolism 73, 74, 76, 79, 113, 212
MetaCyc Metabolic Pathway Database 307
metal binding sites 214–216
$2mF_o$-DF_c density map 154
mitogen activated protein kinase (MAPK) signaling pathway 208
mmCIF format 3, 4, 218, 278
ModelArchive 176, 177, 180–181, 192, 193

molecular mechanics-generalized Born surface area (MM-GBSA) strategy 94
molecule-based discovery 68
MONDO disease 261
morpholine 104, 105, 129

n

NCATS Predictor 241, 252, 253
non-classical *vs.* classical bioisostere 102–105
NorA efflux pump, inhibitor design of 118
normalized ratios of principal moments of inertia (NPR) 115
Nucleic Acid Database (NDB) 304
Nucleic Acid Knowledge Base (NAKB) 304

o

OneDep 145–146, 150, 151, 154
OpenEye 147
OpenTargets 233

p

papain-like protease (PLpro) 94
Patent collection 43
Pathways 73, 79, 246, 251
PDBeChem service 158
PDBe-KnowledgeBase (PDBe-KB) 142
PDBe tools for ligand analysis 155–158
PDB identifier (PDB ID) 278
PDB-REDO databank 278
  automated model completion approaches 204–205
  automatic rebuilding of protein backbone and side chains 203–204
  building new compounds into density 212–213
  creating datasets 222
  data available in PDB-REDO entries 220
  downloading and inspecting individual PDB-REDO entries 218–220

PDB-REDO databank (*contd.*)
  FAIR validation data 222
  first uniformity 203
  glycoprotein structure model rebuilding 214
  histidine flip and improved ligand parameterization 208–210
  loop building
    completes a binding site region 210, 211
    results in improved binding sites 211–212
  metal binding sites 214–216
  nucleic acid improvements 213
  overview of pipeline 205–206
  re-refinement improves ligand conformation 206–207
  side chain rebuilding improves ligand binding sites 207–208
  structure models 223
  systematic integration of structural knowledge 205
  uniform data 222
peptide-based chromophores 146
Peptide Reference Dictionary (PRD) 147–148
pharmacodynamics 72, 122
pharmacogenomic effects/ADRs 73
pharmacogenomics/pharmacogenetics (PGx) 96
Pharmacological Action field 76, 77
pharmacology 71–73, 96
pharmacophores 3, 113, 275–276
PharmaGist 275
Pharos 232–264, 306
  chemical compound 251–260
  dark target 246, 247
    downloading Data 251
    List Analysis 247–248
    primary documentation 242–247
    variations 251
  investigating diseases 260–262
phenotypic-based discovery 68

phosphodiesterase 5 (PDE5) inhibitor 310
pLDDT 179–181, 279
Ponatinib 122–124
programmatic access routes 52
Protein Data Bank (PDB) 2–4, 42, 141–166, 175–178, 181, 182, 189, 192, 278, 304, 307, 311
  additional ligand annotations 148–150
  drug discovery 164–165
  ligand-related annotations 158–164
  models 201
  PDBe tools for ligand analysis 155–158
  small molecule data 142–146
  small molecule dictionaries 146–148
  wwPDB 150–155
Protein Data Bank in Europe (PDBe) 57, 141, 142, 154–156, 158
Protein Data Bank Japan (PDBj) 141, 304
protein–ligand docking 271, 274–276, 280
protein–protein interactions 181, 206, 234, 244, 245, 248, 263
protein-structure databases
  AlphaFold DB 279
  PDB-REDO databank 278
  Protein Data Bank (PDB) 278
  SWISS-MODEL Repository 279
Protein Summary component 238, 242
PubChem 2, 41, 283, 284
  biological activity data 56–57
  Classification Browser 51–52
  2D and 3D neighbors 50, 51
  data collections 43
  data content and organization 42–44
  data for drug discovery 58–59
  data organization 43
  drug-likeness and lead-likeness of compounds in 54–55
  Identifier Exchange Service 52
  Literature Knowledge Panels 49–50
  programmatic access routes 52

range of users 41
spectral information 42
substance and compound records 44
Summary page 48, 49
tools and services 45–54
PubChem Data Sources page 43
PubChem FTP Site 53, 54
PubChem Help site 45
PubChem home page 42, 45
PubChemRDF 53, 54
PubChem Search 45–48
PUG-REST 53
PUG-View 53

q
quantitative structure–activity
 relationship (QSAR) models 2,
 241

r
Reactome Pathway 246, 263
Real Space Correlation Coefficient
 (RSCC) 153, 154, 214
Reaxys 299, 300
ReCore 310
Resource Description Framework (RDF)
 53, 54
RNA-dependent RNA polymerase (RdRp)
 94
ROC curves 287

s
SARS-CoV-2 M-pro inhibitors 288
scaffold hopping 106, 117, 310–311
SciFinder 299, 300
shape-Tanimoto (ST) score 46, 48
Similarity Ensemble Approach (SEA) 3
small molecule data 142–146
small molecule dictionaries 146–148
Small Molecule Pathway Database
 (SMPDB) 79, 307
SMILES format 3, 4, 147, 274
SoftFocus® Libraries 306
spike (S) protein 94
structure-based approaches 1, 3

Structure-Based VS (SBVS) 272
Substituents field 73
Summary page for PubChem 48, 49, 53,
 57, 59, 60
SwissBioisostere
 bioactivity data 107
 biological context 112–113
 blood–brain barrier diffusion 122, 124
 chemical context 113
 construction workflow 107
 database 108
 escape from flatland strategy 128–132
 flexibility reduction 124–128
 fragments
  chemical nature and composition of
   113, 114
 global content 111
 molecular shape distribution 116
 most frequent user requests 117
 nonsupervised matched molecular
  pair analysis 108
 NorA efflux pump, inhibitor design
  of 118
 reduction of aromaticity 128–132
 rigidification of linkers 126
 rigidification of scaffolds 127
 rigidification of side chains 125
 scaffold replacement request,
  analysis and interoperability
  117–119
 shape diversity 113, 115
 web interface 109–111
 Website usage 115
 novel antibiotic and insecticide design
  guided by 120
 passive absorption, optimization of
  122, 124
 replacing unwanted chemical groups
  118–122
Swiss Federal Institute of Intellectual
 Property (IGE-IPI) 302
SWISS-MODEL 3, 177–179
SWISS-MODEL Repository (SMR)
 279
 associated tools 182–183

SWISS-MODEL Repository (SMR) (*contd.*)
    binding site conformational states 189–190
    Computer-Aided Structure-based Drug Design 190–191
    ModelArchive 180–181
    quality estimates and benchmarking 188–189
    structural features, ligands and oligomers 181–182
    Web and API access 183–187
SwissTargetPrediction 3, 118

t

Tanimoto coefficient 240, 241, 254
Tanimoto equation 46
Target Assessment (TA) 300
target-based discovery 67
Target Central Resource Database (TCRD) 232
    analysis methods within Pharos
        amino acid sequence 241
        Enrichment scores 241
        Find Similar Targets 241
        search for ligands 240
        targets predicted 241
    data organization
        data and UI Updates 235
        Disease Alignment 234
        Ligand Alignment 234
        Target Alignment 234
        primary resources 233
        UI Organization 235–236
target-centric paradigm 67
Target Development Level (TDL) 231, 232
Target Illumination GWAS Analytics (TIGA) 246
Targets 79
Targets, Enzymes, Carriers, and Transporters 73, 75–77
Tchem proteins 232
Tclin proteins 232
Tdark proteins 232
tetrahydro-1,4-benzoxazepin-5-one 104
three-dimensional protein complexes 280, 281
Tipranavir 122
Toxicology and Environmental Health Information Program (TEHIP) 307
TOXicology Data NETwork (TOXNET) 307
tutorials 109, 110, 240
tyclopyrazoflor 118, 120
type IIA DNA topoisomerases 206, 207

u

UI organization 235–240
UniProt 4, 75, 77, 162, 178, 233, 234, 242, 246, 261, 279, 307
UniProt human protein database 241
UniProt ID 4, 75, 79, 83, 234, 284
UniProt Knowledgebase (UniProtKB) 176–178, 181–183, 187, 191, 279, 280, 283, 285
United States Patent and Trademark Office (USPTO) 302
user support, on SwissBioisostere website 110

v

Validation HElper for LIgands and Binding Sites (VHELIBS) program 278, 280, 281
virtual screening (VS) 311–312
    bioactive molecules
        BindingDB database 283
        ChEMBL 284
        PubChem 283–284
    biological activity 286
    definition 271
    inactive/decoy molecules database
        building custom-based decoy sets 286
        collecting experimentally inactive compounds from PubChem 285

collecting presumed inactive
compounds from decoy databases
285–286
new drugs
COCONUT 281
Generated DataBases (GDBs) 282
ZINC20 282
protein-structure databases 277–278
tools for 272–274
pharmacophore search 275–276
protein-ligand docking 274–275
shape/electrostatic similarity
276–277

w

Worldwide Protein Data Bank (wwPDB)
3, 141, 150–155
wwPDB Chemical Component Dictionary
(CCD) 146–147

x

X-ray structure models 201–202, 206, 224

z

ZINC20 2, 115, 282, 286